Personality Disorders: Diagnosis, Management and Course
Second edition

Edited by

Peter Tyrer MD FRCP FRCPsych FFPHM FMedSci

Head, Department of Public Mental Health, Division of Neurosciences and Psychological Medicine, Imperial School of Medicine, London, UK

With a Foreword by

Erik Simonsen
Medical Director, Institute of Personality Theory and Psychopathology

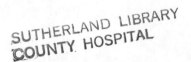
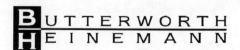
BUTTERWORTH HEINEMANN

OXFORD AUCKLAND BOSTON JOHANNESBURG MELBOURNE NEW DELHI

Butterworth-Heinemann
Linacre House, Jordan Hill, Oxford OX2 8DP
225 Wildwood Avenue, Woburn, MA 01801-2041
A division of Reed Educational and Professional Publishing Ltd

A member of the Reed Elsevier plc group

First published 1988
Second edition 2000

British Library Cataloguing in Publication Data
Personality disorders:diagnosis, management and course.
  2nd ed.
  1. Personality disorders
  I. Tyrer, Peter, 1940–
  616.8'58

Library of Congress Cataloguing in Publication Data
A catalogue record for this book is available from the Library of Congress.

ISBN 0 7506 3433 2

Typeset by Keytec Typesetting Ltd, Bridport, Dorset, UK
Printed and bound by MPG Books Ltd, Bodmin, Cornwall

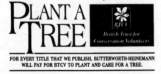

Contents

Preface to first edition

Not much is known about personality disorders and much that is written about them is speculative and anecdotal. Nevertheless, all psychiatrists, whatever their views on the merits and demerits of the term, are aware that many abnormal clinical states cannot be described adequately in the language of mental illness. Psychiatry has made great strides in the last 50 years in honing down the important mental disorders and defining their main characteristics, natural histories and preferred treatments. Personality disorders have not achieved this precision and remain in the shadows, regarded as much as terms of criticism and prejudice as of diagnostic description.

This book attempts to redress the balance by showing that personality disorders can be described adequately and fairly, and that assessment of personality status is an essential part of the mental examination. The separation of personality disorder from other forms of mental illness in current classification, pioneered by DSM-III in the USA, is important because it prevents clinicians thinking of the terms as mutually exclusive. The value of making the separation is emphasized by the frequent coexistence of mental state abnormalities and personality disorder in clinical practice. Nonetheless, the act of separation has given rise to its own problems and the difficulties in constructing the boundary between personality disorder and mental illness is admitted freely throughout this book.

The landscape of personality disorder is also unfamiliar. It is like the other side of the moon, puzzled about for centuries but hidden from view until recently, while the visible side of mental state abnormality has been scrutinized in minute detail. A large part of the book, perhaps too large a part for many readers, is therefore devoted to the description and classification of personality disorders. Without agreement on the classification and definition of the condition, research studies of treatment, course and relationship to mental illness are rendered inadequate. We hope to have demonstrated that, despite the many terms used for the description of personality disorder, there is a surprising degree of agreement on what constitutes personality disorder and the nature of its main diagnostic groups. Although the personality of an individual is unique, with increasing severity of abnormality boundaries coalesce and the major personality disorders can be described economically and comprehensively. The language of description and classification lacks literary merit and makes tedious reading beside the colourful descriptions of Theophrastus, Pinel, Kraepelin and Schneider. We have nonetheless limited individual descriptions of personality disorder because, until recently, they have constituted the only literature on personality disorders and their usefulness as scientific data is limited.

Throughout the book we have tried to maintain a clinical perspective and most of the contributors are practising clinicians as well as research workers. The clinical useful-ness of many of the new categories of per-sonality disorder has yet to be demonstrated but it is important for practitioners to be familiar with these and to understand the arguments for their inclusion. There are no satisfactory laboratory aids to the diagnosis of personality disorder and clinical skills are essential. These have been formalized in structured interview schedules and several of these are now available. The measurement and assessment of personality disorder is an expanding enterprise and a more detailed account of the recently introduced instru-ments is given to familiarize the reader with these developments. One of these instru-ments, the Personality Assessment Schedule, is described in more detail as the personality data in succeeding chapters are largely de-rived from this. One of the reasons why previous classifications of personality disor-der have proved unsatisfactory is their poor reliability; a separate chapter is therefore devoted to this issue.

Once valid and reliable assessments of personality disorder are established, many other questions can be addressed. How com-mon is personality disorder in different clin-ical settings? What is the relationship between personality disorder and mental ill-ness? What is the natural history of person-ality disorder and how does it affect the outcome of other mental illness? Are there any effective treatments of personality disor-der? How is personality disorder caused and how can it be prevented? Some of these are at least partly answered in the latter half of the book. The results indicate that personal-ity disorder is extremely common in psychia-tric practice and that this has a major, and largely negative, effect on the outcome of mental illness. If there are any doubters left who dispute the value of assessing personal-ity disorder, they should be persuaded by the evidence that the presence of a personal-ity disorder has significant implications for the patient, therapists, service planners and society as a whole. The old idea that person-ality disorder was a relatively uncommon problem confined to those in penal institu-tions and others on the fringes of society can no longer be maintained. Personality ab-normality in its many forms is an intrinsic part of all psychiatric practice and cannot be ignored by the clinician or the research worker. A chapter on life events and person-ality by Dr Seivewright illustrates how the ramifications of personality disorder have extended to encompass many other aspects of clinical work and research, and show that if personality status is not taken into account much important information is lost.

We are well aware of omissions in the book. In particular we have skirted round the nat-ure–nurture controversy over the cause of personality disorder and have not discussed the early developmental aspects that seem to have an important bearing on the adult ex-pression of disorder. We have avoided these issues because there are inadequate data available at present, partly because of the difficulties in assessing personality disorder in the young. We are consequently unable to discuss issues concerning the prevention of personality disorder. We may have appeared to ignore much of the important psychologi-cal literature in the field of abnormal person-ality. This is because we have concentrated here on personality disorder rather than ab-normal personality. This is not just a semantic issue and to equate the two would lead to unnecessary confusion. We are also well aware that some of our own conclusions rest uneasily on speculation and guesswork and need supporting data before they can be ac-cepted.

Nevertheless, if this book succeeds in sti-mulating further enquiry in what remains a neglected field of scientific endeavour, it will have served some purpose. There are prob-ably elements of Cressida's 'unkind self' in all forms of mental illness and understanding and identifying those that are more serious is likely to be a major task in the next decade.

We should like to thank the American Psy-chiatric Association and the World Health Organization for permission to quote from DSM-III-R and the 1987 draft of ICD-10, Chapter V 'Mental, behavioural and develop-mental disorders', Sarah White PhD, for sta-tistical and programming assistance, Dr Steven Greer and Professor Cawley for per-mission to reproduce *Figure 11.1*, and Wim van der Brink, Lee Anna Clark, Assem Jablen-sky, Armand Loranger, Philip McLean, Alfred Minto, Bruce Pfohl, Michael Rutter and Charles Shawcross for their stimulating discussions that are partly responsible for the writing of this book. Finally, we should like to thank the Research Committee of the Trent Regional Health Authority for their courage, and possibly their wisdom, for recommending the financial support that has enabled most of the original studies described in this book to be completed.

Peter Tyrer, Nottingham
September, 1987

Preface to second edition

Since this book was first published in 1988 personality disorder appears to have been promoted to the premier league of psychiatric concerns from its former position languishing somewhere near the middle of forensic psychiatry. This heady movement has revealed the need for more research-based evidence in the subject and the time is now ripe for new and energetic minds to take up the challenges of this exciting time. We have tried to give a flavour of this excitement in the second edition. There are extensive revisions to the chapters on classification and epidemiology, with a new chapter on the vexed subject of comorbidity; there are now two chapters on treatment aspects, and substantially more information from outcome studies. The notion of severe personality disorder is raised and attempts made to define and examine the implications of the term. Three versions of the Personality Assessment Schedule are given in a form suitable for reproduction and details of other assessment instruments given.

In the first edition of this book we suggested that studying personality disorder was like looking at the other side of the moon, the part that is always hidden from Earth. We now have a better view of its landscape and it is not so unfamiliar as we expected, but it does have unusual peaks and valleys that are not found in the landscape of mental illness alone. In the past we either ignored the landscape of personality disorder or were lost in it. Today we have some maps, which however primitive, help us to know where we are going and the paths we need to follow to discover more. We hope this book will be a suitable guidebook for your journey.

We thank Catherine Manley, Obioha Ukoumunne and Elizabeth Van Horn for help with work on the Personality Assessment Schedule, and particularly John Alexander, who carried out the original cluster and factor analyses with the schedule, Alex Antoniades for secretarial assistance, Ann Tyrer for help with illustrations, and Jeremy Coid for stimulating arguments.

Peter Tyrer, London
November 1999

Foreword

The foundations of psychiatry are to be laid on the ground of natural sciences and should apply the methods and resources of a common scientific approach to solve problems of clinical psychiatry. It is only from the organic connection between natural science, biology, psychology, medicine and psychiatry and from arduous but reliable methods of investigation that lasting advances can be made. These clear and firm statements are drawn from the introduction of the classical English textbook *Clinical Psychiatry* by Eliot Slater and Martin Roth (Third edition, 1969). Their approach was to some extent influenced by the German tradition in development of phenomenology i.e. the exact study and precise description of psychic events as a primary requisite for their understanding. The study of personality disorders in clinical psychiatry was at that time far from obtaining this level of scientific demands for exactness. The classification of personality disorders were based on astute, discriminating portrayals of characters and personalities described by Freud, Abraham, Kretschmer, Reich and Schneider. But the rapprochement between clinical psychology and psychiatry paved the way for new scientific landmarks for exactness by using psychometrics techniques to define the concept of basic dimensions of personality (Eysenck, 1960 and Cattell, 1965). Peter Tyrer and his associates have carried on this sound and keen striving for an evidence-based approach to personality and its disorders.

There is a long gap from the original text-books of psychopathic personalities by Schneider (1923) and Henderson (1939) to the next important English language textbook in Europe on personality disorders – the first edition of Peter Tyrer's book of 1988. Schneider used the concept psychopathy as a broad term and he included all types of personality disorders (defined as extreme cases of normal variants) based on a simple case description method. Henderson and the later British tradition became narrower in their approach to personality disorders, which mostly became synonymous with the antisocial personalities. The Mental Health Act of 1959 reinforced this standpoint, that the psychopathic states were the only significant personality disorders ('persistent disorders of the mind'). Tyrer's book coined a modern tradition for a both scientifically based and clinically significant approach in which personality disorders should be described adequately. He also argued that assessment of personality status should be an essential part of the mental examination. Personality disorders should be studied after the same principles and scientific demands as schizophrenia, depression and other mental disorders.

This became possible as the status of personality disorder in general grew in significance in the 1970s and 1980s. Peter Tyrer valued at that time the separation of personality disorders on a separate axis by the introduction of the DSM III system in 1980, as this approach emphasized the frequent coexistence of major mental disorders and personality disorder in clinical practice. However, this second edition of the book is very frank and honest about the difficulties and challenges we have to meet in our efforts to study personality disorders. Nothing is swept under the carpet. Tyrer is now in favour of debating the axis I and axis II distinction and that the limitations with regard to defining and delineating the personality disorders are the same. But still, it is a more optimistic book than the first edition from 1988. The basic questions are the same: What is the clinical importance of a personality disorder concept? Can personality disorders be assessed in a reliable way? Can they be separated clearly from other mental disorders and can they be treated successfully? Tyrer is clearly very disappointed with the categorical approach of classifying personality disorders. It is true that most clinicians are very reluctant to classify personality disorders after ICD-10 or DSM-IV. There is all too much overlap in their diagnostic criteria and extensive comorbidity between the different groups of personality disorders. And the categories are also often of very limited clinical value when it comes to treatment planning and execution.

Most textbooks on personality disorders start from the standpoint of theory or in the official classification system. Both the theory and the classification systems need verification. This book sticks to the facts and keeps the focus on the unsolved questions, not least regarding those formulated from the clinician's point of view. It is clearly stated in the book that classification of personality disorder is unreliable, that the diagnostic criteria are not specific, that there is a huge overlap between the personality disorder categories and that it is difficult to separate personality status from mental state on the one hand and normality on the other. It is suggested by Tyrer that one way of solving more of these problems is to work only with three or four clusters of personality disorders based on lower and higher order of dimensions: 1. the odd and eccentric; 2. the flamboyant and dramatic; and 3. the anxious and fearful as drawn from cluster A, B and C in the DSM system. He also argues strongly for the validity of a fourth cluster of anankastic or obsessive-compulsive personalities. In Peter Tyrer's opinion, severity should be added to this classification of major traits and a hier-

archical system to classify level of personality abnormality. This would minimize the inappropriate overlap and still keep the personality disorder as a different dimension from mental state disorders. New ideas, but whether they will work in a reliable way in a clinical setting depends on validation.

This second edition of the 1988 book should also be particularly valued for its extensive revisions of the chapters on epidemiology and outcome and for new chapters on treatment aspects. The chapter on comorbidity digs deep into the above mentioned difficulties of delineation between personality disorders and other mental disorders. The chapter on epidemiology underlines how the paucity of adequate measures, and the confusion about how valid and well demarcated these disorders really are, influences the lack of sufficient studies on incidence and prevalence of personality disorders. But the shift to community based service has generated new interest, both in general practice and community psychiatry, and the use of more valid personality assessment by instruments and use of informants will provide more clinical data for epidemiological studies. The updated data on assessment in the chapter on classification is very useful for those who want to know more about the available instruments. The chapter on psychosocial treatment is mostly an introduction to the cognitive models and the more psychodynamically oriented reader would have liked more attention to psychodynamic management in the treatment of personality disorders. The excuse is probably that this book is primarily faithful to psychometrics and the empirical approach to the study of personality disorders, also referring to my introduction.

The book clearly does not give much room for more philosophical considerations or 'soft data thinking'. Wisdom is not only what we know, but also what we sense, we don't know and never will know.

Nevertheless, I think this book is one of the most sophisticated European contributions to the fast growing number of textbooks on personality disorders. It is based on a number of years of research from Peter Tyrer and his associates. As I have touched upon, it has clear personal angles and viewpoints, but it never shows a we-know-better attitude. Very few centres in Europe have kept the same persistence in this personality disorder research as Peter Tyrer and his associates.

We need reliable instruments to support our clinical judgement and guide us in treatment.

Tyrer and his associates have worked on the Personality Assessment Schedule (PAS) for around two decades. Since the first edition of this book the PAS has been extended also to cover the personality disorders in ICD-10 and it is available in a short form for screening (Quick personality assessment, PAS-Q). It is very useful to have the schedules and instruments printed in the book. I fully agree with Peter Tyrer when he calls for more research with international well accepted personality disorder instruments. It is only by cross-national studies in different settings that we achieve the gold standard of diagnostic tests, as we know from medicine in general. PAS should definitely be one of these instruments to be tested cross-nationally.

We are now in a new millennium. Since the publication of the first edition of this book several initiatives have added to the growing status and cross-cultural importance of personality as a clinical science – the organization of the International Society for the Study of Personality Disorders (ISSPD) and its official journal the *Journal of Personality Disorders*, the sponsorship of several international and national congresses on personality disorders and the establishment of several institutes for personality study. Peter Tyrer has played a major role in strengthening the international collaboration for the study of personality disorders. He was the key person organizing the last European Congress for the Study of Personality Disorders in 1998, where he was instrumental in coining targets for clinical

work and science in the personality field for the first ten years of the new millennium (here in abbreviated form):

a. routine assessment of personality status using an internationally accepted procedure should be provided for all psychiatric patients,
b. establishment of centres devoted to study and treatment of personality disorders,
c. national research centres and centres to train all staff involved in treatment of severe personality disorders to achieve common standards and competence
d. rules for audit and monitoring systems to maintain standards of care of personality disorders.

The optimism in this book plays well together with these visionary targets for the next ten years. For those interested in following our strivings to obtain these targets, this book is a fair judgement of our starting point, our current knowledge, the controversies and our hopes for the future in clinical science of personality and its disorders. Tyrer's own writing in this book is forceful, highly lucid, often provocative, witty and full of deep insight in the field. The book has now become a well-established source book on personality disorders, a distinction which is more remarkable as the subject is so new to scientific study.

Erik Simonsen

Medical Director
Institute of Personality Theory and
Psychopathology (IPTP)
January 2000

Contributors

Patricia Casey FRCPsych FRCPI MD
Professor, Mater Misericordiae Hospital, Dublin, Ireland

Domenic Cicchetti PhD
Senior Research Scientist, Senior Biostatistician and Senior Research Psychologist, Yale Child Study Center, North Branford, CT., USA

Kate M. Davidson MA MPhil PhD
Consultant Clinical Psychologist and Research Tutor, Department of Psychological Medicine, Gartnavel Royal Hospital, Glasgow, UK

Brian Ferguson MRCGP MRCPsych
Consultant Psychiatrist, Stonebridge Centre, Nottingham, UK

John Gunn MD FRCPsych CBE
Professor of Forensic Psychiatry, Institute of Psychiatry, Camberwell, London, UK

Helen Seivewright MBCHB MRCGP
Clinical Research Fellow, Imperial College School of Medicine, London, UK

Peter Tyrer MD FRCP FRCPsych FFPHM FMedSci
Head, Department of Public Mental Health, Division of Neurosciences and Psychological Medicine, Imperial School of Medicine, London, UK

1

History of the concept of personality disorder

Brian Ferguson and Peter Tyrer

Speculation on the nature of personality is a time-honoured practice enjoyed by every culture since man gained the ability to commit his thoughts to a permanent record. Why people have such different characters and dispositions has fascinated writers over centuries and to provide a chronological account of their deliberations or even a reasonable précis would be impossible. This chapter therefore focuses on the concept of personality as a disorder and cannot attempt to chronicle the descriptions and lessons to be gleaned from general literature, or explore the history of psychology and mind. The modern usage of the concept of personality disorder can be traced to the mid-eighteenth century and relies on distinguishing between features of an abnormal personality and those of a mental illness. Prior to this time, it was rare to make such a distinction, principally because it served little use. Treatments for abnormal mental states, whatever their nature, were limited and there was no point in trying to make distinctions which could have no useful impact on the subject or society in general. The exception to this was the legal arena, where it gradually became useful to make distinctions between different mental states on the basis of personal responsibility and allow for property laws and inheritance rules to deal with circumstances in which the subject was considered to be mentally deranged. When exploring the concept of personality disorder, therefore, it is useful to examine the criminal and civil codes that have been estab-

lished in various societies and cultures. When doing so, it becomes quickly apparent how much the elaboration of personality theory owes its source to changes in society at large. Linking the development of the concept of personality disorder to the political and philosophical notions of the day produces a far greater understanding of these conditions when compared to the psychiatric perspective of modern times.

It is worth restating the earliest medical views on personality and temperament. Hippocrates suggested that the body contained four humours: yellow and black bile, phlegm and blood. This led to four types of personality, determined by relative excesses of each of these humours. Thus, yellow bile was associated with a choleric temperament and black bile with a melancholy disposition. The phlegmatic personality derived from those with an excess of phlegm and similarly the sanguine personality had an excess of blood. These words are still in frequent use in our everyday language; indeed, we can all, at times, be said to be in 'bad humour'. The implication in this description is that temperament is a dimensional construct; all people have a mixture of these four humours and it is their *relative* amounts that lead to the type of temperament or personality. However, doctors, as we shall find many times in the course of this book, much prefer categories to dimensions and immediately translated these descriptions into personality types. The distinctions between trait and type and the comparative value of categorical vs dimensional constructs has led to separate traditions in psychology and psychiatry which are still very much in evidence.

Aristotle's pupil Theophrastus (Adlington, 1925) appears to have been the first to set out to describe personality in a systematic way, and indeed his work is still the envy of many twentieth century typologists struggling with the complexities of personality classification in a more scientific age. He described a series of characters in a way that suggests a description of personality rather than of clinical syndromes (*Table 1.1*). Even if some of his 'characters' appear, at times, to be no more than crude caricatures with no real distinction between type and trait, the similarities with some of the major ICD and DSM-III personality disorders are striking (*Table 1.1*). Theophrastus begins each of his characters with a brief description of the core element of personality disturbance and goes on to provide details of how this might be expressed in social behaviour. In all, 30 characters are portrayed, some of which when combined resemble modern descriptions of personality disorder. Others seem almost complete in

themselves, one of the best examples being the account of 'distrustful man' who in many ways resembles the paranoid category of ICD-10 and DSM-IV. The distrustful man, according to Theophrastus, suspects everyone of trying to cheat him. His home life is so dominated by his fear of dishonesty in others and his need for security that he refuses to accept his wife's assurances and has to check his property for himself in the middle of the night, being unable to get back to sleep as a result. Relationships with friends and acquaintances are affected to the extent that he will trust very few of them with as much as a drinking cup. Were he to do so the cups would have to go through a process of rigorous testing on their return to ensure that the originals had not been exchanged for copies. 'When he has sent one of his slaves to buy provisions he sends another one after the first to find out exactly what they cost. He tells the slave who accompanies him to walk in front and not behind so that he can watch him and prevent him from escaping on the way.' (*Table 1.1*).

The 'superstitious man' on the other hand reflects some of the features of the schizotypal

Table 1.1 Theophrastus' characters

Dissimulator – affectation in acts and words	*Gross man* – obtrusive and objectionable jesting	*Vain man* – paltry desire for distinction
Flatterer – degrading self-profiting intercourse	*Unseasonable man* – inopportune attitude	*Boaster* – pretending to have advantages not personally possessed
Chatterer – mania of talking hugely without thinking	*Officious man* – presumptuous benevolence in word and deed	*Arrogant man* – contempt for everyone except himself
Rustic – grossness which is ignorant of good manners	*Stupid man* – sluggishness of mind	*Coward* – shrinking of the soul caused by fear
Complaisant – agreeable intercourse without good motives	*Surly man* – lack of amenity in speech	*Oligarch* – domination in power and wealth
Reckless cynic – effrontery of doing or saying shameful things	*Superstitious man* – cowardice towards divine power	*Late learner* – pursues knowledge at too advanced an age
Loquacious man – incontinence of speech	*Grumbler* – complaining too much of one's lot	*Slanderer* – malevolent disposition of the soul
Newsmonger – inventing false events	*Distrustful man* – suspects all men of dishonesty	*Friend of the rabble* – has a taste for vice
Unscrupulous man – disregard of reputation for sake of base gain	*Offensive man* – repulsive neglect of the person	*Avaricious man* – pursues sordid gain
Penurious man – economy beyond all measure	*Unpleasant man* – annoyance without being really harmful	*Mean man* – lack of generosity

personality, appearing to exhibit 'cowardice towards divine power'. Even when the soothsayer tells him that the mouse hole in his sack has no mystic significance and should be repaired by an ordinary cobbler, he proceeds to offer a sacrifice in expiation. The anti-social personality (the friend of the rabble) is well described, although it should probably be combined with others to be equivalent to the ICD entity. Perhaps the one which almost certainly irritated Theophrastus the most is the 'offensive man' who neglects his person and who is not afraid to show off his filthy nails and sores, offering the explanation that 'his father and grandfather had them so it would not be easy to smuggle a stranger into the house. At a sacrifice he gets splashed with the victim's blood. In conversation he sprinkles you with spittle. After drinking he belches in your face. He sleeps in a dirty bed with his wife. . .'.

It should be said that some criticism has been levelled at these characters alleging that they were intended principally as afterdinner stories. Despite the later Byzantine distortion of the text it is clear that Theophrastus was seeking to focus on people who are different from the average, rather than simply describe the attributes of normal personality. He did not, however, consider aetiology in the way postulated within the *Opus Hippocraticum*. In essence, he stopped at the descriptive stage.

Assessments and description of personality disorder were not, however, confined to the Mediterranean Basin. Caraka, an Indian physician who is believed to have lived sometime during the first and second centuries AD in what is now Peshawar in Pakistan (Rao, 1975), provided detailed description of the features he considered to be characteristic of 16 personality types. Nine of these might today be taken as examples of personality disorder, although there is clearly some overlap with subnormality of intelligence in his account. Many other cultures, for example the Celts, used concepts which distinguish between various forms of mental disorder including subnormality, mental illness and abnormal personality (Robins, 1986). Unfortunately, much information has been lost over the intervening years and it is not possible to appreciate the subtleties of some of these distinctions.

The Greek view of personality and temperament persisted within the Western tradition for many years. Madness, in its myriad forms, was well recognized. The legal services began to develop concepts to be used in cases where the person before the court was clearly deranged and incomprehensible. For centuries, the concept of unsound mind proved a useful one but it was some time before sub-categories of madness, lunacy or idiocy could be introduced in a legal setting (Walker, 1968). The eighteenth century juror was sometimes faced with pleas of insanity and was beginning to accept them. But the same generosity was refused for cases of poverty or plain misfortune. The number of capital crimes, however, was large and there was a desire to move to more humanitarian practices (Porter, 1987).

There are a number of well documented cases from the English courts of the late eighteenth century which are now recognizable as examples of personality disorder. One of the most celebrated was that of Earl Ferrers, who was tried before the House of Lords in April 1760 for the murder of a steward. Lord Ferrers was obliged to defend himself and it was the first case in which medical evidence was called. Dr John Munro, Physician Superintendent of Bethlem, did not examine Ferrers, but testified on the subject of insanity in general and on treatment he had provided to Ferrers' uncle. Ferrers had fallen out with the victim over financial matters, and having invited him to his house, shot him while he was on his knees. The penalty for such a crime was death, but insanity could result in a lesser punishment. Ferrers outlined the criteria for lunacy in this case, and they included 'uncommon fury not caused by liquor, violence against other persons or against themselves, jealousy, quarrelling with friends without cause, being naturally suspicious and going out armed when there is no danger'. Ferrers went on to describe a number of abnormal behaviours, but his principal argument was that he did not know the difference between a moral and an immoral action. The Lords, however, would not accept that this was a reasonable excuse. On reading the transcripts (Walker, 1968) it was clear that the court was being invited to accept immoral behaviour as a form of insanity. They rejected that course of action out of hand and the Earl was duly hanged. But similar arguments put in other cases were accepted. In 1795, the London Times reported a case of a Miss Broderick who had murdered her ex-lover (*London Times*, 1795). Admittedly she was very agitated when she came to Court and nearly fainted. Later on 'she showed great presence of mind with great propriety', and was acquitted on grounds of insanity. The symptoms of her disorder, which were recounted by various witnesses, were 'whimsical conduct, maddish-like behaviour, odd conversations about the best way of dying, and an account of how she had refused change when she had overpaid the baker'. On Christmas Day, she had poured boiling water over her maid, who had failed to clean the stairs to her liking. There were no descriptions of conventional symptoms of lunacy, and the behaviour described fits more closely with that of a personality disorder. She was declared a lunatic and it was of interest to note that she was ordered to be detained on that basis. After the verdict was delivered, there was a 'kind of tumultuous emotion in court'. It was obvious that the jury had felt a great deal of sympathy and wanted to avoid capital punishment. In this instance, the court was able to regard a woman we now conclude was suffering personality disorder as showing signs of insanity, primarily for the motive of clemency.

Throughout this time, great social change was happening across Europe. Men were no longer seen as being born to their condition, but had rights to freedom and self-expression. Pinel, working in the Bicêtre, became famous for releasing the lunatics from their chains. He took an observational approach to his work and described the various cases he came across. One of the most celebrated is that of the nobleman who pushed a female servant down a well in a fit of rage. The nobleman was described as being spoilt and subject to every caprice imaginable. Try as he could, Pinel could not identify the usual symptoms of delusions or hallucinations and coined the term 'manie sans delire'. The patient was rational and coherent but behaved in a manner similar to those who suffered from madness. The outcome of this case was that the nobleman was 'sentenced' to the Bicêtre, which presumably constituted a punitive disposal. It must also be remembered that a great number of diseases were not found to have a recognizable neurological pathology at death and policy was influenced more by philanthropic and humanitarian ideas (Quaersall, 1985).

By the early nineteenth century, therefore, clinicians were beginning to distinguish between personality disorder as distinct from mental states and syndromes. Even before they were properly categorized and described, both were being used in the courts as a way of exonerating the perpetrators of crime. The work of Benjamin Rush in the USA was influential in this regard. Before long, Prichard (1837) coined the term 'moral insanity'; a condition in which there was no apparent illness but gross disturbance of behaviour. It was 'a form of mental derangement in whom the moral and active principles of the mind are strongly perverted or depraved, the power of self-government is lost or greatly impaired, and the individual is found incapable, not of talking or reasoning on any subject proposed to him, but of conducting himself with decency and propriety in the business of life'. Moral insanity was quickly recognized to be an important part of psychiatric practice and became a common diagnostic label from 1840 onwards. Prichard's real contribution was to invent the term which led to the further development of the concept itself. In reality, many of his cases would now be described as forms of mental illness. For example, one of his patients was a girl aged 7 who suddenly became foul-mouthed and abusive, would only eat raw vegetables and her own faeces, and was only satisfied when she was offending others. This extremely abnormal behaviour lasted only 2 months after which time she recovered. Prichard's account, therefore, included all forms of unsociable behaviour occurring without an obvious reason and was insufficiently precise, given that many of the conditions he observed are now understandable as examples of organic states or mental illness. His description can, however, be loosely equated with the term 'psychopathy' used to describe similar disturbances over much of the last 50 years.

Morel (1852), a French psychiatrist, went further in suggesting a hierarchical classification of mental disorders that shows resemblance to today's classifications. He divided all mental disorders into six main groups and the more severe and persistent the extent of the mental disorder, the higher the group of classification. Thus dementia (from all causes) constituted the sixth group. His first group would be regarded as personality accentuation. According to Morel these patients 'have a congenital nervous temperament in consequence of hereditary causes, and who easily become insane under influences which, but for the hereditary taint, would not give rise to insanity'. The second group constitutes one of the best early definitions of personality disorders. He describes such patients who 'in consequence of their hereditary taint, display their insanity in actions rather than words – in eccentricities, incoherence, irregularity and often extreme immorality of conduct'.

At about this time, Briquet (1859) wrote his well-known book that was subsequently taken up by the St Louis group in redefining hysteria 100 years later. He described a clinical syndrome and, although he regarded the condition as a consequence of nervous dysfunction, his descriptions were similar to those of hysterical personality. Later, Maudsley, in the second edition of his important textbook (Maudsley, 1868) was to describe the characteristic features of shallowness and suggestibility in his description of personality disorder, 'They have no well formed will of their own, and they become the easy victims of ideas forcibly presented to them by others'. Their spasmodic temperament 'is eminently favourable to the morbid exaggeration of some feeling or idea' (p. 343). Maudsley continued to pursue the study of moral insanity, which led him to some important conclusions that still hold true. He emphasized that close examination of the mental state (of patients with personality disorder) often revealed no abnormalities whatsoever. This was because outward behaviour and thinking appeared so normal that it was 'difficult to induce the public to entertain the idea that moral insanity is anything more than wilful and witting vice' (p. 356). He also gave an accurate, if somewhat pejorative, description of aggressive and sadistic personality features, describing a group that was 'inherently vicious, instinctive liars and thieves, stealing and deceiving with a cunning and a skill which could never be acquired; they display no trace of affection for their parents, or of feelings for others; the only care which they evince is to contrive the means of indulging their passions and vicious propensities.' (p. 329).

Maudsley also recognized that these individuals were dealt with both by medicine and the law and fully appreciated the dilemma arising from the exercise of personal responsibility which so concerns psychiatrists when accounting for the behaviour of antisocial personalities. Although he considered moral insanity to be a degenerative disease that led to 'the resemblance of these beings in moral character to the lowest savages', he also recognized that this did not excuse their behaviour. Thus he commented, 'to call these cases of moral insanity the results of disease is not to explain them, nor to cancel the need of an explanation; and to designate them as unnatural is not to remove them from the domain of natural law' (p. 328). Thus 'when they belong to the lower classes, they find their way to prison many times; indeed they contribute their quota to the criminal population of the country' (p. 330).

By this time, Darwinian theories were influential in many branches of science. Personality disorders gradually came to be regarded as due to the degeneration of the nervous system of constitutional origin. Koch (1891) developed the concept of psychopathic inferiority and, ever since his time, personality disorders have carried with them a trait of degeneration that makes them much less respectable than mental illness.

The first years of the twentieth century were associated with major advances in psychiatric knowledge. In addition to the explosive growth of psychoanalysis stimulated by Freud, there was the first satisfactory classification of psychiatric illness deriving in the main from Kraepelin's identification of manic depressive psychosis and schizophrenia as separate disorders. Kraepelin also influenced the classification of personality disorder and developed Koch's idea of psychopathic inferiority further. He regarded personality disorders as 'morbid mental states in which the peculiar disposition of the personality must be considered the real foundation of the malady'. In his lectures (Kraepelin, 1905), he also described good examples of paranoia, antisocial and hypochondriacal personality disorders. In his descriptions he emphasized the persistence of the problems caused by the abnormal personality, a feature that has continued to dominate the European classifications of personality disorder. Examination of individual patient histories established in the case of personality disorders that 'the disease is deeply rooted in the general personality. It usually develops early in adult life, and lasts with greater or less fluctuation throughout the whole of life' (p. 272).

The First World War led to great advances in the understanding of psychiatric disorders, particularly into the traumatic conditions created in abundance by the horrors of war. It also led to what might be the first example of what is now known as comorbidity, or dual diagnosis of a mental state and personality disorder, in a paper by Elliot Smith on shellshock. 'The claim has been made by certain workers that the soldiers who become affected by shock are weaklings and are descended from mentally afflicted or nervous parents. It is, of course, unquestionable that in a large army there must be many soldiers with tainted family histories, and it is probably equally certain that such factors play some part in determining the greater susceptibility of certain men to shock' (Smith, 1916, pp. 854–855). These observations have since widened into the extensive literature on post-traumatic stress disorder, personality vulnerability and life events.

Kraepelin's work established the importance of careful case histories in determining the classification of mental disorders and established the German school as the most influential in the next quarter of the century. Schneider (1923) and Kretschmer (1922) produced the first acceptable subclassification of personality disorder through the case description method. Schneider grouped all personality disorders under the label of 'psychopathic' and formulated a classic definition that is still used today: 'Psychopathic personalities are such abnormal personalities who suffer through their abnormalities or through whose abnormalities society suffers'.

Schneider described 10 personality types: the hyperthymic, depressive, insecure (comprising sensitive and anankastic), the fanatic, the self-seeking, the emotionally unstable, the explosive, the affectless, the weak-willed and the asthenic psychopathic personality. Each of these personality types was formulated by clinical description and it is easy to see from reading these how they were accepted as

valid, as the descriptions have a freshness and accuracy that makes them just as apposite today.

Kretschmer showed that there was a link between physique and mental illness, those with manic depressive illness being more likely to be short and stout (pyknic) and those with schizophrenia being more likely to be tall and thin (asthenic). He concentrated mainly on descriptions of temperament (Wesenart) and character rather than personality and it was difficult to know whether he was describing abnormal personality in his work. He did not define personality disorder but described character as 'the totality of all possibilities that are affective and voluntary reactions of any given individual'. Kretschmer's hope was that by correlating physique with temperament and character together with 'chemistry of the blood' abnormal psychology could be predicted and, if possible, prevented.

Jaspers (1946) took a much broader view of personality disorders and included a wide variety of neurotic disorders and adjustment reactions. His most valuable contribution comes in the discussion of normal and abnormal personalities. Jaspers looks beyond mere description in an attempt to provide an understanding of the aetiology of these conditions. He distinguishes between two real types. The first are the 'abnormal personalities that simply represent dispositions which deviate from average and appear as extreme variations of human nature'. The second category are personalities which Jaspers regards as being genuinely ill, and where change has taken place as the result of some additional process. The most common example of the latter was a development of abnormal personalities after experience of a psychotic or dementing illness. The fault lines which still run through this area of psychiatric practice were thereby well delineated. Personality disorder was conceptualized by some as a form of mental illness and by others simply as the extreme end of normal variation, with obvious implications for the exercise of personal responsibility previously alluded to.

Much of the literature of the first half of the twentieth century, particularly from American sources, adopted a very judgemental view of personality disorders. Partridge (1930) classified personality disorders as belonging to three categories. The terms used are remarkably pejorative. The first category was labelled as being inadequate and included people with insecure, depressive, weak-willed and asthenic characteristics. The second group were the egocentrics. These were contentious, paranoid, explosive and excitable individuals. Subjects enter Partridge's final category simply on the basis of criminal behaviour. He describes them as liars, swindlers, vagabonds and sexual perverts. Partly as a result of these influences, there developed a further schism between those who endeavoured to classify personality disorder narrowly and those who took a much broader view. The European school retained this approach. In English-speaking countries, psychopathy came to be regarded as equivalent to one group only, that of anti-social personality disorders. Henderson (1939) separated them into three groups: those who were predominantly aggressive, inadequate or passive, and creative. An example of the third group was Lawrence of Arabia, who was able to read the *London Times* upside down at the age of 5. The emphasis on degeneration was less than that of the European psychiatrists, and they were regarded as states of delayed emotional maturity by many authorities. This notion received support from studies of the electroencephalogram (EEG) in patients described as excessive psychopaths, which showed that 65% of them had abnormal EEGs compared with 15% of normal controls (Hill and Watterson, 1942). The abnormality in most cases consisted of an excessive amount of slow (theta) waves in the temporal region, which are common in children but not in adults.

This somewhat organic view was helpful in explaining some of the clinical features of psychopathic personality. Such personalities could be perceived as overgrown school children whose proclivity to vice could be excused on the grounds of neurological immaturity, and thereby diminish their responsibility for any criminal acts. Despite the burgeoning literature and classification scheme, common understandings were rarely achieved. As late as 1944, Curran and Mallinson stated that there was no real agreement as to how to classify the large and heterogeneous mass of abnormal and unusual people who are not suffering from the more formally recognized type of mental disorder (Curran and Mallin-

son, 1944). They concluded that psychopathic personality at that time was the preferred term and was used to avoid a moral judgement or an unproven theory of aetiology. The term was rapidly incorporated into mental health legislation and acquired a new restrictive meaning. The United Kingdom Mental Health Act (1959) included the concept of psychopathic disorders among the population of patients who could be compulsorily admitted to hospital. Necessity is the mother of invention, but the definition begged more questions than it answered. Patients with psychopathic disorder had 'persistent disorders of mind (whether or not accompanied by subnormality of intelligence) which resulted in abnormally aggressive or seriously irresponsible conduct on the part of the patients, and require or are susceptible to medical treatment'. The implication for this definition was that any mental disorder could be described as psychopathy if persistent aggression or irresponsibility resulted from it. There was also no evidence that treatment was of particular benefit in this group of disorders and the latter part of the definition was more optimistic than accurate. In time, the concept of treatment was broadened to include any form of milieu which provided control and public safety, as long as it contained some element of nursing, psychological or medical care. Such concepts rarely remain static. If treatment is proposed as an effective intervention, then the therapist must be held responsible for its success or failure (Coid, 1993). By extension, the therapist in the latter half of the twentieth century must be ready to accept responsibility for the commission of acts so much decried by his predecessors.

In the USA, Hervey Cleckley (1941) and McCord and McCord (1964) contributed important accounts of the clinical status of psychopathic personality disorder. Cleckley maintained that psychopathic personality disorders were the only important group of abnormal personalities and that these should be placed together with other mental disorders such as depression and schizophrenia. However, this attempt to join personality abnormality and mental state disorders on a single axis of classification has now virtually been abandoned and in the last 30 years personality disorders have been regarded together as a single group. Cleckley's approach has been developed further by Hare (1980), who developed an instrument (Psychopathy Check List) based on a structured clinical interview which provides a robust diagnosis of psychopathic disorder. Its value is in its predictive power. The Hare checklist is widely used in penal institutions to identify those among the criminal population who exhibit the core traits of psychopathic personality. Unfortunately, high scoring subjects have a very poor prognosis in terms of future recidivism and dangerousness and the concept is being used to justify preventative detention for those who are judged to be highly dangerous at an unspecified future date.

Psychodynamic theory has also made an important contribution to the understanding of personality disorders, particularly those that were not associated with disorders of conduct. Although early Freudian theory formulated neurosis as a discrete phenomenon that affected people who were generally well but vulnerable because of early life experience, it was quickly realized that many patients presenting with neurotic problems had personality abnormality. This led to the description of the neurotic character (Alexander, 1930). This perceived a neurosis as alien to normal personal function (egodystonic), whereas the neurotic character might at times show similar behaviour, but this was in keeping with his normal ego function (egosyntonic). It was recognized that the neurotic character was less responsive to psychotherapy than neurotic symptomatology and could be associated with persistent, if not life-long, dependence and insecurity (Horney, 1939; Fromm, 1942).

Ego psychology has continued to have an influence on the description and classification of personality disorders and has attempted to provide explanations for apparently irrational and unpredictable behaviour. It has had an important influence on the development of narcissistic, borderline and passive–aggressive personality disorders in DSM-III.

Separation of Axis I (mental state) from Axis II (personality disorders)

Despite the influential views of Kraepelin, Kretschmer and Cleckley, there remained a strong undercurrent of opinion that personality disorders were quite separate from the

major psychoses and neurotic disorders. This extended right back to the time of Prichard who emphasized that people with 'moral insanity' were rational and usually showed no abnormality of mental state; their disorder was one of behaviour. The argument that personality disorders might be the earlier stages of formes frustes of psychotic disorder did not receive support from follow-up studies as there was no evidence that these disorders progressed to psychotic ones.

The other characteristic that differentiated personality disorders from other abnormal mental states was the persisting pattern of abnormal behaviour, usually beginning late in adolescence and continuing throughout most of adult life. For these reasons the two major classificatory systems in psychiatry, the *International Classification of Disease* (ICD; *see* World Health Organization, 1949, 1968, 1979) and the *Diagnostic and Statistical Manual of Mental Disorders* (DSM; *see* American Psychiatric Association, 1952, 1968, 1980, 1987) have regarded personality disorders as a separate axis of diagnosis that is independent of other mental disorders. The abbreviations ICD and DSM will be used frequently throughout this book to indicate these classifications and the suffix (in Arabic numerals for ICD and Roman numerals for DSM) indicate to which revision the text refers.

The key reasons for separating personality disorder from mental state diagnosis were all incorporated in the definition of personality disorder in the eighth revision of the *International Classification of Disease*. They are described as:

'deeply ingrained maladaptive patterns of behaviour generally recognisable by the time of adolescence or earlier and continuing throughout most of adult life, although often becoming less obvious in middle or old age. The personality is abnormal either in the balance of its components, their quality and expression or in its total aspect. Because of this deviation or psychopathy the patient suffers or others have to suffer and there is an adverse effect upon the individual or on society.'

However, the *International Classification of Disease* has continued to retain personality disorder within the rubric of the main axis of mental disorders, whilst the American classification, *Diagnostic and Statistical Manual of Mental Disorders*, has argued since the third revision in 1980 that personality disorders should be placed in a separate axis, since this 'ensures that consideration to the possible presence of personality disorder that might otherwise be overlooked when attention is directed to the usually more florid Axis I disorders' (American Psychiatric Association, 1994). The debate over the place of personality disorders in psychiatric classification is far from decided but it is perhaps fair to point out that the separation is more a consequence of practical utility than fundamental theory.

The arguments about the placing of personality disorder in relationship to other mental illness continue to be shown in the changes that have been made in the classification of personality disorder over the years. These are discussed in detail in the next chapter but, just to take one example, the loss of cyclothymic personality disorder from DSM-II and its equivalent, affective personality disorder, from ICD-9 in the latest classifications, illustrates that the distinction between mental illness and personality disorder is still somewhat arbitrary. It is now felt that cyclothymic personality disorder represents a version, or forme fruste, of manic depressive psychosis and therefore belongs with mental illness, either as cyclothymic disorder or as manic depressive psychosis. Since 1980 it has therefore been omitted from the list of personality disorders, although is still defended by some powerful protagonists (von Zerssen and Akiskal, 1998; von Zerssen *et al.*, 1998).

Personality accentuation

An additional diagnosis was introduced in the draft tenth revision of the *International Classification of Disease* (World Health Organization, 1987) – that of personality accentuation. This formalizes a component of classification in European psychiatry that has been present for many years. It has already been mentioned that Morel emphasized that those with 'congenital nervous temperament' could become mentally ill under influences which, under normal circumstances, would not give rise to illness. Later, Curran and Mallinson (1944) formalized the description of 'vulnerable personalities' who showed a relatively mild de-

gree of abnormality but who were liable to develop formal mental illness 'when pinched by circumstances'. Thus the stage was set for the formal description of personality accentuation as abnormalities of personality that are intermediate between normal personality and personality disorder.

Leonhard (1968) first used the term 'accentuated personality', although many of the ideas he expressed had already appeared earlier in his book on normal and abnormal personalities (Leonhard, 1963). He differentiated between normal, accentuated and abnormal personalities by reference to both personality and setting. Normal personalities are able to adapt to all kinds of environmental situations, those with personality accentuation show no problem in adapting to a *positive* setting but are maladaptive in a demanding or stressful environment, and abnormal personalities (equivalent to personality disorder) are maladaptive in all situations. Unfortunately, Leonhard does not define maladaptation or positive and negative environments. He further makes a distinction between accentuated characters and temperamental traits and classifies them into single and mixed types.

One advantage of using the term 'accentuated personality' is that it allows personality disorder to be defined more rigorously and confined to persistent maladaptive functioning that is completely independent of situation. Personality accentuation shows more links to normal personality than personality disorder. Integrated function is possible, social malfunction is specific to certain situations and tends to be less in degree than other personality disorders. Unfortunately, Leonhard does not help us to define the boundaries between personality accentuation and normal personality on the one hand and with personality disorder on the other. Implicitly, he conceives of them as a continuum but this may not be assumed. This concept is discussed later under 'Personality Difficulty'.

Relationship between temperament, personality and personality disorders

There is some confusion in the literature about the definition of temperament, character and personality. Many authors (particularly from the German school) use them interchangeably but, in general, temperament and character tend to be regarded as basic substrates on which personality is fashioned. In keeping with this notion are the results of studies that show that heredity has a strong influence in determining temperament. Twin studies (Shields and Slater, 1960) have demonstrated significantly higher concordance rates from monozygotic (MZ; $r = 0.8$) compared with dizygotic (DZ; $r = 0.3$) twins for temperamental and personality features. Buss and Plomin (1975) most forcefully make the argument that temperament is a genetically determined characteristic that shows marked stability over time and which subsequently affects personality development.

Because of the difficulty in reliably diagnosing personality disorder, there are no systematic genetic studies in this group and this remains a major deficiency in our knowledge. Nevertheless there is reasonable evidence from family studies in the USA that the flamboyant cluster of personality disorders, particularly the antisocial, histrionic and borderline categories, probably have a hereditary component in their aetiology (Robins, 1966; Guze *et al.*, 1967; Cloninger and Guze, 1970, 1973; Loranger *et al.*, 1982). However, the twin and adoptee studies that are necessary to show genetic predisposition are few in number. Christiansen (1970) found that monozygotic twins had a concordance rate of 36% for antisocial personality disorder and dizygotic twins only a 12% concordance. However, in most studies the MZ–DZ differences for personality disorder are not as large as this and often not significant. By comparison with other mental disorders, the genetic contribution appears to be relatively low (Slater and Cowie, 1971; Schulsinger, 1972). However, these studies were carried out many years ago before reliable assessment of personality disorder was made and so it would be unwise to conclude too much from them.

Rutter (1987), in his 1986 Maudsley lecture, surveyed the spectrum of personality from temperament to personality disorder. He has the advantage, being a child psychiatrist, of studying personality in developmental terms and viewing personality disorder from a broader perspective. In particular, there are many studies of temperament in children that are pertinent to personality development. These demonstrate individual differences between children that are significant in terms of later psychiatric disorder. Children with 'difficult' temperamental features are more likely to have behaviour problems later in childhood and to lead to hostility and criticism from their parents. Temperament is more difficult to assess than behaviour as Rutter *et al.* (1964) have pointed out that it is an abstraction based on external assessment of the child's behaviour rather than direct observation. As such it is likely to be less reliably assessed than direct observation, partly because of bias in interpreting the behaviour by the assessor and partly because behaviour is situation specific, as the work of Mischel (1979) has shown. Personality, according to Rutter, involves the integration of relationships, certain habitual cognitive sets and motivating traits that go beyond the dispositional aspects of temperament. Personality disorders differ mainly through the persistence of maladaptive personality features from adolescence onwards.

This description might imply a continuum from temperament at one end through to severe personality disorder at the other, with normal personality variation and accentuation in-between. Thus, for example, the conduct disorder demonstrated by Robins (1966) in her classic study to be a precursor of antisocial personality disorder in adult life, has all the ingredients of antisocial behaviour in bud and it is only in adult life that these are seen in full flower.

However, Rutter rejects this model of personality variation because he is unable to identify any common features that apply across this postulated range. Temperament is concerned with 'a relatively small number of simple, non-motivational, non-cognitive factors', personality with 'coherence of functioning' of traits with processes involving cognitive, emotional and social mechanisms, and personality disorders with 'persistent, pervasive abnormality in social relationships and social functioning generally' (Rutter, 1987).

This view differs from much implicit thinking about the relationship between personality and personality disorder. The nomenclature of trait theorists and personality disorder match fairly closely and it is assumed that, for example, a subject with obsessional personality traits present to a mild degree without an impairment in social adjustment is not different fundamentally from another whose marked rigidity and obsessionality create handicaps in most parts of his personal and occupational life.

Graham and Stevenson (1987a,b) argue that extremes of temperamental difficulties are themselves disorder, at least in child psychiatry, and that the distinction between temperament, personality and disorder made by Rutter is not a fundamental one. Taken together, the evidence from genetic, clinical and follow-up studies shows that personality and its disorders are more complex than temperament and involves influences of a range of environmental factors. This acknowledgement does not argue necessarily for a *qualitative* distinction between temperament and personality disorder and, in the studies described elsewhere in this book, the initial hypothesis taken is that temperament and character are part of the same personality spectrum. This view was expressed in the first edition of this book and we see little reason to change in the light of new evidence.

Cloninger (1987) postulated a biosocial theory of personality that incorporates clinical, pharmacological and biological data. He hypothesizes that there are three dimensions of personality called novelty seeking, harm avoidance and reward dependence, and has developed an instrument, the Tridimensional Personality Questionnaire (TPQ), for recording these dimensions. He cites pharmacological evidence that novelty seeking is principally concerned with dopamine modulation, harm avoidance with serotonin (5-hydroxytryptamine, 5-HT) and reward dependence with noradrenaline. By viewing personality disorders as extreme variants of, or imbalance between, these three dimensions, Cloninger aims to identify the main characteristics of eight categories of personality disorder (including the cyclothymic one that has now been abandoned) and gives a convincing account of these in terms of his dimensional approach. The eight disorders he identifies are antisocial, histrionic, passive–aggressive and passive–dependent, explosive, obsessional, schizoid and cyclothymic ones.

This is an interesting theory that has face validity and been extensively studied. It is certainly a useful tool in investigating pathology, particularly in non-psychotic disorders (Mulder *et al.*, 1994) and has now incorporated character into its system (Cloninger *et al.*, 1993). However, research findings have not always supported the tridimensional system (Howard *et al.*, 1997) and its value, as well as its validity, remains an open question. This should not decry its potential, however, because any explanation of personality abnormality that can draw on more than a set of empirical findings (which is currently the major contribution to our knowledge) is worthy of close attention as it could represent a major breakthrough.

Summary

This review of the concept of personality disorder demonstrates the many difficulties it has evoked. It belongs to psychiatry and yet is strangely apart, and at various times we have tried to dismiss it from our professional consciousness. It is a concept like body odour, indubitably affected by constitution and environment, a source of distress to both sufferer and society, yet imbued with ideas of degeneracy and inferiority so that its possession is also a personal criticism.

Nevertheless, it is now well established as a defined group of psychiatric disorders that needs to be studied independently of other psychiatric states. Our own definition of personality disorder is, as in the first edition of this book, 'a persistent abnormality of personal and social functioning that is independent of mental integration', where 'mental integration' is used to describe abnormalities of mental state. This harks back to Prichard's original description of moral insanity but also allows for the co-occurrence of personality disorder with abnormalities of mental state. However, their independence is proved by the persistence of the personality abnormalities when the mental state returns to normal. The extent of this co-occurrence (now called, not always correctly, comorbidity) will be a theme that is returned to repeatedly in future chapters. The prevalence, severity, course and influence on other mental disorders of each type of personality aberration forms the main part of this book. We think it best to retain the notion of personality disorder and mental state diagnoses as belonging to separate axes within the classification and this appears to be the main lesson that this historical review has taught us. It has helped research enormously to have personality disorder evaluated separately from mental state problems and, even if the solution is found eventually to be a recommendation for a single grouping, the exercise of separation has been a fruitful and productive one.

2

Classification of personality disorder

Peter Tyrer and Brian Ferguson

The diagnosis and classification of personality disorder has long been a subject of dispute and has led many in the past to question the whole value of the concept. However, despite these difficulties, the notion of personality disorder is too valuable to be casually cast aside and most effort now is devoted to describing personality disorder more effectively instead of rejecting the concept. However, until a robust and reliable classification of personality disorder can be demonstrated, the argument that personality disorder is a pejorative label, best summarized by the title of a paper by Lewis and Appleby (1988) 'Personality disorder, the patients psychiatrists dislike', can be regarded as an equally valid alternative. The relationship of personality disorders to other variations of personality status is also important and similarly controversial. There are those who maintain that personality disorder is fundamentally distinct from the range of normal personality whereas others, with equal conviction, believe that they are positioned on a continuum in which the decision whether or not to make a formal diagnosis of personality disorder is to some extent arbitrary. As if these difficulties were not enough, the final debate is between those who feel that these disorders can be classified and those who regard personality as a combination of characteristics that separates individuals from each other and thereby makes them unique. For this latter group, any classification which lumps personalities together will destroy the features that make personality the fingerprint of individuality. It is worthwhile exploring this conflict in a little more detail.

Nomothetic and idiographic approaches

Psychologists have characteristically studied personality in large groups and looked for common features, whereas the main psychiatric assessment of personality disorder until recently has been the case history based on clinical judgement. This is a good example of the difference between the nomothetic and idiographic approaches to classification and diagnosis. These terms were originally used by the German philosopher, Wilhelm Windelband, to distinguish between the study of individuals (hence idiographic) and the whole (universal) (hence nomothetic) populations. The idiographic approach focuses on the uniqueness of the individual and as such can provide a rich, multifaceted description of subtle areas of personal attributes and behaviour. Numerous strands are brought together to build up a portrait which cannot be confused with any other. The case history is the most obvious example and has been used with effect to describe processes, which can then be generalized to explain similar psychological mechanisms in others. The terms 'morphogenic' in place of idiographic and 'dimensional' in place of nomothetic were subsequently introduced by Allport (1937) but have not supplanted the originals. Psychoanalytical theories of personality have largely been developed from this source, although the close study of individual dynamics in a small number of individuals has been regarded as a source of universal truths that can be applied in a nomothetic way.

The nomothetic approach uses laws and set parameters such as operational criteria in order to measure the specific aspects of a condition that separate it from others. Yardsticks are established in advance by which the collective measurement of personality is carried out. The chief value in studying groups of subjects comes from our ability to generalize in a more confident way. It, therefore, becomes possible to predict the future behaviour of one individual on the basis of his resemblance to the group in specific and well-described dimensions. The process of applying these laws, however, inevitably leads to the loss of precision and may indeed lead us to ignore important areas of personality not measured by the set parameters. Allport (1937) has succinctly expressed this concern that, by using the nomothetic approach, psychology stands 'in danger of losing the human person in everyday life as we know him'. On the other hand, the subjectivity of the idiographic approach is its greatest weakness. Considerable difficulty is encountered in organizing or classifying material obtained in this way so that exchange of information between professionals is often impeded. For example, projective techniques for assessing personality (e.g. the Rorschach Test), have been said to 'measure a little bit of everything and not enough of anything to give dependable and quantifiable samples of the personality' (MacFarlane and Tuddenham, 1951).

For many years, the assessment of personality disorder by psychiatrists took second place to the equally important arguments about the correct classification of the major mental disorders. The classification of personality disorder in, for example, the eighth revision of the *International Classification of Disease* (ICD-8) was little used and when tested (e.g. Walton and Presly, 1973) it was found that psychiatrists found it very hard to agree on a common diagnosis even when they had criteria defined in advance. Contributions by psychologists, on the other hand, using instruments tested by good statistical methods, seemed best suited to measuring personality traits in normal populations. The whole process of assessment became confused during the controversy, which arose in relation to *situation specificity*, the impact that a situation has on a person's behaviour and the extent to which behaviour is independent of this. In its most extreme form, the situationist view would be that personality traits do not exist as broad dispositions, as it is the setting that is the most important determinant of behaviour and personality (Mischel, 1968). It is doubtful whether any psychologist holds this view any longer. Mischel subsequently altered his viewpoint. In his latest book he suggests that the question 'are persons or situations more important?' in determining behaviour and personality is misleading and unanswerable. The right question is '*when* are situations most likely to exert powerful effects, and conversely, when are person variables likely to be more influential' (Mischel, 1986). The arguments in favour of personality disorder as a separate group of mental conditions hinges on the argument that in such disorders 'person variables' are indeed the most influential characteristics. It is when they dominate a person's behaviour so that they are present in almost all situations of conflict, that serious impairment of relationships and general disintegration of social functioning is liable to occur.

The work of the trait psychologists

Three principal measuring instruments have emerged from the large corpus of psychological work of the twentieth century: the Eysenck Personality Inventory (EPI), the Minnesota Multiphasic Personality Inventory (MMPI) and the 16 Personality Factor Questionnaire (16-PF). There are many other questionnaires that have been introduced for the assessment of personality and several of these are discussed elsewhere in this book but these three have been the major influence in assessing personality within normal populations.

The Eysenck inventories

There are three of these inventories, and all are closely related. These are the Maudsley

Personality Inventory (MPI), the Eysenck Personality Inventory (EPI) and the Eysenck Personality Questionnaire (EPQ). The theoretical concept underlying these instruments is that of organization of personality at four levels. The first level, called stimulus response (SR), is reflected by the subject's response to the demands of a particular situation which may or may not be characteristic of the person. The habitual response (HR) is at the second level of personality organization and reflects the likelihood that the behaviour will be repeated. The third or trait level is based on the intercorrelation of habitual responses, these traits being further organized into the fourth level, namely that of personality type. Eysenck's work has focused principally on personality types and has identified three dimensions of personality: N (neuroticism–stability), E (extraversion–introversion) and P (psychoticism–normality). The first inventory designed to measure neuroticism was developed in 1952 and called the Maudsley Medical Questionnaire (MMQ) and was found to be capable of differentiating between normal and neurotic soldiers. Using this and further items derived from the Guilford Scales (Guilford and Guilford, 1939), Eysenck went on to develop the Maudsley Personality Inventory (MPI), designed to measure both neuroticism and extraversion. The EPI is essentially an improved version of the MPI. It has 108 questions concerning the E and N aspects of personality and contains a separate lie scale based on a very detailed statistical analysis of numerous studies using the earlier instruments (Eysenck and Eysenck, 1969). With the help of these inventories the relationship between personality type and physiological and hereditary factors has been investigated. In general, much of the available evidence supports Eysenck's theoretical construct of personality dimensions, although the third dimension defined by the P scale has attracted controversy. The most used version of the instrument is the Eysenck Personality Questionnaire (Eysenck and Eysenck, 1975).

Eysenck's questionnaires have been used more in the assessment of personality than the instruments of other psychologists. His dimensional perspective has been supported by other workers approaching personality from completely different standpoints (e.g. Tellegen, 1985; Cloninger, 1987). In the USA,

the concept of neuroticism is now less acceptable and negative affectivity has been proposed as an alternative (Watson and Clark, 1984).

Despite early optimism, Eysenck's work has not been of much value to psychiatrists. After publication of Eysenck's first book on personality classification (1947), Eliot Slater predicted that 'one consequence of this work will be that our text books of psychiatry will have to be largely rewritten' (Slater, 1948). No such revision has taken place and, instead of Eysenck's comparatively simple classification, the categorization of both personality and neurosis has become more detailed in the succeeding years. However, subsequent research has established that the trait grouping constituting neuroticism is remarkably useful as a general predictor and is relatively stable.

One of the main concerns that psychiatrists have about Eysenck's inventories is the validity of the questionnaire taken at a single point in time. However, this is true of all such questionnaires and there is little doubt that mental state abnormalities distort the findings of such questionnaires to a significant degree. In large population studies this is not particularly important. However, when the instruments are used in defined psychiatric populations it becomes much more so. Although Eysenck included questions to determine the 'lie score' it does not account for mental state distortion and only partly compensates for 'social desirability', the recognition that most abnormal personality features are not desirable ones and the natural tendency to deny these in ourselves.

Cattell and the 16 Personality Factor Questionnaire

The work of Raymond Cattell, an English psychologist who later emigrated to the USA, is similarly based on multivariate analysis. It also emphasizes the importance of traits in personality assessment. Information is classified according to its source: 'L data' or life record because it deals with real life actual behaviour and can be objectively measured, 'Q data' being the type of data elicited by questionnaire and liable to distortion by imperfect self-knowledge, and 'T data', so-called because this information is based on data obtained from 'objective tests'.

Personality is envisaged as being organized on several levels. When a set of personality variables correlates one with another, then they are regarded as surface traits. A source trait on the other hand is so defined because it is identified as having an influence on the underlying cause. There is a further cross-classification depending on whether behaviour deals with abilities, general personality and temperament traits, and dynamic interest and maturation traits.

Cattell began his work by condensing the list of over 3000 personality trait names supplied by Allport and Odbert (1936). The 16 Personality Factor Questionnaire was then derived from the factor patterns of ratings on these personality dimensions and the factor structure checked independently by further analysis. Cattell resorted to neologisms in labelling the 16 dimensions in order to avoid conceptual contamination through association with previous usage.

Several of Cattell's dimensions are intercorrelated and so can be reduced to second-order factors. The first two of these resemble Eysenck's types to a large degree. Cattell's work has had many applications in areas of educational and industrial selection and organization and in the treatment of neurotic and delinquent patients. At first glance it might appear that Cattell and Eysenck are in total opposition to one another in the number of personality dimensions that each propose. The difficulty stems principally from the methods of factor analysis chosen by either school. Eysenck's personality dimensions are orthogonal, so the factors are independent of one another. Cattell, on the other hand, relies on the rotation of factors to oblique simple structure; in other words, factors may be correlated with one another but nonetheless are distinct dimensions of personality.

Cattell's work, although extremely thorough, careful and antedating Eysenck, has had even less impact on psychiatric thinking. The use of neologisms in describing his 16 dimensions was probably a mistake, although his reasons for choosing them were understandable. Psychiatric opinion has probably changed little since its earliest verdict on his work published in response to his first study

in Leicester in the 1930s. After describing Cattell's dimensions of personality the author writing for the *Lancet* concluded, somewhat unfairly in retrospect, that 'Dr Cattell's study is more interesting in itself than for any possible immediate practical application' (Editorial, 1934). As we shall see later, Cattell's descriptions do correlate well with much of the current descriptions of abnormal personality and it is perhaps unfortunate that his work has been somewhat neglected by the profession.

The Minnesota Multiphasic Personality Inventory

The MMPI was derived through a process of empirical construction. It was developed as a clinical tool to differentiate between abnormal personalities although subsequently it has been used with normal populations. For example, identical questions were put to separate groups of paranoid and non-paranoid individuals: the items which had the most discriminating power were then chosen to be incorporated into the inventory. In all, a total of over 550 statements are presented to the subject to which he responds with a true or false reply. A considerable body of information has now been collected on the individual scales, which show a considerable degree of intercorrelation. The scales themselves have unfortunately been labelled using standard psychiatric nosology (e.g. paranoia, schizophrenia and hypomania) which can lead to confusion with Axis I diagnosis. They should more properly be regarded as indicative of the presence of specific personality attributes. Although the MMPI is currently used in candidate-selection procedures, its principal value would appear to be in the study of clinically abnormal personalities where interpretation by an experienced psychologist is required.

The MMPI still appears to be of considerable value despite being a hoary veteran in personality terms. Morey and his colleagues (1985) have developed 11 scales, which match with the DSM personality disorders, and so the instrument could also be used (see later in this chapter) to classify personality disorders using the current system.

Use of questionnaires in personality assessment

As we have seen, the nomothetic approach emphasizes the standardization of character evaluation. This can be done using one or all of the three types of databanks (Cattell, 1965), i.e. the data derived from observable behaviour (L) (life record), questionnaires (Q) or objective tests (T). L data are valued for their objectivity as the past record can be checked for accuracy, for example, if measuring the number of times prosecuted for drunkenness. Objective testing is obviously time-consuming and difficult to validate and is very much influenced by the conditions under which the test is carried out. Not surprisingly, therefore, the questionnaire method is the most frequently chosen one for personality assessment irrespective of the theoretical bias of the assessor.

Questionnaires, however, have certain well-described drawbacks, in particular their susceptibility to response sets. The acquiescent response set may lead the subject to agree with items simply on the basis of their perceived desirability (Vernon, 1963). The opposite may also be true; the MMPI depression scales have been shown to be significantly related to social undesirability response scores (Langevin and Stoner, 1979). In general, subjects tend to answer personality questionnaires defensively, a problem which naturally assumes greater importance when self-interest is paramount. Compulsorily detained patients and applicants for jobs are especially suspect and in these populations self-ratings are almost valueless (although many who make a living selling these approaches would disagree). Deliberate faking is possible and many questionnaires now include lie scales to test this phenomenon. It is far from clear what the assessor can do with the remaining replies following the discovery that particular ones are manifestly untrue. Less than honest replies may of course be immaterial in empirically derived inventories such as the MMPI which simply rely on the actual responses to the items to differentiate one group from another whether or not those responses are actually true. Specific techniques such as the introduction of forced choice options in questionnaire construction are discussed in detail by Vernon (1963).

The main handicap of questionnaires in assessing personality is their susceptibility to contamination by relatively minor changes in the mental state, of which depression is the most widely studied. The similarity between the dimension of neuroticism or emotionality and affective state has been highlighted by Watson and Clark (1984) and so it is hardly surprising that a temporary change in mood as a consequence of mental illness is likely to alter ratings on this dimension. This has been known for many years (Coppen and Metcalfe, 1965; Knowles and Kreitman, 1965). Ratings for neuroticism increase during illness and return to lower levels on recovery. Although there are many instruments that attempt to separate 'state' affect from 'trait' affect, of which the State–Trait Anxiety Inventory (Spielberger *et al.*, 1970) is perhaps the best known, in practice it is very difficult to separate the two. As a consequence, any studies that purport to demonstrate improvement in personality pathology when there is concurrent mental state disorder (e.g. Ekselius and von Knorring, 1998) cannot do so with any confidence.

Kendell and DiScipio (1968) suggested that if the subjects were specifically asked to ignore their current state when using questionnaires such as the EPI, the results would be more likely to show long-standing personality characteristics. However, Hirschfeld and his colleagues have shown that this instruction does not remove the tendency for scores on this dimension to increase during a depressive illness (Hirschfeld and Klerman, 1979; Hirschfeld *et al.*, 1983). Although the difficulty in separating personality status from mental illness is acknowledged, the change in scores produced by even a relatively brief period of affective disturbance is disturbing and tends to invalidate claims that, for example, high neuroticism scores are predictive of psychiatric disorder (Eysenck and Eysenck, 1964). If the rating of the personality trait is increased by a disorder, the rating can hardly be said to be predictive.

Similar increase in the emotional stability (E) and objectivity (O) scales of the Guilford–Zimmerman Temperament Survey has been noted during anxiety disorders in which panic is the major symptom (Reich *et al.*, 1986) and which fall again on recovery. As the E and O scales of the Guilford–Zimmerman Temperament Survey are highly correlated with neuroticism in the MPI (Guilford *et al.*, 1976) they are probably measuring the same dimension. It seems reasonable to conclude from these findings that any scale concerned with neuroticism or negative affectivity would be unsuitable for the assessment of personality traits in someone with any form of affective illness.

The other major problem with most questionnaires developed by psychologists to measure personality is that the dimensions chosen are difficult to relate to the categories of personality disorder used by psychiatrists (except when special attempts have been made to them such as that described above (Morey *et al.*, 1985)). This may be merely a problem of nomenclature and the fact that most personality scales have been used with people with personalities within the normal range. Nevertheless, all questionnaires used to record personality status before the introduction of DSM-III can be used to record personality as a dimension with no particular reference to personality disorder as a clinical concept. Those who were interested in measuring personality disorder therefore felt that the work of the trait psychologists was going to be of little relevance to them and they set about constructing their own instruments. The need for such instruments has been demonstrated by the dramatic growth of questionnaires used specifically for the assessment of personality disorder in recent years. These are discussed later in this chapter.

The main advantages stemming from the use of questionnaires are the standardization of replies and the resultant ease of analysis of large numbers of subjects. It is theoretically possible to establish good reliability (but has not been achieved as often as might be expected), although validity will obviously be more problematic. This is inevitably true when it is dependent on concurrent measurements that in turn may have unproven or shaky validity despite being widely accepted. The danger, as with all potentially reliable instruments, is that reliability becomes confused with validity. 'If it can be measured it must exist' can be repeated so often it can be believed. Cattell's verdict of the value of questionnaires in personality assessment, that they are 'tolerably useful if intelligently de-

signed', is a modest and realistic assessment of their value. Their main use has been in large populations in which other forms of rating are impractical.

Psychodynamic influences on personality classification

Psychoanalysis has had a major influence on personality classification. Freud's original concepts of the *id*, *ego* and *superego* were subsequently developed into personalities or characters by him and others, particularly Reich (1933) and Fenichel (1945). All individuals were postulated to go through three dynamic stages of development: the oral stage, which corresponds to the period when gratification is achieved largely by taking things by mouth, the anal phase, during which the child develops pleasure from controlling, and sometimes thwarting, the basic needs of his or her sphincters, and the sexual or phallic phase in which attention is focused on the genital areas. Freud (1932) developed these concepts further and suggested that those who became fixed at the oral stage and demanded immediate gratification of the id developed an 'erotic' personality type which could now be roughly correlated with the impulsive and antisocial personality disorders. Secondly, those fixed at the anal stage became anankastic or compulsive personalities, and those who were dominated by the ego became narcissistic personalities.

Alexander (1930) made an important contribution in separating character or personality from neurosis. Those who developed neurotic disorder were said to be *egodystonic* in that their symptoms were alien to their normal personality, thinking and mode of functioning, whereas those with character disorder were *egosyntonic* in that their neurotic mechanisms of functioning were incorporated into their personality and regarded as necessary.

The latest psychoanalytical literature has been more confusing and difficult to integrate easily. Many different subtypes have been proposed but most have not received any common acceptance. In the USA, Otto Kernberg (1967, 1975) has been a major influence. He has largely abandoned the psychosexual model of earlier theorists and introduced the concept of structural organization to personality. Depending on the level of organization, different personalities are assigned to higher, intermediate or lower levels. The lower levels are often referred to as 'borderline' personalities because they are less well formed. Thus antisocial, impulsive and narcissistic personalities are placed in the borderline group and histrionic and compulsive ones at the higher level of structural organization.

Kernberg's views have influenced the current classification of personality disorder in DSM-III and DSM-IV. In particular, the most common cluster of DSM-III personality disorders, commonly known as the flamboyant, emotional or dramatic (cluster B), includes histrionic, narcissistic, antisocial and borderline personalities. The other two clusters, the eccentric one containing the paranoid, schizoid and schizotypal disorders (cluster A), and the anxious or fearful one, including the avoidant, dependent, compulsive and passive–aggressive personality disorders (cluster C), belong to Kernberg's higher level of structural organization.

Current classification of personality disorder and its assessment

It is only in the last 30 years that the classification and assessment of personality disorder has achieved the degree of scrutiny appropriate for a mental science. Before then, clinical psychiatry was largely unaffected by the great strides made by psychologists throughout the twentieth century in the understanding of personality. There appear to have been two reasons for this. Clinical psychiatrists who are not psychotherapists traditionally operated within the framework of personality descriptions elaborated by Kretschmer, Schneider, Henderson and Cleckley, which are based on intuitive understanding and critical observation. This essentially idiographic approach has not lent itself to good reliability and the subclassification of personality disorder has been so handicapped by this that it was hardly taken seriously. Psychotherapists worked within their own specific school of personality development in which precise measurement was often lacking

and considered relatively unimportant. Although the questionnaires of psychologists had some interest, much of the information derived had little obvious clinical relevance and could not be used to predict prognosis or provide adequate guidelines in the choice of treatment. The evidence that questionnaire scores were different when measured during the active phase of a psychiatric illness and after recovery also limited their value. It is also fair to add that almost all the psychologists who developed the questionnaires for personality assessment had no knowledge of personality disorder and very few of them had any direct contact with psychiatric patients. Unfortunately this latter fact was often considered a virtue; it was only when the inventor was uncontaminated by experience that he could build personality castles in the air.

The clinician's reluctance to take the classification and assessment of personality disorder seriously was highlighted by important studies in the 1970s. Walton *et al.* (1970) and Walton and Presly (1973) showed that not only was inter-rater reliability of personality disorder poor, but that the individual diagnoses of personality disorder were more related to personal idiosyncrasy than any objective criteria. Australian colleagues encountered similar difficulties when looking at the clinical diagnoses of Axis II disorders (the personality disorder group in DSM-III) (Mellsop *et al.*, 1982). They went on to observe that, although a standardized interview schedule would help in respect of reliability, it would not carry over into ordinary clinical use. This is unfortunately still true.

Since the introduction of structured interview schedules for assessing personality disorders in the last 20 years the assessment of personality disorder has undoubtedly improved in research practice. Although most clinicians do not define personality disorder with the help of such instruments the awareness of the importance of making an independent assessment of the personality domain has become appreciated to a much greater extent. What is sorely missing is an instrument that is easy to use and carries a wide degree of acceptance so it could be employed in ordinary clinical use. The alternative of ordinary clinical use coming to resemble the use of a structured interview is also equally acceptable. At the third European Congress on Personality Disorders held in Sheffield 1998, a set of six targets was agreed for personality disorder by the year 2010 in all European countries. The first of these targets was that 'an internationally accepted instrument for diagnosing personality disorders' would be used in all patients being assessed by mental health services by the year 2010. This is an ambitious target and we can only hope that it will be achieved in at least some countries.

Specific questionnaires for the diagnosis and assessment of personality disorder

There are now many of these questionnaires, most of them using the DSM classification as their reference criteria. The many that exist indicates a disturbing fact; none of them can be regarded as satisfactory. Despite this it is useful to look at each of them in some detail to assess their relative merits and disadvantages.

Dichotomous versus categorical classification

Although doctors and decision-makers in all parts of medicine prefer categorical classifications to dimensional ones there is increasing evidence from research studies in personality disorder that the dimensional system of classifying personality disorder is more valid and reliable (Livesley *et al.*, 1994; Clark *et al.*, 1995). The major problem appears to be with the specific personality disorder diagnoses rather than the broad concept of personality disorder as a whole. Thus the ICD-10 and DSM-IV definitions of personality disorder as 'deviations of personal characteristics and behaviour patterns from the norm', manifest mainly as dysfunctional behaviour which is 'pervasive', and which leads to distress or impairment in social, occupational and personal function, is more reliably rated than any of the individual personality disorders (listed in *Table 2.1*) (Bronisch, 1992; Bronisch and Mombour, 1994). The inadequacy of the specificity of the individual personality disorders is demonstrated by the degree of overlap between different personality disorders, particularly for disorders within the flamboyant

Table 2.1 Levels of agreement between a checklist and a structured interview (International Personality Disorder Examination) in rating ICD-10 and DSM-III-R personality disorders (from Bronisch and Mombour, 1994)

Classification system	Personality disorder	Level of agreement (K_w)	Level of clinical significance (after Cicchetti and Sparrow, 1981)
ICD-10	Paranoid	0.63	Good
	Schizoid	−0.03	Poor
	Impulsive	0.54	Fair
	Histrionic	0.38	Poor
	Anankastic	0.48	Fair
	Anxious	0.68	Good
	Dependent	0.63	Good
	Any personality disorder	0.75	Excellent
DSM-III-R	Paranoid	0.63	Good
	Schizoid	−0.03	Poor
	Schizotypal	−0.03	Poor
	Borderline	0.55	Fair
	Histrionic	−0.07	Poor
	Narcissistic	0.54	Fair
	Avoidant	0.71	Good
	Dependent	0.27	Poor
	Obsessive–compulsive	0.30	Poor
	Passive–aggressive	0.66	Good
	Self-defeating	0.0	Poor
	Sadistic	0.0	Poor
	Any personality disorder	0.52	Fair

personality cluster (Pfohl *et al.*, 1986; Fyer *et al.*, 1988; Flick *et al.*, 1993). This overlap is often inflated with the description of 'comorbidity', implying that two or more separate disorders exist in the same person, when it is more likely that the person has one disorder than is inadequately defined (Tyrer, 1992, 1996).

Nevertheless, the fact remains that categorical diagnosis is still the preferred option for clinicians and, in the field of forensic psychiatry in particular, this is often imperative since the presence of a specific defined disorder has been the cornerstone of treatment and detention decisions ever since the Lunacy Act of 1890 was introduced. The diagnostic importance of personality disorder became even more important with the introduction of 'psychopathy' as a reason for special management of mental disorder (Dolan and Coid, 1993). It is therefore sad that the criteria for making these diagnostic decisions were, until so recently, so poorly defined that the diagnosis of personality disorder was influenced more by subjective judgement than any independent assessment.

The next section of this chapter describes the main principles lying behind the diagnosis of personality disorder; this is followed by description of categories of personality disorder and their assessment (and in which special attention will be paid to those disorders that are common in forensic psychiatric practice) and the last discusses the dimensional assessment of severity.

General principles of diagnosis and assessment

A good diagnosis is one that should be relatively easy to obtain, preferably in the course of a clinical interview. Increasingly, formal means of obtaining diagnosis in all parts of psychiatry are being recommended, most frequently in the form of structured or semi-structured interviews, but it is important to realize that these only consist of good comprehensive clinical interviews together with a formal scoring system. There are several important differences between the assessment of personality disorder and mental state disorders. In the case of personality disorder the assessor is not primarily interested in recording symptoms and clinical features in a standardized way as is the case with most mental disorders, but in assessing maladaptive behaviour and its effects on the subject and others, attitudes and relationships with other people, and social functioning in all its areas (at work, at home, with family and friends, and with society in general). The second important difference is that in assessing personality disorder the present state is not necessarily important; the normal functioning of the subject over a much longer time scale, ideally since adolescence, is being determined.

These differences immediately give rise to problems that make it more difficult to diagnose personality disorder than mental state disorders and those who make personality assessments should not be too apologetic about them. The reliability and validity of assessment is clearly going to be less when a hypothetical (or more strictly, a past norm) is being determined instead of present mental state, and the important elements of observation of the subject and describing the phenomenology of the mental state are spurious to the clinician assessing personality disorder (except in helping to discount mental state elements). The reliability problems are accentuated by the tendency for those with some forms of personality disorder, particularly in the flamboyant group, to exaggerate, minimize or deny aspects of their personality.

Because of these problems there are arguments for using much more than an interview with the patient in order to make a diagnosis of personality disorder. This has led to the suggestion that the best form of diagnosis is what has been called the LEAD standard (the longitudinal expert evaluation that includes all data) (Spitzer, 1983; Skodol *et al.*, 1988). This may be true, but unfortunately there is no good way of deciding which source of information is more reliable when different sources disagree. Informants are often considered on theoretical grounds to be more accurate assessors than subjects but unfortunately there is no fundamental evidence that they are more valid assessors (Zimmerman *et al.*, 1988). However, in comparisons of types of informant there are important differences and women, particularly if they are closely involved with the subject and spend much time with them, are generally superior to other sources (Brothwell *et al.*, 1992; Pilgrim *et al.*, 1993).

Most of the instruments used for assessing personality disorder are subject-based and, bearing in mind that the assessment covers a long period, it is understandable that subjects are generally preferred by investigators. There remains a worry that in the most severe cases of personality disorder that the subject is inherently inaccurate or deliberately deceitful in an interview situation and that other forms of data are needed to corroborate the information obtained. Such information should always be obtained if a comprehensive assessment of personality is to be made.

Categorical diagnosis of personality disorder

The current categorical diagnoses of personality disorder are shown in *Table 2.2*. Although these are now well known to most clinicians, mainly because of the well-oiled publicity that always accompanies a new edition of the *Diagnostic and Statistical Manual of Mental Disorders* (DSM) they, in the current language of medical science, have little evidence base. They illustrate the best and the worst of current classification procedures. Because they are created by consensus by a democratic process they command broad accep-

Table 2.2 Summary of ICD-10 and DSM-IV classifications of personality disorder

Code	ICD-10 (World Health Organization, 1992)	DSM-IV (American Psychiatric Association, 1994)	Code
F 60.0	Paranoid – excessive sensitivity, suspiciousness, preoccupation with conspiratorial explanation of events, persistent tendency to self-reference	Paranoid – interpretation of people's actions as deliberately demeaning or threatening	301.0
F 60.1	Schizoid – emotional coldness, detachment, lack of interest in other people, eccentricity and introspective fantasy	Schizoid – indifference to social relationships and restricted range of emotional experience and expression	301.20
	No equivalent	Schizotypal – deficit in interpersonal relatedness with peculiarities of ideation, odd beliefs and thinking, unusual appearance and behaviour	301.22
F 60.5	Anankastic – indecisiveness, doubt, excessive caution, pedantry, rigidity and need to plan in immaculate detail	Obsessive–compulsive – preoccupation with orderliness, perfectionism and inflexibility that leads to inefficiency	301.4
F 60.4	Histrionic – self-dramatization, shallow mood, egocentricity and craving for excitement with persistent manipulative behaviour	Histrionic – excessive emotionality and attention-seeking, suggestibility, and superficiality	301.50
F 60.7	Dependent – failure to take responsibility for actions, with subordination of personal needs to those of others, excessive dependence with need for constant reassurance and feelings of helplessness when a close relationship ends	Dependent – persistent dependent and sub-missive behaviour	301.60
F 60.2	Dyssocial – callous unconcern for others, with irresponsibility, irritability and aggression, and incapacity to maintain enduring relationships	Antisocial – pervasive pattern of disregard for and violation of the rights of others occurring since the age of 15	301.7
	No equivalent	Narcissistic – pervasive grandiosity, lack of empathy, arrogance, and requirement for excessive admiration	301.81
F 60.6	Anxious – persistent tension, self-consciousness, exaggeration of risks and dangers, hypersensitivity to rejection, and restricted lifestyle because of insecurity	Avoidant – pervasive social discomfort, fear of negative evaluation and timidity, with feelings of inadequacy in social situations	301.82
F 60.3	Impulsive – inability to control anger, to plan ahead, or to think before acts, with unpredictable mood and quarrelsome behaviour Borderline – impulsivity with uncertainty over self-image, liability to become involved in intense and unstable relationships, and recurrent threats of self-harm	Borderline – pervasive instability of mood, interpersonal relationships and self-image associated with marked impulsivity, fear of abandonment, identity disturbance and recurrent suicidal behaviour	301.83

tance and are used internationally, but the process also means that contradictory elements are commonplace and there is no overall integration of the classification, best summarized in the statement 'a camel is a horse created by a committee'.

The personality disorders are generally less well described in the classification than any other group of disorders (Sartorius *et al.*, 1993). This is largely because although each disorder has face validity when considered separately the degree of overlap between them is so great that there is little value in each diagnosis individually. This phenomenon, which really indicates bad diagnosis, is reified in the literature by the word 'comorbidity', which is a respectable term to describe the presence of two or more coexisting diseases (Feinstein, 1970). In the case of personality disorders comorbidity is more often consanguinity, the same basic disorder described in different forms and by different titles (Tyrer, 1996).

The research evidence is different. Personality disorders, and personality variation in normal subjects, naturally fall into three or four major groups: a risk-taking, irresponsible one with a tendency to behaviour which, in colloquial terms, is 'over the top'; a converse one which is withdrawn and avoids social contact; a third which is timid, fearful and lacking in confidence; and the last (sometimes incorporated into the previous group) which is abnormally rigid and fastidious in its dealings with the world (Walton and Presly, 1973; Tyrer and Alexander, 1979; Cloninger, 1987). These groupings have now been formalized into a three-cluster system in the DSM system, cluster A consisting of the odd or eccentric cluster (comprising schizoid, schizotypal (in DSM) and paranoid personality disorders, cluster B consisting of the flamboyant or dramatic group (antisocial (dissocial), borderline, impulsive, narcissistic (in DSM), and histrionic personality disorders), and cluster C comprising anxious (avoidant), anankastic (obsessive–compulsive), and dependent personality disorders (Reich and Thompson, 1987). However, the cluster classification is not entirely satisfactory and has led to debate, mainly because it has little theoretical basis.

Factor and cluster analytical approaches were originally involved in getting the notion of clusters developed. There is some doubt as to whether there are three or four natural clusters. The four possibilities comprise the odd/eccentric cluster (cluster A), the flamboyant or dramatic one (cluster B), the anxious/fearful one (cluster C), or a fourth cluster (called here cluster D but not described as such by most authorities) dominated by obsessional characteristics. The support for the cluster system has almost entirely derived from empirical research (e.g. Zimmerman and Coryell (1990) using dimensional scores from the Structured Interview for DSM-III Personality Disorders (SIDP) (Stangl *et al.*, 1985)) but in this three cluster model passive–aggressive and compulsive personality disorders did not load strongly with any factor. Kass *et al.* (1985) factor-analysed the ratings of 609 outpatients made on four-point severity scales and found four clear groupings (the three Axis II clusters and a fourth consisting entirely of obsessive–compulsive personality disorder). The same four groups were identified by Tyrer and Alexander (1979) using cluster analysis and by Hyler and Lyons (1988) using factor analysis.

However, both the three or four cluster concept have limitations. Thus, although there is good evidence of close affinities between the flamboyant diagnoses in cluster B (histrionic, borderline, narcissistic, antisocial personality disorders), avoidant personality disorder links as much to cluster A as cluster C (Oldham *et al.*, 1992) and the histrionic and dependent groups overlap considerably.

There is also considerable argument over the place of avoidant personality disorder, which is in a hinterland between cluster A and cluster C as it has characteristics of both (Stuart *et al.*, 1998).

There have also been arguments in favour of abandoning all forms of categorization of personality disorder in favour of a global concept of persistent abnormality in social functioning and impaired relationships (Rutter, 1987). This has led to the development of an interview schedule that records all personality in terms of social function, the Adult Personality Functioning Assessment interview (APFA) (Hill *et al.*, 1989). Although this approach has its merits, the notion of equating all personality variation within a common framework is not generally popular, and in the field of forensic psychiatry in particular it would seem unhelpful to equate the kinds of personality disturbance seen in special hospitals (where they are often categorized as severe personality disorder) with the very different personality disturbance of conditions such as typical anankastic personality disorder. We personally favour the cluster model as the best compromise for categorical classification at present as it represents reasonably homogeneous entities that separate important groups.

Current classification of personality disorder

Most readers will be familiar with the two major classification systems in psychiatry; the *International Classification of Disease* (ICD-10), now in its tenth revision (World Health Organization, 1992), and the *Diagnostic and Statistical Manual of Mental Disorders* (DSM-IV) now in its fourth revision (American Psychiatric Association, 1994). Although the ICD is the world classification, and therefore takes pre-eminence, most of the changes made in the last 20 years have been a direct consequence of the introduction of the third revision of DSM in 1980. To refine and improve diagnosis DSM-III introduced the concept of operational criteria, central core features of the condition which can be defined clearly and together represent a distillate of the diagnostic core features. The introduction of operational criteria followed good evidence that the two major research classification systems before 1980, the Feighner criteria (Feighner *et al.*, 1972) and the Research Diagnostic Criteria (Spitzer *et al.*, 1978), were a major advance. ICD has imitated the DSM classification in many respects, although is less rigid about operational criteria and calls them *diagnostic guidelines*. These 'indicate the number and balance of symptoms usually required before confident diagnosis can be made, but they are phrased so that a degree of flexibility is retained in the diagnostic decision'. Conditions, therefore, can overrule a guideline if it conflicts with their diagnostic impression in a particular case.

Both ICD and DSM classification systems are consensual in development and dissemi-

nation. Task forces and work groups examine draft guidelines in field trials and from the results of these the final classification is developed. A democratic vote decides whether a diagnosis is included or excluded.

Although the individual diagnostic categories of personality disorder are very similar in ICD-10 and DSM-IV there is one fundamental difference between them that is sometimes forgotten. DSM recorded personality disorder as a separate axis of classification (Axis II) from mental state disorders (Axis I) because personality was considered to be in a completely different domain from that of mental state disorder. ICD-10 (and indeed all other ICD classifications) regards personality disorders as one of the mental state disorders and both are recorded amongst Axis I of the classification system. Axis II in ICD-10 records disability and level of functioning.

There are now many in the North American continent who feel that personality disorder should not have been given its own axis of classification, except possibly as a trait measure (Livesley, 1991; Clark, 1992). Most of the contributors to this book disagree and think that the decision was a sound one and should be maintained, largely because it does not allow personality assessment to be forgotten or subsumed to a far corner of the evaluation of psychopathology.

The reasons for making the separation are summarized in *Table 2.3*. The main difference stems from the fact that personality is an integral and ingrained component of a person; it is not drafted on from outside. It is therefore in a completely different domain from that of mental state disorders, which may become persistent and even alter the personality in time, but are not intrinsic to the normal functioning of the person. Because personality is intrinsic to normal functioning it is generative rather than reactive; this is illustrated later in this book when discussing life events and personality disorders. The importance of personality disorders being persistent is also an important difference, as is the fact that they tend to early in life and are normally manifest by the time of late adolescence. The evidence that personality disorders are best measured by functioning and behaviour rather than symptoms is also an important difference from mental state disorders.

Table 2.3 Differences between mental state and personality disorders

Mental state disorders	Personality disorders
Temporary (usually)	Permanent (or at least long-standing)
Reactive	Generative
Dominated more by symptoms than behaviour	Dominated mainly by behaviour and relationships with others
Diagnosed mainly on present state	Diagnosed on basis of long-term function
May develop into other mental state disorders	Tends to remain stable

These differences are important and perhaps have been lost sight of by some who have made classifications of personality disorder in both ICD-10 and DSM-IV. In particular, the diagnosis of borderline personality disorder, a condition which is often temporary, reactive, associated with major mental state disturbance, and which leads to variable impairment of function, satisfies most of the criteria in *Table 2.3* for a mental state disorder rather than a personality one, and its inclusion as a personality disorder seems to be a consequence of a large number of other factors – historical, psychodynamic and biological models, and need for care provision – that are quite independent of simple nosological ones (Simonsen, 1994).

One of the other reasons for separating personality and mental state disorders into separate axes is that the problem of comorbidity becomes much less of a diagnostic problem once this decision is made. If we regard all individuals as having a mental state and a personality then it is quite possible for someone to have a mental state and a personality disorder without it necessarily being regarded as a defective diagnosis. Subsequently it might be appropriate to define a group of 'co-axial syndromes' in which certain mental state disorders are found in association with personality ones (e.g. Tyrer *et al.*, 1992). If this is so then the nomenclature might change but the first stage is to allow both axes to exist so that assessment of both mental state and personality can be made in everybody presenting to psychiatric services.

Categorical diagnosis of personality disorder

The current guidelines for the diagnosis of the personality disorder group category (*Table 2.4*) and individual categorical description in ICD-10 and DSM-IV (*Table 2.2*) are shown. In both classifications the first stage is to decide whether an individual has personality disorder before then deciding on his classification type. This dichotomous process

Table 2.4 General diagnostic criteria for a personality disorder (derived from ICD-10 and DSM-IV guidelines)

A.	An enduring pattern of inner experience that deviates markedly from the expectations of the individual's culture. This pattern is manifested in two (or more) of the following areas: i) Cognition, i.e. ways of perceiving and interpreting self, other people and events ii) Affectivity, i.e. the range, intensity, lability, and appropriateness of emotional response iii) Interpersonal functioning iv) Impulse control.
B.	This pattern is inflexible and pervasive across a broad range of personal and social situations.
C.	The pattern leads to clinically significant distress and/or impairment in social, occupational, or other important areas of functioning.
D.	The pattern is stable and of long duration and its onset can be traced back at least to adolescence or early childhood.
E.	The enduring pattern is not better accounted for as a manifestational consequence of another mental disorder.

is far from ideal because it allows for no shades of personality abnormality short of actual disorder and the dividing line is far from clear. Although as noted in the previous chapter there was a move to have personality accentuation included as a sub-category in ICD-10 this was subsequently rejected and both classification systems are similar in having no mechanism for rating the severity of personality disturbance.

Individual categories of personality disorder

Many of the personality disorders described in ICD-10 and DSM-IV are equivalent (*Table 2.2*). Many have a well-established pedigree with what can be described as good temporal reliability; they have been described consistently over a long period of time by authorities from several different cultural settings. Others are of more recent origin and far less well established.

Paranoid personality disorder

This category is a well-established one. It combines sensitive personality, first described by Kretschmer (1918), and the paranoid personality proper. Thus, it includes the sensitive features of excessive reactions to setbacks and rebuffs, litigiousness with an excessive sense of personal rights and persistent self-reference, as well as the paranoid features of excessive suspiciousness, persistent bearing of grudges, a tendency to morbid jealousy and a tendency to find conspiracy behind innocent events. The diagnostic guidelines and operational criteria for ICD and DSM show a remarkable degree of congruence in the description of this personality disorder. It is also very long lasting; Theophrastus' 'distrustful man' seems to be the first description of paranoid personality disorder.

It is sometimes difficult to distinguish paranoid personality from other paranoid conditions, particularly paranoid schizophrenia and with paraphrenia in the elderly. The distinction may be particularly difficult if schizophrenia has developed early in life as it is almost impossible to decide what constituted 'pre-morbid personality' in such conditions.

Under these circumstances pre-morbid personality classification tends to have low reliability (Tyrer *et al.*, 1983a). It is sometimes even more difficult to distinguish some of the conditions within the schizophrenia spectrum, such as persistent delusional disorder, from paranoid personality disorder. In persistent delusional disorder a single paranoid delusion is held over a long time-period, sometimes since adolescence, and has a major influence on behaviour. The main distinguishing feature between the personality disorder and the mental state ones is that in the paranoid personality there is long-standing general suspiciousness and mistrust quite unrelated to the presence of any psychiatric symptoms. This has a major influence on the development and maintenance of relationships and very few of these individuals will trust more than one person intimately.

Schizoid personality disorder

The concept of the schizoid personality is also well established. It has usually been linked to the presence of schizophrenia and Kretschmer (1922) regarded the schizoid personality, or constitution, as an intrinsic part of the schizophrenic syndrome. Most other writers have regarded schizoid personality as independent, although present in a substantial proportion (20–40%) of patients with schizophrenia (Bleuler, 1941). Most of the key features of schizoid personality disorder are negative ones. They include lack of emotional responsivity, reluctance to achieve any close relationship, including a sexual one, a preference for isolation and eccentric behaviour. In DSM-IV the presence of 'constricted affect' (i.e. cold detachment with no emotional expression) is also an operational criterion. The presence of such a range of negative features has been a concern; this is the only individual personality disorder that comprises a list of negative features that to many smacks of the old diagnosis of simple schizophrenia, an entity that has never been properly validated.

In the preparation of DSM-III-R (R=revised) and DSM-IV, consideration was given to dropping the category of schizoid personality disorder altogether because of the growing importance of schizotypal personality disorder, which overlaps considerably with the schizoid one. However, in addition to eccentric behaviour, absence of close friends and constricted affect, the schizotypal personality is characterized by the positive features of odd speech, peculiar beliefs with magical thinking, unusual perceptual experiences and ideas of reference.

To European psychiatrists, these features are remarkably like those of schizophrenia and so, in ICD-10, schizotypal disorder is described as latent schizophrenia and placed within the schizophrenic group of disorders. Schizotypal personality disorder as a diagnostic category has developed from genetic evidence that the relatives of schizophrenic patients have these bizarre, schizophreniform features but do not satisfy the diagnosis of schizophrenia. The Danish–American adoption studies (Rosenthal *et al.*, 1971; Kety *et al.*, 1975) have perhaps had the greatest influence. These demonstrated that a significant proportion of children of schizophrenic parents had bizarre thinking and behaviour that was sufficient to place them within a grouping which they called schizophrenia spectrum disorder, but not schizophrenia itself. There are many parallels between the personality characteristics of the schizophrenia spectrum and the old descriptions of pseudoneurotic schizophrenia (Hoch and Polatin, 1949), a diagnosis that has always been frowned upon in Europe, but which includes the elements of affective disability, looseness of thinking and social anxiety, but are all described in the operational criteria for DSM-IV schizotypal personality disorder. The concept of the schizotype that lies behind schizotypal personality disorder was introduced by Rado (1956) and subsequently elaborated by Meehl (1962). However, the stability of the diagnosis over time has yet to be demonstrated and its separation from other personality disorders, particularly the borderline group, is extremely difficult (Spitzer and Endicott, 1979).

Two other conditions are relevant to schizoid and schizotypal personality disorder; Asperger's syndrome and schizoid personality disorder of childhood.

Asperger's syndrome appears to be a minor form of childhood autism but has important differences. Unlike autism, it is not associated with any speech delay or impairment of language. It begins in early childhood, is more common in boys, and includes problems in relationships with others, particularly peer groups, circumstantial repetitive speech, a tendency to be rigid in activities, sometimes involving the development of intense but rather strange interests (e.g. railway time-tables) and specific aversion of gaze (Mawson *et al.*, 1985; Tantam *et al.*, 1993). These features tend to persist into adult life but are somewhat less marked than in childhood.

Schizoid personality disorder of childhood is characterized by solitary behaviour, emotional detachment, rigid interests, peculiar forms of communication, strange fantasies and strange gestures. Unlike childhood autism, most such children are either of average or superior intelligence. Follow-up studies have suggested that schizoid personality disorder of childhood is more closely related to schizoid and schizotypal personality disorders, and indeed to schizophrenia, possibly through varying degrees of genetic penetrance (Wolff and Chick, 1980; Wolff, 1991).

Anankastic and obsessive–compulsive personality disorders

The ICD-10 and DSM-IV descriptions of anankastic and obsessive–compulsive personality disorders are almost identical. In European psychiatry, the adjective 'anankastic' was used by Kahn (1928) to describe the obsessional personality. The term has persisted, probably because it is useful to have a separate term for obsessional personality to separate it from obsessional neurosis. Unfortunately the adjective anankastic has not been successful in emigrating to North America, where the more clumsy 'obsessive–compulsive' is used both to describe the related personality and neurotic disorders.

Obsessional personality was first identified most clearly by Freud in his important paper on the 'anal character' (Freud, 1908). He emphasized the relationship between the child postponing gratification over bowel action and the adult obsessional's control of his environment by excessive orderliness. In Freud's terminology, the id is being tamed by the superego. Freud's descriptions are paraphrased in more mundane language in both ICD-10 and DSM-IV. Thus perfectionism, indecisiveness, excessive scrupulousness, rigidity and hoarding are all included. Although on the important characteristics it differentiates the anankastic personality from obsessional neurosis by the absence of true obsessional symptoms (i.e. thoughts or actions that the subject feels compelled to entertain despite subjective resistance), in DSM-IV minor examples of those that do not qualify for an obsessional syndrome may be included here. This is a change that deviates from the ICD concept of anankastic personality disorder.

The criteria for diagnosing anankastic or obsessive–compulsive personality disorder are ones that are considered desirable by many individuals when present to a small degree. The criteria include perfectionism (but only when it interferes with getting tasks completed), preoccupation with excessive detail, excessive devotion to work to the exclusion of leisure and friendships, difficulty in making decisions, excessive scrupulousness over morality, ethics or values, a general lack of generosity (mean-mindedness) and a tendency to hoard. In making assessments of this type of personality it is therefore important to realize that many would like to think that they have very mild degrees of this disorder as it is these qualities that make us all good citizens.

Histrionic personality disorder

Histrionic personality disorder is a frequently described but controversial category, which is similar in both ICD-10 and DSM-IV. Its cardinal features, self-dramatization, egocentricity, lability of mood, sexual provocativeness and excessive demands for reassurance, approval or praise, are perhaps so well known as to be a clichéd stereotype. Although, as mentioned in Chapter 1, Victorian authorities such as Maudsley and Briquet described many features typical of hysterical personality, stimulation to its separate description came from Freud's description of the oral character. This was refined into the concept of the hysterical character by Reich (1933). Perhaps the central feature is more the absence of a coherent and consistent personality. Theatricality is all embracing and, in Jaspers' words (1946), the 'personality seems to have lost its core and it consists entirely of a series of shifting masks'.

Unfortunately, histrionic personality disorder can be criticized because it has strong overtones of sexism (Chodoff and Lyons, 1958; Lerner, 1974; Kaplan, 1983). This is a serious charge because it implies that the diagnosis of histrionic personality disorder is invalid as it represents a prejudiced male view of women or, in the words of Chodoff and Lyons (1958), 'a caricature of femininity'. The charge is reinforced by evidence that histrionic personality disorder is much more frequently diagnosed in women than men (Halleck, 1967; Walton and Presly, 1973) although with better refinement of descriptions this difference is becoming less marked (Singleton *et al.*, 1998).

Because many of the features of histrionic personality disorder may be present in interviews with medical attendants (e.g. manipulative and seductive behaviour, impressionistic style of speech, seeking of approval or praise) but not necessarily present in other settings, there is concern that the diagnosis might represent an interaction between therapist and patient rather than a long-standing and persistent personality disorder. The high degree of association between histrionic personality disorder and other mental state and personality disorders (e.g. Cloninger and Guze, 1970; Lilienfeld *et al.*, 1986), together with a generally better function of patients with this disorder compared with other personality disorders (Gunderson and Zanarini, 1987) leads us to agree with Dowson and Grounds (1995) that this particular diagnosis 'requires further research to determine whether it merits a separate category'.

Dependent personality disorder

Although ICD-10 and DSM-IV largely agree on the criteria for dependent personality disorder, it is one of the categories that has changed frequently over the years. Such personalities used to be labelled with pejorative terms such as 'inadequate' and its Greek translation, 'asthenic', and in DSM-I was incorporated into the passive–aggressive personality (American Psychiatric Association, 1952). The passive–aggressive personality was separated into the three subtypes: passive–aggressive (more or less equivalent to the DSM-III passive–aggressive personality disorder), passive–dependent subtype (similar to dependent personality disorder in DSM-III) and the aggressive subtype (showing many of the characteristics of current borderline personality disorder). The operational criteria for dependent personality disorder in DSM-III-R emphasize the presence of dependent and submissive behaviour which, by implication, follow from subjective choice rather than from inability to act differently. They include the need for excessive advice and transfer of responsibility to others, inability to initiate tasks, and a constant preoccupation with being abandoned or rejected that leads to submissive and acquiescent attitudes. The diagnostic guidelines of ICD-10 are almost identical to these.

Dissocial and antisocial personality disorders

This group is the most extensively studied of the personality disorders and its validity is better established than all other types. A great deal of the credit for this is due to the St Louis group at the Washington University School of Medicine who have consistently relied on follow-up studies before reaching firm diagnostic criteria about psychiatric disorders. These studies have established clearly that antisocial personality disorder becomes manifest earlier than most others, usually during the time of secondary schooling. Delinquent behaviour, truancy, running away from home and aggressive behaviour are frequent before the age of 15 and persist into adult life and through to middle age (Robins, 1966; Guze and Goodwin, 1971; Guze, 1976; Harrington *et al.*, 1991).

The operational criteria for antisocial personality disorder therefore concentrate heavily on evidence of conduct disorder before the age of 15, as well as continuation of this pattern of behaviour beyond that age. Thus the operational criteria before 15 'include persistent truancy, suspension from school, use of weapons in fights, forced sexual activity, cruelty to animals and other people, and persistent lying'. The criteria after the age of 15 include significant unemployment (when expected to work and work was available), antisocial behaviour that leads to arrest, failure to plan ahead, and inability to function responsibly as a parent. In DSM-III the operational criteria, in effect, were the antisocial acts. Not surprisingly, therefore, inter-rater reliability was much higher for antisocial personality disorder than for other categories

(Mellsop *et al.*, 1982). The criticisms of this approach (e.g. Frances, 1980) have led to modifications of the criteria in DSM-III-R and DSM-IV, so that they are more in line with the criteria for other disorders.

Dissocial and antisocial personality disorders have more impact on society than any of the others in the classification and they therefore figure prominently in definitions of severe personality disorder.

Impulsive and borderline personality disorder

These categories, subgroups of emotionally unstable personality disorder, replaced explosive personality disorder in ICD-9 and DSM-II. The ICD change is really one of nomenclature only because the main characteristics of impulsive personality disorder – inability to plan ahead, unpredictable mood and behaviour, and constant need for an immediate reward – are all subsumed within explosive personality disorder but not fully described. Explosive personality disorder has been taken out of DSM-II because 'the explosiveness itself was in contrast to the individual's normal mode of behaviour and represented a paroxysmal deviation from what was usually a quiescent baseline state' (Lion, 1981). This raises an interesting semantic point about what constitutes persistent personality attributes, and suggests that any characteristic that is not shown more or less continuously should not be regarded as part of the personality disorder.

In spite of this, there are many characteristics of borderline personality disorder that are equivalent to those of explosive and impulsive personality type. The concept of borderline personality is well established in the USA but continues to cause bemusement elsewhere, not least because 'borderline' has so many meanings (Simonsen, 1994). Although the original description of 'borderline' by Gunderson and Singer (1975) was fairly clear, there is still confusion over whether it refers to the hinterland between neurosis and psychosis, between egodystonicity and egosyntonicity, or between normal personality organization and personality deviance. This point has been put even more forcefully by Millon (1981) who writes 'I find the word, borderline, to mean, at best, a level of severity and not a descriptive type . . . Unless the word is used to signify a class that borders on something, then it has no clinical or descriptive meaning at all' (p. 332). The diagnostic criteria for borderline disorder include these disparate psychodynamic, behavioural and mental state elements. They are (American Psychiatric Association, 1994):

1. A pattern of unstable and intense interpersonal relationships characterized by alternating between extremes of idealization and devaluation.
2. Impulsivity in at least two areas that are potentially self-damaging (e.g. spending, sex, substance misuse, reckless driving, binge eating) (but not suicidal behaviour which is covered by point 5 below).
3. Affective instability due to marked reactivity of mood (e.g. intense episodic dysphoria, irritability, or anxiety usually lasting a few hours and only rarely more than a few days).
4. Inappropriate, intense anger or lack of control of anger (e.g. frequent displays of temper, constant anger, recurrent physical fights).
5. Recurrent suicidal behaviour, gestures or threats, or self-mutilating behaviour.
6. Identity disturbance; persistent and markedly disturbed, distorted, or unstable self-image or sense of self.
7. Chronic feelings of emptiness.
8. Frantic efforts to avoid real or imagined abandonment.
9. Transient, stress-related paranoid ideation or severe dissociative symptoms.

After reading this list and the full literature on borderline personality disorder, it is easy to see how so many patients fall into its net and why it is associated with so much comorbidity. Choose a symptom and the borderline patient will demonstrate it at one time or another. So many of the operational criteria necessary for the definition of the syndrome are similar to the criteria for other personality disorders (e.g. unstable relationships in antisocial personality disorder, affective instability in histrionic personality disorder, persistent identity disturbance in schizotypal personality disorder). It is, therefore, not surprising that it is extremely difficult to separate the diagnosis of borderline personality from these others (Kroll *et al.*, 1981; Barrash *et al.*, 1983) and this absence of specificity is a major criticism of the category.

Borderline personality disorder is the only DSM-III diagnosis that includes a significant affective component to the disorder. Although the links between it and depression are not specially marked (Gunderson and Phillips, 1991) whilst the criteria for definition include affective disturbance it is going to be a continuing source of difficulty in diagnosis. Indeed, the new diagnosis of brief recurrent depression in ICD-10 appears uncannily like the description of borderline personality disorder with only the affective component included. If the diagnosis cannot do without its mental state components it would be more appropriately described as a clinical syndrome rather than as a personality disorder (Tyrer, 1994, 1999).

In contrast with the great body of work on borderline personality disorder, there has been very little research carried out into the validity of impulsive personality disorder. The degree of overlap between this and borderline personality disorder is likely to be considerable.

Anxious and avoidant personality disorder

Although these two categories appear somewhat different, their descriptions are very similar and the word *avoidant* can be ascribed to the anxious personality disorder in ICD-10. The main characteristics of both categories are persistent self-consciousness, hypersensitivity to rejection, exaggeration of risks in everyday activities, which lead to persistent avoidance, and reluctance to enter into relationships unless there is certainty of acceptance.

Although these criteria include many of the attributes of anxiousness and self-consciousness that have been argued to be persistent personality features by many authorities (e.g. Mann *et al.*, 1981; Watson and Clark, 1984), care has been taken not to make this category an equivalent of chronic anxiety which would be indistinguishable from a mental state diagnosis. Even then there is considerable overlap between the characteristics of avoidant personality disorder and the clinical symptoms of phobic anxiety and avoidance, particularly with social phobia (Herbert *et al.*, 1992) and a consensus is beginning to develop that the two diagnoses cannot be regarded as truly separate (Dahl, 1996). The term was derived as a theoretical construct by Millon (1969) and is one of the few categories of personality disorder that has not been introduced through the acceptance of a long-standing clinical description. This has yet to prove its worth.

Narcissistic personality disorder

This has no equivalent category in ICD-9 or ICD-10 and is rarely used outside the USA. Although it has only been used in the last 20 years, it is one of the categories of personality disorder that owes its origins to psychoanalysis and again originates from Sigmund Freud (1914). However, the category owes its inclusion in DSM-III-R and DSM-IV primarily to the work of Kohut (1971) and Kernberg (1975). They emphasized the common constellation of features that have now become the operational criteria for the diagnosis of narcissistic personality disorder. These are based on the triad of self-importance, the need for admiration, and the inability to empathize with others. The first two of these are well exemplified by the story of Narcissus in Greek mythology. The operational criteria include excessive reaction to criticism, manipulative behaviour, exaggerated sense of achievements and special abilities, a strong sense of entitlement and requirement for constant attention while being indifferent to the feelings of others.

Kernberg and Kohut have different standpoints that are important with regard to therapy. Kohut claims that the understanding of narcissistic personality has changed psychoanalysis and offered new hope for treatment (Kohut, 1975). This remains to be confirmed. There are no clear links between narcissistic personality disorder and any specific mental state disorders but there are relatively high associations with bipolar disorder and substance misuse, depression and anorexia nervosa (Ronningstam, 1996).

Passive–aggressive personality disorder

This category has persisted throughout the various editions of DSM but was excluded in DSM-IV; it has never gained acceptance in Europe. It too has developed largely from psychodynamic theory (cynically summarized as 'those who withhold their fees to their psychoanalyst until the last possible moment'). It is now included under the heading of 'other personality disorder'. Despite this the term is still used widely, never as a friendly term, referring to passive resistance, and includes persistent procrastination, sulking and irritability as responses to unwelcome requests, obstruction and excessive slowness in tasks, and other examples of rather childish resentment. It is possible to recognize many of these characteristics in all of us (e.g. 'puts off things that need to be done so the deadlines are not met'), but it is argued that in passive–aggressive personality disorder they are persistent patterns of behaviour. There is also concern that it may overlap considerably with many mental state diagnoses (Small *et al.*, 1970). Its temporal stability is also in doubt (Hyler *et al.*, 1983).

Self-defeating and sadistic personality disorders

These are also categories that were included in the appendix to DSM-III-R but have been removed from DSM-IV. Again there is no equivalent in ICD. Considerable debate took place in the American Psychiatric Association about the inclusion of these two additional personality disorders. Although there were strong points in favour of their inclusion (Simons, 1987), there were equally strong arguments, particularly from the feminist lobby, for excluding them (Caplan, 1987; Walker, 1987). Indeed, the original description of self-defeating personality disorder, that of masochistic, was dropped because of these pressures.

According to DSM-III-R, self-defeating personality disorders 'avoid or undermine pleasurable experiences, be drawn to situations or relationships in which he or she will suffer, and prevent others from helping him or her'. Thus the sufferer both prevents others from helping with their problems and tends to choose those as friends who are bound to disappoint. Achievements are considerably less than potential and the person engages in 'excessive self-sacrifice'. As one of the examples given in DSM-III-R a student may 'help fellow students to write papers but is unable to write his or her own'.

Some forensic psychologists and psychiatrists may mourn the departure of these two 'almost diagnoses' but they seem to have added little more than more comorbidity to the literature on personality disorders.

Assessment of personality disorder in the presence of a major psychiatric syndrome

Before discussing different instruments to measure personality disorder, it is worth highlighting two important issues: the difficulty in assessing abnormal personality in the presence of other psychiatric disorders and the relative merits of informants and subjects in assessing abnormal personality.

The problems of attempting to assess personality in the presence of an Axis I disorder have already been mentioned. Coppen and Metcalfe (1965) found that N scores on the MPI decreased on recovery in depressed patients whereas E scores had increased. Furthermore the mean score of depressed patients after recovery was similar to that obtained from normal subjects. The work of Bianchi and Fergusson (1977) also underlines the susceptibility of the N scale to changes in mental state and, interestingly, these workers felt unable to suggest modifications which could eradicate the resultant contamination. They concluded that the N scores in clinical samples should be approached with some caution. Snaith (1976) has gone so far as to argue that, in this group of patients, personality scores should be interpreted principally as a measure of illness.

Most subsequent assessment procedures have attempted to heed our earlier warning of the dangers of attaching labels to personality during periods of illness. In the Personality Assessment Schedule (PAS), for example, every effort is made during the informant or subject interview to elicit the premorbid personality by obtaining examples of aberrant behaviour at a time when the subject was clearly well. Difficulties of course arise when a prolonged illness results in changes in personality as in the case of chronic schizophrenia. The question arises as to whether the assessor should focus on personality before illness; for example, what procedure should be followed when a 40-year-old man whose onset of illness was at the age of 18 is being assessed. The Structured Interview for DSM-III (SIDP-IV) deals with this difficulty by instructing the rater to consider the personality that predominated for the greatest period of time in the last 5 years. Other schedules have avoided this contentious area altogether by excluding patients with some major Axis I disorders (Loranger *et al.*, 1985). A great deal of further work is required in this area before definite recommendations can be made.

Sources of personality data

Since the diagnosis of personality disorder is inevitably linked to the possession of socially undesirable attributes, self-inventory data are liable to distortion both overtly and in more subtle ways. Projective techniques obviously have the advantage of reducing the influence of this factor, but as Masling has pointed out, subjects tend to make use of all sorts of cues from the tester when many of these techniques are actually administered (Masling, 1960). Tyrer and Ferguson (1987) have argued that, although all the variation in personality may be rated correctly by the subject, the level of impaired social functioning is probably best determined by those close to him. The nature and quality of information obtained from an informant would of course be significantly influenced by the personality of the informant. Should this prove to be abnormal, as for example when assortative mating has taken place, then the whole process of assessment would have limited value. Sears (1936) demonstrated a tendency for informants to project the undesirable traits, which they themselves were considered to possess by independent raters. Similarly, if the relationship between informant and subject is dysfunctional as a result of the social impairment caused by the subject's abnormal personality, one might reasonably expect similar distortions in the assessment procedure, for example this might be expected to happen in a couple undergoing dissolution of marriage as a direct consequence of the antisocial personality of one of the partners. On the other hand, Guze (1976) has contested the view that most antisocial personalities are untrustworthy historians. Several present-day personality schedules attempt to overcome this difficulty by using all available information and seeking to clarify discrepancies before the diagnostic procedures are applied (PAS, SIDP). It is clear, however, that relatively little is known about the effect different types of informant have on the assessment procedure. Preliminary evidence from over 200 patients suggests that close informants (e.g. spouses and co-habitees) are judged to be better assessors of personality than more distant informants and that women are thought to be superior to men in the validity of their assessments (Brothwell *et al.*, 1992).

Assessment of personality disorders

One major advantage of the new DSM and ICD classification systems is that they are amenable to measurement, and this applies as much to personality disorder (Axis II) as to mental state disorder (Axis I). The operational criteria given for each diagnosis may be correct inferences from good research data, inspired guesswork from missing or inadequate data, or wild shots in the dark that are way off target, but at least all are measurable. It should, therefore, be possible to record reliably each of the personality disorder categories in DSM-IV, and only further testing using these instruments can establish whether these categories are valid. The authors of DSM-III made this clear in formulating their

classification, but the popularity of the classification has become such that some regard the DSM-III categories as valid purely because they appear in the classification. Such biblical faith is unwise.

Formal assessments of categorical personality disorder

There are an increasing number of instruments for recording the presence or absence of the main categorical personality disorders (*Table 2.5* and *Table 2.6*). These are particularly focused on the DSM personality disorders and so their success is largely dependent on the validity of this classification. Questionnaires are always more convenient than other measures in the assessment of personality but their value is limited by the tendency for those with severe personality disorder to answer dishonestly.

Self-report inventories

Inventories for clinical and research use, however, have been available for some time and have been of value in examining the relationship between personality disorder and neurotic illness. The Lazare–Klerman–Armor Self-report Inventory (Lazare *et al.*, 1966) identified three personality styles: ob-

Table 2.5 Instruments for measuring DSM-IV personality disorders

Intended use	Questionnaires	Interview schedules
All personality disorders	Millon Clinical Multiaxial Inventory (MCMI; Millon *et al.*, 1997) Personality Disorder Questionnaire (PDQ-IV; Hyler, 1994) Wisconsin Personality Inventory (WISPI) (Klein *et al.*, 1993)	Structured Interview for DSM-III Personality Disorders (SIDP-IV; Pfohl *et al.*, 1995) Structured Clinical Interview for DSM-III Personality Disorders (SCID-II; First *et al.*, 1995) International Personality Disorder Examination (PDE; Loranger *et al.*, 1994) Diagnostic Interview for DSM-IV Personality Disorders (DIPD-IV) (Zanarini *et al.*, 1994)
Borderline personality disorder	Borderline Syndrome Index (BSI; Conte *et al.*, 1980) Bell Object Relations Self-report Scale (Bell, 1981)	Schedule for Interviewing Borderlines (SIB) (Baron, 1981) Diagnostic Interview for Borderline Patients (DIB; Gunderson, Kolb and Austin 1981) Borderline Personality Disorder Scale (BPD-Scale; Perry, 1982)
Antisocial personality disorder		Schedule of Affective Disorders (SADS; Spitzer and Endicott, 1983) Diagnostic Interview Schedule (DIS; Robins *et al.*, 1979)
Schizotypal personality disorder		Schedule for Schizotypal Personalities (SSP; Baron *et al.*, 1981)

Table 2.6 Comparison of structured interview schedules for assessing personality disorder

Title	Author	Main features
Standardized Assessment of Personality (SAP)	Mann *et al.*, 1981	Trained clinical interviewer Short verbatim personality profile from informant followed by seven probe questions designed to elicit key words in eight areas of personality attributes Takes about 10 minutes ICD diagnosis
Structured Interview for the DSM-III Personality Disorders (SIDP-IV)	Pfohl *et al.*, 1995	Administered by psychologist or psychiatrist 107 questions in 16 areas of personality functioning Four levels of severity for each item 60–90 minute patient interview and 30 minute informant interview
Structured Clinical Interview for DSM-III-R – personality disorder (SCID-II)	First *et al.*, 1995	Clinician interview of subject Overview followed by specific questions in each category of DSM-IV Positive replies summate to reach threshold for diagnosis 60–90 minutes Accompanying personality questionnaire
Personality Assessment Schedule (PAS)	Tyrer and Alexander, 1979 Revised (Tyrer, Alexander and Ferguson, 1988b – *see* Appendix)	Trained clinical interviewer 24 dimensions of personality assessed Five main personality classes empirically derived with five levels of severity (computer program available) Revised classification yields 13 classes Takes 25–40 minutes Interview can be with subject or informant and composite score obtained
International Personality Disorder Examination (IPDE) for DSM-IV and ICD-10 personality disorders	Loranger *et al.*, 1994	Trained personnel Highly structured Questions cover both operational criteria for ICD-10 and DSM-IV, may take up to three hours to complete

sessive, hysterical and oral dependent. Nyman and Marke (1962) developed a 60-item questionnaire to measure personality attributes defined by Henrick Sjöbring's differential psychology (1973) and was able to demonstrate its ability to assess the dimensions of validity, stability and solidity, the original work being carried out both on student groups and a large selection of car owners. Perris (1966) shortened this instrument to 10 questions for each of the three dimensions and used it to examine the relationship between premorbid personality and manic depressive illness.

The Millon Clinical Multiaxial Inventory III (MCMI-III) is a self-report inventory of 175 items that produces scores for both basic personality patterns and severe personality disorder. It takes around 30 minutes to complete, can only be used under copyright and costs £120 (Millon *et al.*, 1997). It is a good instrument for recording personality styles but not well suited for the assessment of

personality disorder. The Wisconsin Personality Disorders Inventory (WISPI) is a self-rated questionnaire with 224 questions scored on a 10-point scale and this range allows personality to be scored dimensionally (Klein *et al.* 1993). It is of greatest use in the psychotherapeutic treatment of patients with and without personality disorder. The Personality Diagnostic Questionnaire (PDP-Q), an instrument which has followed the four revisions of DSM (Hyler and Reider, 1984; Hyler *et al.*, 1988; Hyler, 1994), is frequently used because of its convenience in administration. The latest version (PDQ-IV) asks the subject to rate their personality in 85 questions with a time frame of several years. A total score of 50 or more suggests personality disorder, but no more, as there is evidence that the instrument is too catholic in its attribution of personality disorder and may be assisted by an informant version (Dowson, 1992b). In many studies the PDP-Q is used as a screening instrument.

Structured clinical interviews

Structured interview schedules are now the instruments of choice in assessing personality disorder, mainly because their reliability and differing types of validity are superior to those of questionnaires. In recognizing this it is also important to note that the level of agreement between the diagnosis of personality disorder made by both interviews and self-report is remarkably poor, with overall agreement being little better than chance (Perry, 1992). Although agreement between interview schedules is a little better than self-report/interview comparisons it seldom reaches the modest level of 0.50 agreement, illustrating that although these interviews achieve better internal reliability their failure to generalize indicates fundamental problems.

There are more than 10 personality interview schedules in current use and more are being developed monthly. The earliest is the Personality Assessment Schedule (PAS) developed in 1976 and first published in 1979 (Tyrer and Alexander, 1979; Tyrer et al., 1979). This identifies the personality traits that create the most severe social dysfunction when present to excessive degree and these are scored on eight-point scales. Further details of the PAS and its several forms are given in Chapter 4.

Although it is natural for instigators of rating scales to want to protect their progeny, I would be more than happy to dispose of the PAS if there were better instruments available. Only one, the Adult Personality Functioning Assessment (APFA) (Hill et al., 1989) and a modified form of the PAS with additional questions (M-PAS) (Piven et al., 1994), have focused specifically on social dysfunction as the key consequence of personality disorder and these are only suitable for assessments in dimensional form.

The other instruments have all pinned their hopes on the definition of personality disorder through the identification of prototypical behaviours that can be fashioned into operational criteria (Blashfield et al., 1985) in the same way that the Research Diagnostic Criteria identified the core features of depressive illness and began the reform of psychiatric classification with the introduction of DSM-III. Four schedules currently compete for priority in assessing DSM personality disorders, the International Personality Disorder Examination (IPDE), the Structured Interview for DSM-IV Personality (SIDP-IV), the Diagnostic Interview for DSM-IV Personality Disorders (DIPD-IV), and the Structured Clinical Interview for DSM-IV Axis II Personality Disorders (SCID-II).

The IPDE (Loranger et al., 1987a, 1994) is a semi-structured clinical interview for both DSM-IV (99 questions) and ICD-10 personality disorders (67 questions). It is available in two versions: a DSM-IV module containing 99 sets of questions and an ICD-10 module containing 67 sets of questions. It scores each question on a three-point scale (absent, exaggerated or pathological) and can therefore be used for dimensional scoring (although the range is somewhat restricted). The SIDP-IV (available in three versions) (Pfohl et al., 1995) also allows both categorical and dimension assessments of DSM-IV and ICD-10 personality disorders and, by using a four-point scale for each of the 107 questions, allows somewhat better dimensional assessments to be made.

The DIPD-IV is a semi-structured clinical interview of 108 sets of questions (three-point scale) with each set designed to assess a specific criterion of the DSM-IV personality disorders (Zanarini et al., 1987, 1994). The SCID-II (First et al., 1995) is a development of Structured Clinical Interview for DSM-III which was developed first with mental state diagnoses before being adapted for personality ones (Spitzer et al., 1987). The schedule is available in screening and full versions and, as the screening version has cut-off points, the schedule may only take 20 minutes to complete. It comprises 119 items in the full version with each scored on a three-point scale to allow for dimensional assessment. The Personality Disorder Interview-IV (PDI-IV) (Widiger et al., 1995) is a similar instrument accompanied by a comprehensive manual.

The Diagnostic Interview for Borderlines (DIB) (Gunderson et al., 1981) and other similar measures for borderline patients for those with specific personality disorders (e.g. Borderline Syndrome Index (BSI) (Conte et al., 1980); Bell Object Relations Self-Report Scale (Bell, 1981) are now much less often used. The DIB is a semi-structured interview with

165 items that takes about 60 minutes to complete. Inter-rater reliability is good to excellent in several studies (Kolb and Gunderson, 1980; Kroll *et al.*, 1981b; Cornell *et al.*, 1983). The DIB preceded DSM-III but there is considerable overlap between them and high correlation between them has been noted (Loranger *et al.*, 1984). This is mainly because of the large degree of overlap between different personality disorders and this is most marked for borderline conditions (Fyer *et al.*, 1988). When assessing personality disorder it is wise to assess all available categories and then select those of special interest. The Borderline Symptom Index, a 52-item questionnaire developed as a screening instrument, has been compared with the Personality Assessment Schedule in a validation study (Marlowe *et al.*, 1996). Whilst the BSI was moderately sensitive at identifying personality disorder (as recorded by the PAS) it was non-specific and seemed to be influenced greatly by symptomatic depression.

Finally, as Dowson and Grounds (1995) have emphasized, when patients do not agree to being interviewed with one of these instruments, which can take between 30 and 180 minutes to administer, other methods will have to be used. One of the most frequently used of these is the Standardized Assessment of Personality (SAP) (Mann *et al.*, 1981) which assesses ICD personality disorders (disorder, abnormal personality or no abnormal personality) using informants and which takes about 15 minutes to complete. The SAP (*see Table 2.2*) was developed in order to improve the reliability of ICD-9 personality diagnosis, but includes two additional categories of anxious and self-conscious personalities (Mann *et al.*, 1981). The interview is carried out with an informant, who is asked to confine his replies to aspects of premorbid personality by an interviewer specifically trained in the technique. Two grades are possible; one of which is regarded as abnormal. The use of a limited number of defined probes is designed to elicit key words on which the diagnosis itself is based. The structure of the inventory, however, is very loose and necessarily depends on cultural factors. Despite this the authors obtained satisfactory reliability for cyclothymic disorder ($\kappa_w = 0.85$) with lower inter-rater agreement for self-conscious, anxious and obsessional groups ($\kappa_w = 0.67$, 0.61 and 0.60, respectively). It has been used to examine patients in general practice and both in- and outpatient psychiatric settings. Its advantages are seen in comparison with other instruments in *Table 2.7*. The SAP is a sensitive but not very specific instrument that may

Table 2.7 Commonly used instruments for diagnosing personality dimensionally

Main purpose	Questionnaires	Interview schedules	Comments
Identification of personality characteristics in general	Eysenck Inventory Questionnaire (EPI and EPQ)	Personality Assessment Schedule (PAS)	It is likely that many more instruments will be including a dimensional component in the future. At present, many of the standard instruments (e.g. IPDE, SCID-II) include a sub-threshold diagnosis that can be coded as personality difficulty (see Table 2.8) but none has a higher level of severe personality disorder
	Karolinska Scales of Personality (KSP)	Personality Disorder Interview-IV (PDI-IV)	
	Karolinska Psychodynamic Profile (KAPP)	Structured Interview for DSM-IV Personality Disorders (SIDP-IV) (Pfohl *et al.*, 1994)	
	Personality Assessment Inventory (PAI)		
	Schedule for Normal and Abnormal Personality (SNAP) (Clark, 1990)	ADP-IV (Schotte *et al.*, 1998)	The ADP-IV is a Dutch instrument that records both trait and distress components of the DSM-IV disorders and so is a combined categorical and dimensional model
	Dimensional Assessment of Personality Pathology – Basic Questionnaire (DAPP-BQ) (Schroeder *et al.*, 1992)		

overdiagnose personality disorder but is suitable as a screening instrument (Mann *et al.*, 1999). The choice of informant is difficult to make with this and with other instruments designed for informants. Evidence from comparison of informant data suggests that close informants (e.g. spouses and cohabitees) are judged to be better assessors of personality than more distant informants and that women are generally superior to men in the validity of their assessments (Brothwell *et al.*, 1992; Pilgrim *et al.*, 1993).

Dimensional assessment of personality disorder

Personality was assessed dimensionally long before any attempt was made to categorize it into disorders and so many of these instruments are old (*Table 2.7*). The Maudsley and related personality inventories (MPI) (Eysenck, 1959), Eysenck Personality Inventory (EPI) (Eysenck and Eysenck, 1964) and Eysenck Personality Questionnaire (EPQ) (Eysenck and Eysenck, 1975) have been widely used in personality research and demonstrate the stability of the concepts of extraversion and neuroticism, although the third dimension, psychoticism, measured in the EPQ, is a less satisfactory measure of what others call psychopathy. The Karolinska Psychodynamic Profile (KAPP) (Weinryb and Rössel, 1991; Weinryb *et al.*, 1992, 1997) is exceptional in that it measures psychodynamic aspects of personality and can be used to record changes in personality over the course of treatment. It is normally stable over time and deserves to be more widely used by those exploring the place of psychotherapy in treating personality pathology. KAPP should not be confused with the Karolinska Scales for Personality, which are felt to underpin the biological basis of personality (Perris *et al.*, 1984; von Knorring *et al.*, 1983) and which are frequently used to record personality variables in drug trials.

Although many of the structured interviews for the DSM personality disorders maintain that they can score all the personality disorders dimensionally their main use is for categorical diagnosis and the dimensional measures are really afterthoughts. However,

the Personality Disorder Interview (PDI-IV) (Widiger *et al.*, 1995) is a semi-structured clinical interview of 93 sets of questions. It has the advantage of being scored both categorically and on a dimensional scale with greater scope than the other DSM structured interviews with all items scored on a six-point scale (absent, traits, sub-threshold, threshold (i.e. presence of the disorder), moderate, or extreme). The DAPP-BQ (Dimensional Assessment of Personality Pathology-Basic Questionnaire) (Schroeder *et al.*, 1992) and Schedule for Normal and Abnormal Personality (SNAP) (Clark, 1990; Clark *et al.*, 1996) are also useful dimensional systems which are best used with people who have less severe personality disorders.

All these DSM instruments, both questionnaires and interview schedules, use the operational criteria of DSM-IV as their yardstick of measurement. Each question in a schedule gives rise to another question: Will the answer be an operational criterion of DSM-IV? If the answer to this second question is no, the first one has to be abandoned, whether or not it is an excellent question discriminating between normal personality and personality disorder. It might, therefore, be expected that all the instruments would show a high level of agreement as they are all attempting to measure the same definitions of disorder. However, in one of the few comparisons between different instruments (two questionnaires, the PDQ and MCMI, and one interview schedule, SIDP (Reich *et al.*, 1988), the agreement between the instruments was uniformly poor. Avoidant personality disorder showed the best correlation between the three instruments ($\kappa_w = 0.51$ for PDQ/SIDP, $\kappa_w = 0.68$ for PDQ/MCMI and $\kappa_w = 0.53$ for MCMI/SIDP) and compulsive disorder the least ($\kappa_w = 0.53$ for MCMI/SIDP, $\kappa_w = -0.47$ for MCMI/PDQ and $\kappa_w = -0.29$ for MCMI/SIDP). For the other personality disorders, agreement was at the level of 0.5 (κ_w) for PDE/SIDP comparisons and 0.3 (r) for the MCMI comparisons. It may be significant that all patients seen in the study also had an Axis I disorder, mainly anxiety or depression in its various forms. The effect of mental state on questionnaire assessments is greater than that with interview schedules and could account for the lack of agreement. However, it seems likely that there are other subtle differences as well between the instruments.

Increasingly, as the inadequacies of the DSM operationalized criteria become apparent, people are trying to develop instruments that go beyond the strict definitional requirements of personality disorder and attempt to get agreement independently of this. One interesting instrument, the Shedler–Westen Assessment Procedure, or SWAP-200, is an assessment tool designed to allow clinicians to provide 'detailed, clinically rich personality descriptions in a systematic and quantifiable form'. Preliminary findings suggest it is effective in this respect and shows high convergent and discriminant validity (Westen and Shedler, 1999).

The Psychopathy Checklist (PCL) (Hare, 1970), now in revised form (HPCL-R) (Hare, 1991) is commonly used with offenders with personality disorder as it aims to assess the concept of psychopathy categorically and dimensionally. It is derived from the notion of psychopathy first formulated clearly by Cleckley (1941) and modified somewhat by Hare (1970). The HPCL-R measure of psychopathy is a checklist of 20 items that includes the standard features of psychopathy; glibness and superficial charm, self-grandiosity, risk-taking behaviour, manipulative behaviour, pathological lying, lack of guilt, callousness and insensitivity, impulsiveness, promiscuity and irresponsibility. It is important to emphasize that psychopathy so defined is different from antisocial personality disorder but this is not necessarily important, particularly if one wishes to chart progress in treatment over time. The ratings may be reinforced by information derived from clinical notes and reports and it could be argued that these need to be studied in all cases because of the plausibility of such individuals.

Classification of severity of personality disorder

The notion of severe personality disorder is central to much of the work of forensic psychiatrists and yet there is no standard way of recording this from the DSM-IV and ICD-10 classifications. However, it has been noticed in many studies that the more severe personality disordered patients tend to have a much greater number of personality disorders than those with less severe disorders (Kass *et al.*, 1985; Oldham *et al.*, 1992; Dolan *et al.*, 1995).

This therefore leads to the suggestion that comorbidity (or, more strictly speaking, overlap) of personality disorder is a measure of severity. There has also been considerable debate about the classification of sub-threshold levels of personality disorder. In the initial draft of the ICD-10 guidelines for personality disorder personality accentuation was included as a category but subsequently omitted in the final description. However, the notion of personality difficulty or accentuation making patients more vulnerable to stresses is a well established one (Leonhard, 1968) and could have a place in formal classifications. The proposal below combines these approaches and also allows the existing classification systems to be adapted for measuring severity. Five levels of severity of classification are allowed, the first four of which were included in the original description (Tyrer and Johnson, 1996) (*Table 2.8*) and the last, or severe category, being added for a special group characterized by 'gross societal disturbance', in which there is gross severity of personality disorder within the flamboyant group and a personality disorder in at least one other cluster also. For the diagnosis of 'gross societal disturbance' we suggest three requirements, spread outside family, significant societal impact, and creation of threat, all of which have to be present:

1. Clear evidence of personality disturbance influencing a wider group than just family and friends (questions over operational criteria for personality disturbance (*Table 2.1*) should include 'the enduring pattern of inner experience creates significant distress not only to immediate friends, family or household members but also to wider society').
2. The creation of significant problems to at least 20 other individuals apart from family members and close friends as a direct consequence of the 'enduring pattern' (*Table 2.1*) (amplifying questions about level of distress to others include 'how many people have been adversely affected to a significant degree by X's behaviour and attitudes?').
3. Clear evidence of threat created by the pattern of personality characteristics in that

Table 2.8 Procedure for converting categorical personality disorders to levels of severity (derived from Tyrer and Johnson, 1996)

Level of severity	ICD-10	DSM-IV	Structured interview schedules
0 – no personality abnormality	No personality abnormality	No personality abnormality	No personality abnormality
1 – personality difficulty	Personality difficulty recorded when general criterion G1 for personality disorders is met and three diagnostic criteria present for either paranoid, schizoid, histrionic, anankastic and/or anxious personality disorders or two criteria present for dissocial, impulsive or borderline personality disorders	Personality difficulty recorded when any of the following are present: four diagnostic criteria present for either schizotypal, borderline, histrionic, narcissistic and dependent personality disorder; three diagnostic criteria present for either paranoid, schizoid, avoidant or obsessive–compulsive personality disorders; or two criteria present for antisocial personality disorder in section 3 of the criteria	Sub-threshold criteria for personality disorder met according to criteria of interview schedule
2 – simple personality disorder	Either a single personality disorder or, if more than one, all personality disorders are within the same cluster. (Cluster 1 – schizoid and paranoid; Cluster 2 – dissocial, impulsive, borderline or histrionic; Cluster 3 – anankastic, anxious and dependent)	Either a single personality disorder or, if more than one, all personality disorders are within the same cluster. (Cluster A – schizotypal, schizoid and paranoid; Cluster B – antisocial, borderline, histrionic and narcissistic; Cluster C – avoidant, dependent and obsessive–compulsive)	One or more personality disorders within the same ICD-10 or DSM-IV cluster
3 – complex personality disorder	Two or more personality disorders from different clusters	Two or more personality disorders present from different clusters	Two or more personality disorders present from different clusters
4 – severe personality disorder	Two or more personality disorders from different clusters that create gross societal disturbance (see text for definition)	Two or more personality disorders from different clusters that create gross societal disturbance	Two or more personality disorders from different clusters that create gross societal disturbance

fear of mental or physical harm is an intrinsic part of the distress or discomfiture created by the personality abnormality (e.g. 'is there anything that you fear about the pattern of behaviour shown by X?', identification of aggressive impulses and irresponsibility that puts others at risk (dissocial and antisocial group), outbursts of anger and violence (emotionally unstable group), insensitivity to social norms (withdrawn group)).

The system has the merit of allowing the existing ICD-10 and DSM-IV systems to be adapted for this new classification of severity (Tyrer and Johnson, 1996). In research assessments using structured clinical interviews this re-classification is also easy to carry out except that only a few measures record gross societal disturbance and these might have to be incorporated.

Screening for personality disorder

Although several instruments have been involved in screening for personality disorder, including the Personality Assessment Schedule and the Standardized Assessment of Personality (*see* Chapter 4) only one (the Iowa Personality Disorder Screen) has been introduced specifically for screening purposes. This is a recently introduced instrument focused on DSM personality disorders (which generally take longer to assess) and which is quicker than any other personality disorder assessment in the USA, taking only 5 minutes to be completed (although in preliminary testing in the UK it can sometimes take longer). This consists of 11 screening items (*Table 2.9*) which cover the range of disturbance in personality disorder and which, when compared with a standard structured clinical interview (Structured Interview for DSM-IV Personality

Table 2.9 The Iowa Personality Disorder Screen, Version 1.2 (reproduced with permission of the *Journal of Personality Disorders* and the University of Iowa Department of Psychiatry)

Name: _____   Number: _____   Date: _____

I'd like to ask you a few questions about some of your thoughts and feelings. Your answers will help me better understand what you are usually like. If the way you have been in recent weeks or months is different from the way you usually are, please look back to when you were your usual self.

1.	**Experiences marked shifts in mood: throughout the course of a typical day, experiences sudden spells of depression, irritability, anxiety or anger.** *(Rate only if both responses are positive)*	Y N

Some people find their mood changes frequently as if they spend every day on an emotional roller coaster. For example, they might switch from feeling angry to depressed to anxious many times a day. Does this sound like you?

(If YES): Have you been this way most of your life?

2.	**Feels uncomfortable in situations where he/she is not the centre of attention.** *(Rate only if both responses are positive)*	Y N

Some people prefer to be the centre of attention, while others are content to remain on the edge of things. How would you describe yourself?

(If CENTRE): Does it bother you when someone else is in the spotlight?

3.	**Actions usually directed toward obtaining immediate satisfaction: difficulty persisting with long-term goals.** *(Rate if either response is positive)*	Y N

Do you frequently insist on having what you want right now, even when waiting a little longer would get you something much better?

Do you often get into trouble at work or with friends because you act excited at first but then lose interest in projects and don't follow through?

4.	**Is reluctant to confide in others because of unwarranted fear that the information will be used against him or her.**	Y N

Do you find that most people will take advantage of you if you let them know too much about you?

5.	**Excessive social anxiety, e.g., extreme discomfort in social situations involving unfamiliar people.** *(Rate if either response is positive)*	Y N

Do you generally feel nervous or anxious around people?

Do you avoid situations where you have to meet new people?

6.	**Unwilling to get involved with people unless certain of being liked such that the number of friends has been limited.** *(Rate only if both responses are positive)*	Y N

Do you avoid getting to know people because you're worried they may not like you?

(IF OFTEN): Has this affected the number of friends you have?

7.	**Lack of stable self image.** *(Rate if either response is positive)*	Y N

Do you keep changing the way you present yourself to people because you don't know who you really are?

Do you often feel like your beliefs change so much that you don't know what you really believe any more?

8. **Prone to discuss and overemphasize importance of own achievements and why he/she should**   Y   N
   be considered a special case.

   Do you often get angry or irritated because people don't recognize your special talents or
   achievements as much as they should?

9. **Expects to be exploited or harmed by others.**   Y   N
   (Rate only if both responses are positive)

   Do you often suspect that people you know may be trying to cheat or take advantage of you?

   (If YES): Do you worry about this a lot?

10. **Bears grudges or is unforgiving of insults or slights.**   Y   N

   Do you tend to hold grudges or give people the silent treatment for days at a time?

11. **Insensitive to the concerns and needs of others.**   Y   N
   (Rate if either response is positive)

   Do you get annoyed when friends or family complain about their problems?

   Do people complain that you're not very sympathetic to their problems?

Disorders (SIDP-IV)) shows a sensitivity of 79% and a specificity rate of 86%. As most of the quick schedules show good sensitivity but poor specificity these findings are impressive. A decision is made whether the item is present or absent after each question. The authors recommend that if an absolute minimum of questions is to be made that the five questions 4 to 8 are asked only.

At present the authors of the Iowa Personality Disorder Screen regard it as 'a promising tool and warrants further study in a variety of clinical and research settings'. The authors are keen to get information about its use in a variety of different clinical settings. Their published study, although it involved preliminary work on over 1200 interviews, was only completed with 52 subjects (42 outpatients and 10 inpatients) and very few had antisocial personality characteristics (Langbehn *et al.*, 1999).

In deciding which method of assessing personality disorder to choose several issues need to be addressed (*Table 2.10*). Whatever

Table 2.10 Choice of instruments for measuring personality disorder (see also Table 4.8)

Purpose of enquiry	Suggested instruments
Screening instruments prior to full survey	Iowa Personality Disorder Screen (Langbehn *et al.*, 1999); Standardized Assessment of Personality (Mann *et al.*, 1981)
Personality questionnaires for traits only	No clear guidance is possible as so many are available. The NEO-Personality Inventory-Revised (NEO-PI-R) (Costa and McCrae, 1992) (commonly known as the Big Five) is perhaps the most used
Self-rating for personality disorders	Personality Disorder Questionnaire (PDQ-IV) (Hyler, 1994) (but also see Table 4.8)
Psychodynamic assessment of personality disorder	Karolinska Psychodynamic Profile (KAPP) (Weinryb and Rössel, 1991)
Forensic populations	Hare Psychopathy Check-list (Revised) (Hare, 1991)
Comprehensive assessment of all personality disorders in ICD and DSM	International Personality Disorder Examination (IPDE) (Loranger *et al.*, 1994)
DSM-IV personality disorders	Difficult to choose from the many available: no firm choice possible

their imperfections, the DSM and ICD classifications are the current gold standard in personality diagnosis and so for purposes of official statistics and international comparisons (e.g. epidemiological surveys) they must be chosen. One of the important advantages of the categorical diagnosis in psychiatry is that many management decisions are dichotomous, and when these are based on diagnosis there is alternative to the categorical description. If, therefore, one of the necessary pre-requisites of treatment in a special institution or using a new type of therapy is the possession of a diagnosis of personality disorder, an assessment that allows categorical assessment is essential.

Categorical diagnosis is also necessary when planning treatment or services for patients with mental state and personality disorders, now commonly called dual (or triple) diagnosis. Although it is possible to use dimensional measures for most practical purposes it is more useful to use categories for ease of communication and efficiency. Lastly, and by no means flippantly, for research workers wishing to obtain grants, the merits of the dimensional approach have not yet penetrated to the personality disorder establishment in most countries, and so it is unwise to plump for the assessment of dimensional personality disorders alone.

Further information about instruments described in this chapter

APFA. This is not copyrighted and further information is available from Professor Jonathan Hill, of the University Department of Psychiatry, Royal Liverpool Children's Hospital, Alder Hey, Eaton Road, Liverpool L12 2AP, UK. It is also available in a form suitable for the assessment of younger people aged between 16 and 25, the Adolescent to Adult Personality Functioning Assessment (ADAPFA) (Naughton *et al.*, 1996).

DIB. The DIB and DIB-R may be obtained, free of charge for the initial copy, from John G. Gunderson, M.D. or Mary C. Zanarini, Ed.D., McLean Hospital, 115 Mill Street, Belmont, MA 02178-9106, USA, tel. 617-855-2293,

fax: 617-855-3299. Neither the DIB or DIB-R are copyrighted.

DIPD-IV. The interview contains 108 sets of questions (yes/no and open-ended), with each set designed to assess a specific DSM-IV personality disorder criterion. The interview also covers passive–aggressive (negativistic) personality disorder and depressive personality disorder, both from DSM-IV's Appendix B (Criteria Sets and Axes Provided for Further Study). Further information is available from Mary C. Zanarini, Ed.D., McLean Hospital, 115 Mill Street, Belmont, MA 02178-9106, USA, tel: 617-855-2293, fax: 617-855-3299.

IPDE. The DSM-IV Module of the IPDE, screen, manual, scoring sheets, and an optional computer scoring program can be obtained from the American Psychiatric Association or from Dr Loranger at The New York Hospital, Cornell Medical Center, Westchester Division, White Plains, New York, 10605 USA. It is copyrighted.

PAS. The Personality Assessment Schedule (together with ICD-10 and PAS-Q versions) is obtainable from Professor Peter Tyrer at the Division of Neurosciences and Psychological Medicine, Imperial College School of Medicine, Paterson Centre, 20 South Wharf Road, London W2 1PD, UK, free of charge. It is not copyrighted. There is also a special version suitable for children which is available from Professor Elena Garralda, Department of Child and Adolescent Psychiatry at Imperial College School of Medicine, St Mary's Campus, Norfolk Place, London W2 1PG, UK. There is also a version for people with learning disability being prepared by Dr Angela Hassiotis, Senior Lecturer in Developmental Disorders and Learning Disability, Academic Department of Psychiatry Behavioural Sciences, Wolfson Building, 48 Riding House Street, London W1N 8AA, UK. There is a computer program to score individual profiles or sets of data (Tyrer and Tyrer, 1997) available for £30. This scores the PAS diagnoses, ICD-10 and DSM-IV personality disorders, and severity of personality disorder.

PDI-IV. The PDI-IV may be obtained from Psychological Assessment Resources, P.O.

Box 998, Odessa, FL 33556, USA. The cost is $85 for an introductory kit (consisting of the manual, two copies of each interview booklet, and 10 profile booklets), $42 for the manual, $11 per copy for either version of the interview booklet ($10 each if ordering five or more), and $19 for a package of 10 profile booklets. Further information is available from Thomas A. Widiger, PhD, University of Kentucky, 115 Kastle Hall, Lexington, KY 40506-0044, USA (606-257-6849; email: widiger@pop.uky.edu). The PDI-IV is copyrighted.

SAP. The Standardized Assessment of Personality (ICD-10 version) is available from Professor Anthony Mann, Institute of Psychiatry, London SE5 8AZ, UK. There is no charge.

SCID-II. The interview, screen, manual and scoring sheets are available from the American Psychiatric Press, 1400 K Street, NW, Washington, DC 20005 (800-368-5777). The cost is $46 for a starter kit including the manual and five instruments. A computer administered version of the screen and interview (Computer-Assisted SCID-II) is available for $450 (unlimited use) from Multi-Health Systems, 908 Niagara Falls Boulevard, North Tonawonda, NY 14120-2060, USA (800-456-3003). A training videotape and training workshops (together with information re-

garding foreign language versions) are available from the Biometrics Research Department, New York State Psychiatric Institute, 722 West 168th Street, New York, NY 10032 (212-960-5524). The SCID-II is copyrighted.

SIDP and IOWA Personality Disorder Screen. All information, including a modular version, Super SIDP, foreign language versions, a computer scoring program, a computer administered interview, a training video and training courses may be obtained from Bruce Pfohl, MD, Department of Psychiatry, University of Iowa College of Medicine, Iowa City, IA 52242, USA (319-356-1350; fax: 319-356-2587; email: bruce-p@compuserve.com).

Conclusion

Personality disorder can be assessed and classified with some degree of success. However, there are too many assessment schedules in the diagnostic kitchen and it is not surprising that the cook gets confused and often cannot produce the right recipe. We urgently need some consensus in both classification and assessment if we are to realize some of the gains we have made in the last few years. Recent efforts to produce internationally accepted instruments should be a major part of this enterprise.

3

Personality disorder: a clinical suggestion

John Gunn

The Shorter Oxford English Dictionary defines personality as 'the quality or fact of being a person; that quality which makes being personal'. Note the use of the singular in this definition, implying that we ascribe to other people a single all-embracing quality which we then call their personality. It may well be this singular attribution which leads us sometimes to think of personality disorder as a single diagnostic entity. However, the uniqueness actually arises from a mixture or collection of psychological characteristics. It is the mixture which is unique. The characteristics include broad concepts such as lifestyle, attitudes, skills, beliefs, affective responses, aggressiveness, intelligence, etc. This list is very long. In turn, each of these characteristics can also be unpacked. Furthermore, it is likely that most of these characteristics can vary independently.

It may be useful to consider how we conceptualize other human characteristics, but characteristics without the mystique of persona. Physique may be a useful analogy. In one sense, a person's physique is unique, but a man or woman is more likely to be described in group terms as being pyknic, corpulent, lanky, a midget or a giant. All these words convey a broad general picture of an individual, but if we wish to give a description that is unique to an individual we have to describe more measurable discrete characteristics such as height, weight, strength, muscularity, fat distribution and body limb ratios. Facial appearance is another higher order, and unique,

attribute we ascribe to human beings which again comprises components such as colour, bone ratios, eye characteristics and mouth characteristics.

In most ways the model of personality being a unique collection of attributes is helpful. Unfortunately, however, it does not help to conceptualize the concept of personality disorder very easily. To pursue the analogy, the only equivalent of physique disorder or a facial disorder might be ugliness, a term which conveys some meaning but requires considerable expansion before we can really understand what the ugly person looks like. It is closer to a term of disparagement than to a description. Obesity is a disorder and so is a hare lip, but these are abnormalities of individual characteristics (weight or palate) rather than global disorders. Personality disorder, too, is a vague and global disparaging term used to label entities that must be capable of more specific designations.

In spite of its limitation, however, the term 'personality disorder' refuses to go away. In practice it seems to be used for persistent major psychological dysfunctions in several important characteristics. This is acknowledged in the definition of personality disorder given in the *International Classification of Disease* (ICD) (World Health Organization, 1992) and the *Diagnostic and Statistical Manual of Mental Disorders* (DSM) (American Psychiatric Association, 1994). Personality disorder is described as 'a severe disturbance in the characterological constitution and behavioural tendencies of the individual, usually involving several areas of the personality, and nearly always associated with considerable personal and social disruption'. The first sub-category defined in ICD-10 is paranoid personality disorder which is an 'excessive sensitivity to setbacks and rebuffs, unforgiveness of insults and injuries, a tendency to bear grudges persistently, suspiciousness and a pervasive tendency to distort experience by misconstruing the neutral or friendly actions of others as hostile or contemptuous, and by a combative and tenacious sense of personal rights'. The definition picks on a mental state characteristic which is both persistent and which affects many important characteristics of the respective individual, including lifestyle, attitudes, beliefs and values, so that one way of viewing an individual afflicted with personality disorder X is to see him or her as having important psychological characteristics coloured by a persistent mental state attribute such a paranoia, depression, obsessionality or anxiety.

Perhaps such a colouring model could lead to a list of personality disorder types which should have the important feature of being discrete from one another. Such a list could then be relatively easily agreed between different practitioners and the diagnoses reliably made. In practice this beguiling idea does not work out. Behaviour, other than speech, is also widely considered to be a central aspect of personality.

Every clinician is aware that diagnostic reliability in this area of psychiatry is very poor and this has been demonstrated in some studies (e.g. Thompson and Goldberg, 1987; Perry, 1992). Thompson and Goldberg urge us to stop using the terms 'hysterical personality' or 'histrionic personality disorder' altogether, for they found they are not only used unreliably, but they distract the diagnostician from other underlying pathology such as alcoholism, drug addiction, epilepsy and especially affective disorder including suicidal ideas. In a review of assessments for personality disorder Perry reported that the average kappa (κ) between any two measuring instruments was 0.25, i.e. very low. Inter-rater (κ)s for the DSM instrument SCID-II are also very low (First *et al.*, 1995). Psychologists are not so stuck with diagnostic categories. They tend to break down the global concept of personality into a number of different characteristics or traits.

The psychological approach which appears to be gaining most ground is the 'big five' factor model (e.g. Watson *et al.*, 1994). The five factors are neuroticism (emotional disorganization), extraversion, conscientiousness, agreeableness (friendly compliance) and openness (*see* Caspi, 1996 for a thorough review). This approach leads to a discussion of the areas of functioning and possible treatments for dysfunctions.

The unreliability is compounded by a considerable overlap between categories within either classification. For example, a study carried out at Parkhurst prison showed that when patients with severe personality disorders were rated carefully on DSM-III criteria, almost all of the subjects fell into several personality disorder categories. Some fulfilled the characteristics of five or six different subtypes (Coid *et al.*, 1991). As pointed out elsewhere in this book, this makes the classification not only unreliable but invalid.

Clinical illogicalities

The desire to draw a sharp boundary round the diagnosis of personality disorder has led to curious anomalies which, in turn, lead to management difficulties. One anomaly is in making a sharp distinction between personality disorders and psychoses. A diagnosis of psychosis is usually made when reality resting is so distorted that either delusions or hallucinations, or both, are present in the patient's mental state. At first sight it seems perfectly reasonable to distinguish in this way between psychotic patients and others. There seems to be a good deal of difference between the mad, deluded individual and the patient who is simply exhibiting abnormalities of behaviour with some neurotic complaints. In practice, the distinction is nowhere as easy to make. First, there is a gradation between so-called normal ideas and so-called delusions; secondly, individual patients show different phenomena at different times, a patient may be deluded one week and rational the next; thirdly, there seems no logic in making a sharp and unbridgeable separation between patient A who has a whole set of neurotic behaviour problems plus a paranoid delusion, and patient B who has a similar set of problems, but without the delusion.

The core psychosis schizophrenia illustrates the point. In ICD-9 (World Health Organization, 1978) it was defined as a psychosis characterized by 'a fundamental disturbance of personality'. This has been dropped in preference for 'fundamental and characteristic distortion of thinking and perception' in ICD-10. The new classification also describes disturbances of 'the most basic functions that give the normal person a feeling of individuality, uniqueness, and self-direction'; i.e. disorders of personality more clearly defined. Simple schizophrenia is defined as the 'development of oddities of conduct, inability to meet the demands of society, and decline in total performance', in other words a disorder of personality. To omit other schizophrenias from the personality disorders is convenient for the nosologists, but it has the distinct disadvantage of implying that there are few similarities. The converse is true and the skills and techniques which are appropriate to the treatment of schizophrenia are also frequently appropriate for patients with personality disorders simply because, in each case, the clinician is dealing with a collection of persistently disordered psychological characteristics.

To separate personality disorders from the neuroses is just as artificial. It can be that a neurotic trait, such as obsessionality, colours all the psychological life of an individual to an extent where the notion of global disorder becomes appropriate. When most severely personality disordered patients are examined, they show many neurotic features, some to the point where 'pan neurosis' might be an equally applicable term.

To attempt to separate personality disorder from other major persistent psychiatric disorders leads to further confusion. Psychotic patients are often described as 'ill', personality disordered patients are different therefore they are 'not ill', or even on occasions 'not suffering from formal mental illness' (whatever that is). This semantic distinction leads to a whole range of attitudinal and management differences because the three-letter word 'ill' carries very large social implications with it. Being ill is a specific social role with a number of special privileges and release from a number of social obligations. In

particular, it entitles the patient to certain sorts of health care, including hospitalization, and degrees of tolerance that are not normally accorded to other people. On the other hand, not being ill is virtually tantamount to being well, responsible and, if behaviourally disordered, bad. This leads to rejection by health care services, the withdrawal of patient privileges and a lack of mitigation in legal circumstances.

This distinction may have important practical consequences. For example, a patient suffering from severe chronic mania was readmitted to hospital after a relapse following his refusal to continue with his medication. On admission he was truculent, alternately aggressive and ingratiating, restless, noisy, teasing to other patients and almost totally lacking in concentration or consistency. He frequently wandered away from the ward and annoyed other patients and members of the public. One option was to nurse him on a closed ward and recover control of his mood and behaviour with either phenothiazines or butyrophenones. This policy met considerable nursing resistance. A senior member of the nursing staff urged that the patient should be discharged forthwith as he was too difficult to manage. It was only after a long discussion that one of the senior nurses paid particular attention to the diagnostic label of chronic mania. She immediately said: 'Oh you mean he is ill, I thought he had a personality disorder'. Thoughts of 'manipulation' and 'lack of motivation' faded into the background, and he was managed successfully without further ado. In fact, before the introduction of ICD-10, he could easily have been labelled as suffering from ICD-9 diagnosis 301.1 (affective personality disorder) for, although his condition fluctuates it is 'characterised by lifelong predominance of a pronounced mood ... persistently elated'. The management techniques required were not changed by the change of label, but the social attitudes were and those attitudes interfered with the delivery of appropriate care.

This example may be regarded as atypical or unfair as the patient showed evidence of affective disorder which, like delusions, is acceptable as illness. However, many patients who are personality disordered are comorbid (to use the current jargon) for a variety of

DSM Axis I disorders, such as depression, paranoia, substance abuse, severe anxiety and post-traumatic stress disorder. For these and other reasons patients with a diagnosis of personality disorder are at risk of premature death. Lee Robins (1966) found that sociopathic youths had a much greater mortality than other youths. Robertson (1987) has also demonstrated, this time in the UK, that patients compulsorily admitted to hospital as mentally disordered offenders with a diagnosis of personality disorder, neurosis or substance abuse, are as likely to die prematurely as schizophrenic patients. A brief case history may illustrate.

> Mr A was brought up roughly and aggressively in an uncaring household, largely without any consistent father figure. By the age of 14 he was a persistent thief and he spent the next 30 years in and out of penal institutions. He found it almost impossible to form long-term relationships. He was a good kitchen porter in prison, but could not sustain employment in free conditions. He drank excessively when free, largely to suppress intense feelings of inadequacy, terror, and misery which he constantly experienced. Another means of relieving unbearable tension was to take a razor blade and inflict deep cuts on himself, usually on his abdomen. Many of these could have been lethal, but he died in prison, at the age of 44, from an alcoholic cardiomyopathy.

A well-documented story of severe personality disorder leading to death by ingestion of foreign bodies is given in the account of 'Harry' in *Born to Trouble* by Lloyd and Williamson (1968). Three medical disasters related to rejecting attitudes have been described in an earlier paper (Gunn, 1974).

It is perhaps not surprising that patients with persistent personality problems are rejected. They are after all extremely troublesome patients who, almost by definition, do not improve rapidly whatever techniques of management are used. They therefore offer us few rewards, at times make us feel impotent and guilty, and are relatively expensive in resource terms. These issues are common to such patients whatever the basis of their personality problems: this description is just as valid for those suffering from chronic schizophrenia as for those suffering from personality disorder. The different use of the word 'ill' protects the schizophrenic patient from rejection to some extent, but eventually most patients with behaviour disorders are rejected, whatever their initial label, if those behaviour disorders prove to be persistent and resistant to treatment. Behaviourally difficult people with schizophrenia will begin to be labelled as suffering from schizophrenia and a personality disorder. Two studies in Brixton remand prison have found that patients labelled in this way are less often accepted for hospital treatment (Bowden, 1978; Taylor and Gunn, 1984). Eventually some patients, whether neurotic, psychotic or brain damaged, will end up with the single label 'personality disorder' and be excluded from treatment (see Thompson and Goldberg, 1987). What seems to happen in these cases is that the therapist's despair is defended against by rejection of the patient (a form of protection). The label switch authenticates the rejection with minimal suffering from guilt. After all the patient is not 'ill' and does not merit medical attention.

A further difficulty with the concept of personality disorder is illustrated by the impeccable definition of personality disorder given by Davis (1987): 'A person with a personality disorder has an enduring way of perceiving, relating to, and thinking about, his environment and himself that causes distress or significant impairment in social and occupational functioning'. This definition neatly sums up the way modern psychiatry perceives the concept of personality disorder – at its heart is the notion of durability and persistence. How would these enduring impairments be measured? By references to such items as work record and marital history. All very reasonable, but in an important respect unhelpful. When trying to assess change in an individual, historical data are only useful in the very long term. A poor work record will remain a poor work record, despite effective treatment, for many years and only show evidence of improvement after a considerable time lag. Furthermore, items such as a work record are very dependent on the environment and on social conditions. An improvement in work record may reflect national employment trends as much as it reflects individual change; a deterioration might be almost entirely due, for example, to a wife's illness. The same considerations apply to many characteristics that are used in the diagnosis of personality disorder. The diagnosis of antisocial personality disorder in DSM-IV is heavily dependent upon items which could be as easily explained in terms of environment as of individual psychology. When studying personality disorder we need to find features that could be amenable to change and can be subject to repeat measurement with a realistic expectation of some change.

Suggestions

Kendell (1975) in his book *The Role of Diagnosis in Psychiatry* argued strongly against a dimensional approach to diagnosis because, in his view, dimensional systems have to be reduced to categories before the information they contain can be utilized. He argued that most scientific statements are concerned with populations rather than with linear distributions and that, once a population has been defined, even if this is done in terms of scores on one or more dimensions, a category has been created. In his view most of the advocates of a dimensional representation of disease are essentially theoreticians, whereas those responsible for day-to-day decisions about the management of individual patients have usually found themselves forced to use some sort of typology.

Clearly, there is a lot in this and the pressure to categorize patients is considerably so great that any attempt to displace the diagnostic process is bound to fail. What might be helpful, however, is to supplement the current diagnostic systems with a non-categorical trait analysis. Different analyses could be used for different purposes; for example, a trait analysis of a series of individuals could be used to determine whether factors emerge which would assist in the diagnostic process. The work of Livesley and his colleagues (Schroeder and Livesley, 1992; Livesley *et al.*, 1998) offers a way forward here but it should be developed more in a clinical context.

Another approach is to use the patient's history and examination to compile a list of deficits and difficulties as well as a list of skills and assets. Each trait in these lists can be examined in some detail to note how truly persistent any disorder is, to note fluctuations and possible precipitants of those fluctuations, and to note areas of potential. From such lists treatment tactics flow. Simply comprising and discussing the list with a patient gives him or her better self-understanding, but the list is particularly important in focusing attention on traits that might be modified or improved and assets that might be capitalized upon.

The American DSM classification has tried to apply a multiaxial system to psychiatric diagnosis. It suggests five axes: Axis I consists of psychiatric syndromes, Axis III is for physical disorders, Axis IV for severity of psychosocial stresses, and Axis V for the highest level of adaptive functioning during the last year. This leaves Axis II for personality disorder and 'mental retardation'. The manual tells us that Axis II may also be used to list prominent maladaptive personality features and defence mechanisms. This approach seems to have a lot of merit and recognizes that personality is a feature of all individuals and must be properly described in an array of features in any psychiatric evaluation. To that extent the DSM system can be advocated. Unfortunately, however, the system does not allow proper recognition of the traits/characteristics which will need to be targeted in any treatment approach. Certainly one end of the spectrum of personality problems could be regarded as 'disordered' and even 'ill', but the attempt to break the disordered part of the spectrum of persistent psychological malfunction into discrete syndromes has produced an unsatisfactory set of alleged diagnoses which are unreliable, overlap, and give no therapeutic guidance.

An analysis of personal functioning may be helpful. It is standard practice in psychiatry to examine the mental state. This turns out to be an assessment by interview of a list of feelings, thoughts and behaviours which have by tradition become associated with psychological illnesses of various kinds. The list includes, for example, anxiety, depression, obsessionality, hypochondriasis, sleeping, eating, thought disorder, delusions and hallucinations. Understanding these psychological functions greatly assists in understanding the patient's disabilities and gives strong clues about treatment. Furthermore such assessments can be repeated serially at fairly short time intervals to monitor progress. However, the list usually omits other important psychological phenomena. It is these others, in the same three categories of feelings, thoughts and behaviour, which could be used to construct a personal function analysis, to assist in the better understanding of all psychiatric disorders, including personality disorders.

There are many ways of assessing personal functioning; they all have their advantages and disadvantages and attempts to cross-validate them are important. It would seem appropriate in this approach to relatively neglect the historical and the social approaches, and to concentrate on the psychological. Of course this cannot be done in any absolute sense; every aspect of our psychology is affected by our history and by our environment. Items can be chosen, however, that are more likely to be personal and concerned with the present. Assessment periods, for example the past week, the past month or even the past year, are appropriate to the item

under consideration and would allow progress to be monitored by serial interviewing.

The suggestion here is that a list of psychological characteristics is drawn up such that it is expected to cover the full range of personal functioning, without too much intercorrelation between characteristics. This is a tall order in itself, but the following list might give some idea of what is meant. The list is somewhat arbitrary, but divided into feelings, behaviour and thinking (*Table 3.1*).

The aim would be to rate each characteristic on a scale (say 0–4) and thus produce a personal function profile. The ratings would preferably be made after some detailed knowledge of the patient, or after close contact with informants. Clearly such a task is too difficult, too onerous for the 1–2 hour outpatient session, but *any* personality assessment is too difficult for such brief encounters and we should face the fact that some of our current problems with personality assessment are related to inadequate ill-digested information. It is highly likely that such a list could be reduced, indeed would have to be reduced

Table 3.1 Characteristics that should be included in assessments of personality functioning

Feelings	depression elation mood instability sensitivity callousness loneliness
Behaviour	stubbornness quarrelsomeness irritability sadism self-destructiveness social withdrawal social isolation compliance tendency to control others low self-esteem dependence upon others theatricality and attention seeking
Thinking	identity problems paranoia grandiosity magical thinking tall story telling consistenty using other people for own ends suggestibility preoccupation with death obsessionality

because of intercorrelations, but this would need to be tested. As with traditional mental state assessments, a timescale could be used for personal functions, perhaps the past few months, or perhaps the last year. For every patient, a personal function analysis would be of considerable value. It would improve communication between psychiatrists and others, it would provide a baseline against which to measure change and, above all, it might loosen some of the negative attitudes towards personality disordered patients, in that it would identify disability in a non-pejorative manner while indicating areas for treatment. For the group of patients currently labelled personality disordered, it would provide understanding of their difficulties.

Conclusion

Our current conceptualization of personality disorder is unsatisfactory. This is partly because it is a global concept which has so much potential variance within it that transmits little meaning between discussants. To improve on it, psychiatrists may have to follow their psychology colleagues and be more content with personality descriptions in terms of separate psychological characteristics, each of which may or may not be disordered.

Nevertheless, the term is very persistent and doctors are very reluctant to view disorder except in terms of a global diagnosis. The idea of diagnosis is frequently a useful one in medicine. If Dr A tells Dr B that patient X has pernicious anaemia then in those two words a great deal of information is transmitted, information relating to aetiology, pathology, treatment and prognosis. In psychiatry, such semantic economy is unusual and if Dr A tells Dr B that patient X also has a personality disorder, Dr B will have very little further information. Dr A will have to amplify, spelling out separate characteristics, perhaps constructing a formulation before Dr B has solid data to go on. However, as Williams suggested in 1979, 'diagnosis' is a separate clinical decision from management and treat-

ment. Williams suggested that there are four or five different models of management in current use, for example, medical, social, behavioural and psychological. If, he postulated, the chosen model is not medical, then diagnosis *per se* is unhelpful and a problem analysis is required. Even with the medical model the predictive power of diagnosis to treatment is low. Williams recommended a problem-oriented approach for most psychiatric conditions. What is being suggested here is one kind of problem-oriented approach.

The suggestions here do not conflict in themselves with the traditional art of personality disorder diagnosis. What is proposed is an addition to the traditional process, an addition which would in effect be an extension of the mental state examination. A series of personal functions would be assessed by interview and observation as they are at the time of interview or in the very recent past. The functions would fall into the three usual categories of feelings, thoughts and behaviour, and would be chosen to cover all the traits which psychiatrists believe to be of clinical importance and which are loaded as little as possible with environmental effects outside the patient's influence. It is suggested that such an analysis should be done on all patients (where time allows) whatever the diagnosis. The purpose of the analysis would be to give better understanding of the difficulties exemplified in the history, to provide a functional baseline against which progress could be managed and to give therapeutic pointers. The belief is that the system would offer an immediate improvement in the understanding of personality aberrations and maybe, in the long term, give clues for the better diagnostic nosology.

Perhaps the suggestion does conflict with the traditional approach in one respect. It could be used to avoid the diagnostic label of personality disorder altogether, thus avoiding the social and attitudinal baggage that such a label brings with it. Even so, a purely dimensional/trait approach for the second axis of the DSM system still seems a long way off.

4

Personality Assessment Schedule

Peter Tyrer and Domenic Cicchetti

Despite criticisms of the system used in DSM classification of psychiatric disorders in many parts of this book – summarized in the explanation that DSM stands for Diagnosis for Simple Minds – there is no doubt that it has been a major stimulus for research and clinical advance. The decision to introduce clearly defined operational criteria for the diagnosis of all psychiatric disorders was a momentous one and, where sufficient information exists to create good definition, these criteria are invaluable. Although the introduction of criteria sometimes appears arbitrary and procrustean to the clinician, they are invaluable for the research worker who wishes to have a reliable assessment of diagnostic status. As we have already seen, operational criteria are now an essential part of the latest classifications of personality disorder. When a great deal is known about a disorder and full assessment can be made at a single point in time by close examination of the patient, operational criteria have major advantages. The assessment of schizophrenia can now be carried out reliably and validly with high specificity and sensitivity.

Nevertheless, despite some assertions to the contrary, personality disorders are different. There is much less agreement about their categorization into types and the requirement of persistence and pervasiveness makes it impossible to make a cross-sectional diagnosis. The operational criteria introduced for the diagnosis of personality disorder are more speculative and, despite their widespread adoption in the past 30 years, represent working hypotheses that have still not been supported by the evidence, as Livesley and his colleagues have established with unerring and unanswerable arguments throughout this time (Livesley, 1986, 1987; Livesley *et al.*, 1994, 1998), arguing that the operational criteria for the current classification of personality disturbance only provide a viable classification through the balletic, but not particularly elegant, contortions of comorbidity (Stuart *et al.*, 1998).

The Personality Assessment Schedule (PAS) was developed in 1976 before operational criteria were introduced and much less had been written about individual categories of personality disorder. It was felt necessary to examine each of the characteristics that were commonly found in personality disorder and determine to what extent they group together in both nature and severity. In developing the schedule, four principles were kept in mind. Some would argue that these represent hypotheses rather than principles but they have been common accompaniments to the descriptions of personality disorder for many years (although we see reason to question the fourth of these now). These are:

1. Personality disorders are only quantitatively different from normal personality variation.
2. Personality is determined primarily by traits or underlying attributes that lead to relative consistency in behaviour.

3. Personality disorder leads to impaired personal and social function because these traits and behaviour are both more prominent and persistent.

4. Personality disorder is enduring and begins early in adult life, so its assessment must be longitudinal.

This theoretical position comes close to many other investigations into 'personology' (Millon's term for the science of this subject). In his words (Millon, 1987) 'each person possesses a small and distinct group of primary traits that persist over time and exhibit a high degree of consistency across situations. These enduring (stable) and pervasive (consistent) traits are the attributes we search for when we consider diagnosing a 'personality disorder' term'.

The primary traits chosen when developing the PAS were ones that recur throughout descriptions of personality disorder and normal personality. Some were derived from Allport's synonyms (Allport and Odbert, 1936) but most came from the descriptions of personality disorder in ICD, DSM and Schneider's original case histories (Schneider, 1923).

It was felt important to keep the list as short as possible so that each trait could be explored in depth at interview. An original list of 45 was reduced to 29 and used in preliminary field studies. These showed some items that were highly correlated with each other. These were removed and the final list of 24 characteristics or traits chosen (*Table 4.1*).

Because it was postulated that those with personality disorder would develop personal and social dysfunction as a consequence of excessive prominence of these traits each was rated on a scale with anchor points defined by the degree of social dysfunction caused by the characteristic in question. A nine-point scale was chosen and subsequent investigations suggest that this was an appropriate number to achieve optimal levels of reliability (Cicchetti *et al.*, 1985). The scale was constructed so that it would be most sensitive in detecting personality disorders. The scoring was skewed so that most people with normal variation would score between 0 and 3 on each characteristic. The interview is a semi-structured one that includes mandatory questions as well as optional probes. In the PAS

Table 4.1 Personality traits investigated in preliminary studies of the Personality Assessment Schedule

	Trait	
Traits found to occur with insufficient frequency or severity to be included in the schedule	Possessiveness Dominance Fickleness Ambivalence Disorderliness Passiveness Stubbornness Humility	Fanaticism Gullibility Foolhardiness Conformity Timidity Carelessness Vanity Self-aggrandisement
Traits which correlated too strongly with other traits (r > 0.65) and so were excluded	Anger Touchiness Insensitivity Shallowness Weakness	
Traits included in PAS – final version	Pessimism Worthlessness Optimism Lability Anxiousness Suspiciousness Introspection Shyness Aloofness Sensitivity Vulnerability Irritability	Impulsiveness Aggression Callousness Irresponsibility Childishness Resourcelessness Dependence Submissiveness Conscientiousness Rigidity Eccentricity Hypochondriasis

only the negative attributes of each characteristic are being rated in order to make the diagnosis of personality disorder. Subsequently an expanded scale, the Comprehensive Assessment of Personality (CAP) (which has never been formally tested but is available from the author PT on request) was introduced to measure both the amount of impairment and advantage created by each characteristic. Subsequent experience with the 24 personality traits included in the PAS have shown them to be reasonably robust and independent. Although examination of inter-trait correlation showed a substantial degree of intercorrelation between many of the items in the first 1000 patients tested, this is to be expected in view of the natural clustering of data into groups of personality disorder. The highest inter-trait correlation ($r = 0.57$) was found between impulsiveness and irresponsibility. Indeed, it is of interest that the inter-trait correlations were higher for the characteristics that can be loosely grouped together as antisocial, and this is the group that has been shown to be the most consistent category of personality disorder in most other investigations.

Several methods of categorizing the scores from the PAS were considered. These included specific criteria (which at the time of development of the schedule were lacking for personality disorder), classification according to Schneider's subtypes along the lines that have been carried out by Standage (1978, 1979), and categorization into the ICD-8 and DSM-II categories which were in existence at that time. Eventually, all these were rejected. It was felt that sufficient was not known about the separation of individual personality disorders to have confidence in any classification. For this reason, an agnostic method of classification was chosen in which personality diagnosis was determined not by the investigators but by the data. This primarily involved cluster analysis, but factor analysis and discriminant function analysis were also included and produced very similar findings (Tyrer and Alexander, 1988).

Analysis of data

Once the initial reliability of the ratings in the PAS was shown to be satisfactory, a study was carried out with 130 patients, 65 with a clinical personality disorder (according to the judgement of the author PT) and 65 with another psychiatric diagnosis without personality disorder. These ratings were first subjected to factor analysis. This revealed two major factors, which matched sociopathic and passive–dependent features and were labelled as such. Additional factors accounting for obsessional, anxious (or dysthymic) and schizoid characteristics were also identified (Tyrer and Alexander, 1979). However, we were primarily interested in identifying characteristics that could group patients into categories and so cluster analysis techniques were used.

Following Everitt (1974) and Garside and Roth (1978), a number of different approaches was used and the results compared for each individual. The rationale of cluster analysis is simply geometric; each observation is thought of as a point located in n-dimensional space, and the clustering algorithm assembles clusters of points that are close according to some predetermined criterion. In hierarchical cluster analysis, a sequence of merging clusters is followed, starting with individual observations. Once two observations cluster they remain together for the whole analysis. Non-hierarchical methods, on the other hand, are more free in that a preset number of clusters is specified, and when the algorithm proceeds to fewer clusters those observations grouped together at a lower level no longer need to remain grouped in this way. One disadvantage of non-hierarchical methods is the heavy computational requirement; hierarchical methods use less computer power, but suffer from the disadvantages that wrongly allocated individuals, or 'strangers', can be included in clusters more easily.

There are many different methods of both forms of cluster analysis and with our data the GENSTAT package (Lawes Agricultural Trust, Rothamstead Experimental Station, Herts) was used, as this provides a number of alternatives. In particular the *nearest neighbour*, *furthest neighbour* and *centroid* methods of merging clusters were all employed in hierarchical analysis, and Wilks' criterion used for non-hierarchical analysis (Tyrer and Alexander, 1988).

When these methods of cluster analysis

were applied to the 130 cases, seven distinct clusters emerged (Tyrer and Alexander, 1979). The clusters defined by different methods showed some variation, as might be expected, but each also contained a core of cases that remained together using all methods. The profiles of mean scores on all 24 items were plotted using an ordering of the variables derived from the factor analysis, and it was found that the two pairs of clusters had similar mean profiles, with differences mainly in the vertical scales. The seven clusters were labelled explosive, paranoid–aggressive, histrionic, asthenic, anankastic, schizoid and normal, or, more accurately, no personality disorder. However, the profiles for the explosive and paranoid–aggressive clusters, and for the histrionic and asthenic ones, were sufficiently similar for the question to be raised as to whether these consisted of patients with the same disorder but of different degree, in which case separate categorization was superfluous.

Strauss *et al.* (1973) discuss this issue at some length and recommend the use of a measure of distance between points which is not simply geometric, but instead relates to the correlation between observations, calculated by treating each pair of 24 ratings of 24 observations on two variables. This was applied to the 130 cases, after standardizing each variable in the usual way, and the resulting hierarchical cluster analysis revealed only five clusters, which were labelled sociopathic, passive–dependent, anankastic, schizoid and normal. In both the distance and correlation analyses, one cluster was comprised largely of the non-personality disorder group (normal), which accounted for 55 of the 65 non-personality disordered patients in the furthest neighbour distance-based analysis, while all but two of the 65 personality disorder cases were grouped into the other personality disorder clusters in the same analysis.

The clusters defined were expected to be *noisy* in the sense that some cases would not fit easily into any cluster. The possibility that other clusters exist but in too small numbers to coalesce in this limited sample could not be discounted. In order to produce operational definitions of clusters, the profiles of each individual were drawn up and compared visually to the cluster mean profile by PT. Individual cases who both geometrically and clinically did not 'group' well were removed and the remaining cases subjected to discriminant function analysis to help further in validating the classification system. This relatively clear identification of four types of personality disorder was supported by further observations and a computer program written to give appropriate weights to each of the 24 personality characteristics (now available in a simple Visual C++ format (Tyrer and Tyrer, 1997)). However, it was also felt appropriate to continue the analysis with a larger population.

Two hundred and fifty-six further cases were therefore examined; 167 (65.2%) of these had a clinical diagnosis of personality disorder. The ratings of these patients were subjected to furthest neighbour cluster analysis with a correlational distance measure applied. This method was used because it had given rise to the most distinct classification in the previous analysis. The hierarchical merging continued smoothly as the distance criterion relaxed until 15 clusters were identified. At this stage, there was a considerable reduction in the merging criteria needed before further merging took place and so these 15 clusters were extracted and scrutinized carefully. One of these clusters (15 cases) appeared to show few positive scores except on conscientiousness and rigidity and was rejected as representing a non-disordered group. Only one other cluster was rejected. This comprised nine cases and had high scores for pessimism, worthlessness, impulsiveness and irresponsibility. This small group was the nearest the analysis came to identifying an equivalent of borderline personality disorder. When the cluster analysis algorithm was allowed to progress beyond this point until just four groups were defined, it was seen that the profiles of these four groups were very similar to the four profiles from the original 130 cases and, moreover, the proportions in the four clusters were also similar to those in the first analysis. This, therefore, not only validated the broad categorization into sociopathic, passive–dependent, anankastic and schizoid groupings, but also allowed a subclassification giving a total of 13 categories (*see* Appendix).

Classification of personality disorders using the PAS

The full PAS is given in Appendix 1 together with scoring instructions. A hierarchical system was employed in which the personality category that has the highest score for social impairment becomes the named personality disorder, although if other major categories reach similar levels of scoring they too can be mentioned in the diagnostic description. Patients who do not reach the scores necessary for the diagnosis of personality disorder may still attain the level required for personality difficulty and be coded as such and severity can also be assessed using the system of Tyrer and Johnson (1996).

The original dimensional system allowed five levels of diagnosis: (1) personality difficulty, (2) personality disorder in one major category only, (3) personality disorder in two or more major categories, (4) severe personality disorder, one only, and (5) gross personality disorder, in which two or more major categories achieve the level of scoring required for the diagnosis of severe personality disorder, but analysis of data using this system shows no evidence of linear relationship and the rating of severity is better determined by overlap of clusters than by severity of an individual personality disorder (Tyrer and Johnson, 1996).

Cluster analysis of the data from the PAS has shown repeatedly that four major types of abnormal personality can be identified (*Figure 4.1*). These are termed socio-pathic, passive–dependent, anankastic and schizoid. It has been noted that these categories bear a close resemblance to the three main clusters of DSM-III personality disorders (Reich and Thompson, 1987). The flamboyant cluster is similar to the socio-pathic category, the eccentric one to the schizoid category, and the anxious or fearful cluster to the passive–dependent category in the PAS. The anankastic category is included (under obsessive–compulsive) in the anxious cluster of DSM-IV personality disorders, but in cluster analyses in the PAS it can be identified as a separate group.

Nine further sub-categories of personality disorder have been identified using cluster analysis and these are illustrated in *Figure 4.1*. However, correlational cluster analysis suggests that these belong as sub-categories to the main groups rather than separate entities and so we are not recommending that each diagnosis is given independent status; they are just felt to require further investigation. Close examination of each of them may reveal important differences between them that justify one or more of the sub-categories being raised to major categories in their own right, but as yet no such evidence is available. There are many resemblances between the main and subsidiary categories of personality disorder in the PAS and those in DSM-IV and ICD-10 and it is valuable to look at each diagnosis separately to discuss its similarities and differences from the two standard classifications.

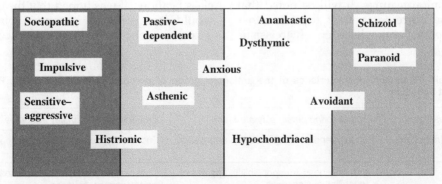

Figure 4.1 Diagnostic categories determined by cluster analysis from the Personality Assessment Schedule. The four major categories are sociopathic, passive–dependent, anankastic and schizoid and these determine the boundaries in the figure. The remaining nine groups are sub–categories and some show overlap as indicated on the figure. The avoidant category also has some overlap with the passive–dependent group

Sociopathic personality disorders (equivalent to cluster B in other classifications)

This group is the most clearly identified cluster in the analysis of PAS data. Together with the explosive and sensitive–aggressive personality disorders they make up a major group (*Table 4.2*). The ratings that contribute mainly to the diagnosis are those of callousness, aggression and impulsiveness, closely followed by irritability and irresponsibility. Conscientiousness, worthlessness and eccentricity usually have low ratings in this group.

Within this group there are two major subcategories, the sensitive–aggressive and impulsive ones. The sensitive–aggressive, also termed 'paranoid–aggressive' (Tyrer and Alexander, 1979) is so named because suspiciousness and sensitivity are so prominent that they are at least equally as important as the aggressive personality features. It is a group that is not identified in current classification disorders but is probably very important because of the current concern over violent people with personality disorders in the community; this group is likely to figure highly amongst these. The explosive group shows its highest ratings on impulsiveness and irresponsibility, closely followed by aggression. There are very close similarities between the explosive sub-category and impulsive personality disorder in ICD-10 and between sociopathic category and antisocial personality disorder in DSM-IV, and examination of *Table 4.2* shows that the three subgroups within the antisocial cluster also show many common features. It will be noted that there is no representation of the two other DSM-III personality disorders (narcissistic

and borderline categories) that make up the flamboyant cluster in DSM-IV. Both of these include beliefs and attitudes that are not always represented in behaviour and therefore would not be detected by the PAS. Nevertheless, important behavioural connotations of each are covered by the PAS variables and it is particularly surprising that a cluster of labile, impulsive and depressed characteristics do not cluster together to form a borderline group.

Passive–dependent personality disorders (equivalent to cluster C in other classifications)

The term 'passive–dependent' was used to describe this group because it includes the range between manipulative and self-dramatic personalities and those which are passive and acquiescent (*Table 4.3*). The term is well described in the psychoanalytical literature and was first proposed as a diagnostic label for personality disorder by Millon (1969). The key characteristics in the PAS that contribute to the diagnosis of passive–dependent personality disorder are childishness, dependence and resourcelessness and, to a lesser extent, lability and vulnerability. The histrionic subgroup has many similarities with both histrionic personality disorders in DSM-III and ICD-10. Self-dramatic, manipulative childish behaviour together with dependence and emotional lability are the main features but, as histrionic behaviour is not specified to quite the same degree as in other classifications, it was hoped that the diagnosis would lose some of its sexual bias. Thus, excessive concern over appearance, seduc-

Table 4.2 Main personality characteristics of the antisocial group of personality disorders in the Personality Assessment Schedule

Personality category	High-scoring personality attributes	Low-scoring personality attributes
Sociopathic (major group member)	Impulsiveness, irresponsibility, aggression, irritability	Eccentricity, conscientiousness, optimism
Impulsive	Impulsiveness, irresponsibility, aggression, irritability, anxiousness	Conscientiousness, submissiveness, worthlessness, shyness
Sensitive–aggressive	Aggression, irritability, sensitivity, suspiciousness	Eccentricity, optimism, dependence

Table 4.3 Main personality characteristics of the dependent group of personality disorders in the Personality Assessment Schedule

Personality category	High-scoring personality attributes	Low-scoring personality attributes
Passive–dependent (major group member)	Dependence, vulnerability, anxiousness, lability	Callousness, rigidity, eccentricity
Histrionic	Dependence, lability, vulnerability, childishness	Callousness, aloofness, eccentricity, rigidity
Asthenic	Anxiousness, sensitivity, submissiveness	Callousness, conscientiousness, rigidity

tiveness and other features that are at least partly dependent on gender, are not included.

The asthenic subgroup shows some similarities with dependent personality disorders in ICD-10 and DSM-III-R but also shows some important differences. Sensitivity, anxiousness and submissiveness are key features and are not represented in other current classifications (*Table 4.2*). Ever since earlier classification included the pejorative label *inadequate personality* there has been concern about any label that suggests incompetence that is independent of personality. Some people are not able to achieve as much as others through no fault of their personalities. Nevertheless, in one study in which asthenic personality disorder was assessed using the Standardized Assessment of Personality (SAP; Mann *et al.,* 1981) in patients with mental handicap, none was found to have satisfied the criteria for asthenic personality disorder (Ballinger and Reid, 1987). It might be thought that all patients with mental handicap would have some asthenic features as a consequence of their intellectual impairment, but it appears

that this can be separated from asthenic personality features.

Anankastic personality disorders (equivalent to the fourth obsessive cluster in some classifications)

This is the largest group of disorders identified by the PAS and includes four categories. These together make up the inhibited group (*Table 4.4*). Like other classifications, the PAS has no difficulty in identifying a rigid, over-conscientious introspective personality type. The other three groups are all different from the categories in ICD-10 and DSM-IV although one of them, anxious, is accorded a similar label in ICD-10. Throughout the use of the PAS, it was noted that anxiousness was one of the most highly rated attributes and, as the second group of cluster analyses revealed a group with high ratings for submissiveness, conscientiousness and shyness as well as anxiety, it was felt appropriate to give the label of anxious personality disorder

Table 4.4 Main personality characteristics of the inhibited group of personality disorders in the Personality Assessment Schedule

Personality category	High-scoring personality attributes	Low-scoring personality attributes
Anankastic (main group member)	Conscientiousness, anxiousness, rigidity	Optimism, irresponsibility, impulsiveness
Anxious	Submissiveness, anxiousness, shyness, conscientiousness	Optimism, aggression, callousness
Dysthymic	Worthlessness, shyness, conscientiousness, aloofness	Aggression, optimism, childishness
Hypochondriacal	Hypochondriasis, conscientiousness, anxiousness	Irresponsibility, submissiveness, eccentricity

to this group and ICD-10 used a similar description subsequently. In some respects it combines both the anxious and self-conscious personalities described by Mann *et al.* (1981).

The dysthymic group is characterized by high ratings for worthlessness, shyness, introspection and aloofness (*Table 4.4*). It is not recognized in any other personality disorder classification, although the concept of dysthymic disorder, first described by Akiskal and his colleagues (1980) is now part of the DSM-IV classification. Interestingly enough, Akiskal regards dysthymia as one of the 'characterological depressions' in which personality disorder coexists with mood disturbance. The dysthymic cluster from the PAS supports this distinction, although it should be emphasized that the personality dimensions of worthlessness and pessimism are scored independently of formal mood disorder. The concept of dysthymic personality disorder is now resurrected in the suggested new category of depressive personality disorder. The evidence (discussed further in Chapter 6) suggests that the degree of comorbidity of this group with depression is much less than might have been expected and argues for its introduction as a personality disorder (Klein and Miller, 1993; Hirschfeld and Holzer, 1994; Phillips *et al.*, 1998).

The last subgroup, hypochondriacal personality disorder, is also not recognized in any existing personality classification. Although, after considerable argument over its diagnostic status (Kenyon, 1965; Bianchi, 1971), hypochondriasis is now recognized as a neurotic disorder, hypochondriasis as a personality characteristic has not previously been identified. In the PAS, as for all other ratings, hypochondriasis is only rated in the absence of mental state disorder. The results identified a cluster in which hypochondriasis is the main component and accompanied by anxiousness and conscientiousness (*Table 4.4*). The persistent preoccupation with physical health shows some similarities with the syndrome described by Briquet (1859), but perhaps it is best described by Emil Kraepelin (1905, pp. 271–272). He gives an excellent account of the type of patient who can only be described as having hypochondriacal personality disorder:

'The patient is quite collected, clear and well ordered in his statements. He says that one of his sisters suffers in the same way as himself …. Gradually he began to fear that he had a serious disease, and was going to die of heart apoplexy. All the assurances and examinations of his doctor could not convince him. For this reason he suddenly left his appointment and went home one day, seven years ago, being afraid that he would die shortly. After this he consulted every possible doctor, and took long holidays repeatedly, always recovering a little, but invariably finding that his fears returned speedily. The whole course of the present case shows that the disease is deeply rooted in the general personality. It usually develops early in adult life, and lasts with greater or lesser fluctuation throughout the whole of life.'

Kraepelin did not refer to this condition as hypochondriasis, instead describing it as 'the insanity of irrepressible ideas', but the hypochondriacal hallmark is unmistakable. We have continued to examine the implications of the diagnosis of hypochondriacal personality disorder and found it to be more predominant in affective and neurotic disorders than other diagnoses (Tyrer *et al.*, 1990a) and to show overlap with hypochondriacal syndromes. In a subsequent study of the impact of hypochondriacal personality disorder in patients with neurotic disorder over 5 years the presence of hypochondriacal personality disorder at baseline was related to persistent somatization (*Figure 4.2*) (Tyrer *et al.*, 1999).

Withdrawn personality disorders (equivalent to cluster A in other classifications)

This group also shows a good correspondence with ICD-10 and DSM-IV equivalent categories. The withdrawn or schizoid personality group is identified by high ratings for eccentricity, suspiciousness, introspection and aloofness and probably covers the range of both schizotypal and schizoid personality disorders in DSM-IV (*Table 4.5*). The subcategory of paranoid personality is virtually identical to both DSM-IV and ICD-10 para-

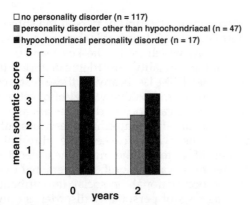

☐ no personality disorder (n = 117)
◨ personality disorder other than hypochondriacal (n = 47)
■ hypochondriacal personality disorder (n = 17)

Figure 4.2 Distribution of somatization scores in 181 patients from the Nottingham study of neurotic disorder over two years separated by initial personality status (PAS) F-ratio (groups) = 2.5; df 2,178; ns F-ratio (groups × times) = 2.8; df 2,178; p = 0.065 (reproduced by permission from the Journal of Psychosomatic Research)

noid personality disorders. The key traits making up this disorder include sensitivity, suspiciousness, vulnerability and anxiousness; patients satisfying the old descriptions of 'sensitive Beziehungswahn' (Kretschmer, 1918) would also be included here.

The additional cluster of avoidant personality disorder, with its main features of lack of self-confidence, shyness, introspection and anxiousness (*Table 4.5*), complicates the terminology of personality disorder. There has long been some uncertainty about the position of a withdrawn, anxious, shy personality disorder in the cluster grouping of personality disorder (Trull *et al.*, 1987). Avoidant personality disorder shows some characteristics of both cluster A (odd/eccentric) and cluster C (shy, inhibited) and in the PAS it came out towards the end of the cluster A spectrum (although it straddles the border between the anankastic and withdrawn groups) (*Figure*

4.1). However, as discussed later (Chapter 6) there is a strong overlap between social phobia and avoidant personality disorder (Herbert *et al.*, 1992; Alpert *et al.*, 1997) and reason to believe that they may be consanguineous rather than merely comorbid (Tyrer, 1996). If so, avoidant personality disorder would be best placed with cluster C as it is in both DSM and ICD classifications (Trull *et al.*, 1987). Nevertheless, because its primary feature is that of withdrawal from social contact, it could in many cases be regarded as part of the schizoid group and retains its place there in the PAS classification.

This makes clear that the cluster system of personality disorders, despite having clear advantages in simplifying the classification, is not without difficulties in classifying some conditions. There is further overlap between disorders with histrionic personality disorder, a condition grouped with the flamboyant (cluster B) group in ICD-10 and DSM-IV but with the dependent group in the PAS system (*Table 4.3*; *Figure 4.1*). Certainly the original work using older diagnostic descriptions of histrionic personality disorder suggested it was the female equivalent of antisocial personality disorder in men (Robins, 1966; Guze *et al.*, 1971). Similarly, the anxious and dysthymic personality disorders overlap into anankastic and passive–dependent groups, respectively. Although the PAS diagnosis is made using a hierarchy, it is perfectly appropriate to use the key trait scores for each of the categories in research studies. Thus, for example, if one wished to know whether schizoid personality features were more common in one group of psychiatric disorders compared with another, it would be appropriate to use the key trait scores for schizoid personality for comparison. An example of this approach is given in Chapter 7.

Table 4.5 Main personality characteristics of the withdrawn group of personality disorders in the Personality Assessment Schedule

Personality category	High-scoring personality attributes	Low-scoring personality attributes
Schizoid (major group member)	Eccentricity, aloofness, introspection, suspiciousness	Lability, irritability, aggression
Paranoid	Sensitivity, anxiousness, suspiciousness, vulnerability	Irresponsibility, callousness, optimism
Avoidant	Shyness, introspection, anxiousness	Eccentricity, irritability, aggression

Although the PAS does not have simple equivalents to DSM-IV personality disorders, it is possible to code it in a way that approximates closely with DSM-IV operational criteria and these, together with the ICD-10 ones, are shown in Appendix 1.

Rapid assessments of personality status

A full comprehensive personality assessment can take up to 4 hours and any quick assessment instrument is bound to be deficient in some respects as John Gunn has pointed out in the previous chapter. Despite this there is a constant demand for short instruments to be used for screening personality disorder and, where possible, identifying major components of personality abnormality. In deciding on the best instrument there is a trade-off between using a questionnaire, which takes the patient a lot longer but involves virtually no time for the clinician, and short interviews that are possibly less affected by subjective bias but which take a much shorter time.

Standardized Assessment of Personality (SAP)

The SAP is a specific semi-structured interview designed for use with an informant who has known the subject for at least 5 years. It is recommended that the instrument is used with a relative or close friend where possible and there is some information that suggests that the closer the contact and relationship the more reliable the data (Brothwell *et al.*, 1992). It is a major advantage using an informant with patients who are difficult to assess because of severe current mental state problems and the instrument takes no longer than 15 minutes to administer and can be carried out by telephone. The later version of the instrument (Pilgrim *et al.*, 1993) includes ICD-10 and DSM-IV versions. The later version of the instrument shows satisfactory inter-rater reliability ($\kappa = 0.76$) (Cicchetti and Sparrow, 1981; Pilgrim *et al.*, 1993) but somewhat less satisfactory test–retest reliability ($\kappa = 0.65$) (Pilgrim *et al.*, 1993).

The interview is in two parts. The first is open-ended in which the informant gives a free account of the kind of person the subject is normally. The informant is then asked a set of questions which probe the key features of the main personality disorder categories in ICD-10 and DSM-IV. If any of these features are responded to positively a set of questions relating to the category of disorder are asked in more detail. If the informant describes sufficient items which exceed the threshold number of criteria, the rater then decides whether these cause significant personal distress or occupational or social impairment. The diagnosis of personality disorder is only made if the subject scores for these criteria and there is associated impairment; one of these alone is not sufficient.

There is some evidence that using an informant to make personality assessment may elicit more pathological aspects of personality than self-report (Zimmerman, 1994). The SAP has been compared with the most comprehensive subject-based interview for personality disorders, the International Personality Disorder Examination (IPDE) (Loranger *et al.*, 1994). Although it was found that the SAP was a suitable screening instrument for the IPDE, having a high negative predictive value of 97%, it tended to over-diagnose the flamboyant (cluster B) personality disorders and so the predictive value of the instrument was poor (47%) (Mann *et al.*, 1999).

Quick Personality Assessment Schedule (PAS-Q)

The Quick Personality Assessment Schedule is a direct development from the longer PAS and has been through several revisions before achieving its current form (Appendix 3). Although it can be completed within 10 minutes it should only be carried out by trained interviewers who have had experience of assessment using the full PAS. It is also possible that those trained in other personality instruments may also be able to use the PAS-Q reliably but this has not been tested. The reason why it is so important to have previous experience is that the threshold level for diagnosis depends on deciding whether not only personality characteristics are present but also whether they cause serious social dysfunction. This is covered by the full PAS and helps the rater to decide to what extent any social dysfunction is created by personality abnormality as well as helping to formulate the degree of social dysfunction created by the disorder.

The instrument is given in two parts. For those who are new to the interviewer preliminary information is obtained about issues that are both relevant to personality assessment and social dysfunction, including occupation and personal history, difficulties with the law, substance misuse problems, and geographical mobility. None of these is necessarily indicative of personality disorder but helps to give information for which questions can be asked later in the interview. The screening questions for 16 of the 24 characteristics of the PAS are then asked and followed up by supplementary questions if the answers are positive. After each of these sections a rating of severity of the relevant personality group is made and scored on a three-point scale. The scoring system for the description of personality disorder is shown in Appendix 3.

Iowa Personality Disorder Screen

This is discussed in more detail in Chapter 2. More information is needed about its properties from other centres outside Iowa.

Reliability of the PAS and associated scales

Personality is one of the most difficult of psychological states to measure and so it follows that reliability of such measures may be less good than for other psychological variables. The difficulties in achieving good reliability, particularly with psychosocial attributes (Cicchetti, 1976), can be discussed under three headings: the subject's behaviour, the assessor's perception of the behaviour and contamination.

Subject's behaviour

Personality comprises a mixture of attitudes, feelings and behaviour and all of these may vary at different times. The work of psychologists such as Eysenck and Cattell emphasizes that certain habits and attitudes are consistent whereas others may vary. Those which are consistent are described as traits and these are recorded by means of suitable tests, mainly questionnaires. However, since that time there has been a reaction in psychology to the uncritical acceptance of traits and more attention has been paid to the situations in which personality characteristics are shown. With most normal people, it is situations rather than personality that determine behaviour and there are few characteristics that are shown in all situations. Thus a shy young school girl with few friends may suddenly blossom when she goes to university and exercises her new-found freedom. Her self-confidence improves and she apparently becomes extraverted and brash. If she later marries and has to give up work her self-confidence may wane, especially if she is confined to the house all day looking after young children. Again, as the children grow up and she takes up her occupational skills again, her level of confidence will most likely increase. For such a person, it is impossible to derive a measure of personality from mere study of behaviour.

Such a superficial examination will have all the disadvantages of looking into a room through a keyhole; only a small area can be surveyed at any one time and it is impossible to synthesize the whole from the image created. When these keyhole images contradict each other, the investigator is tempted to abandon the concept of traits altogether. This inconsistency in behaviour is described well by Mischel (1968) and had led to a study of personality within a broader framework that incorporates cognitive and social factors (Mischel, 1973). Much greater attention has, therefore, been paid to the situations in which these various manifestations of personality occur as these apparently evoke the personality characteristics (Moos, 1973).

The subject may also present a false image because of the wish to present a personality that is expected by others. In most instances the subject tries to project a more impressive and desirable personality than the true one (Goffman, 1956). These displays of personality become incorporated into rituals of behaviour which vary with setting. Sometimes the ritual is recognized as such by the parties involved (e.g. a salesman talking to a customer), but often it goes unrecognized. Berne (1970) has described a large number of ritual interactions that are best perceived as games as they are concerned with one party gaining superiority. This subject has developed into a system of treatment called transactional analysis. Its proponents regard a large proportion of mental distress as caused by faulty and inappropriate rituals of this type. An observer watching these rituals may greatly misinterpret personality characteristics unless he recognizes that a ritual is taking place in which each member has to follow a well-defined role.

Assessor's perception

Even when several observers see the same manifestations of personality and behaviour, they can score them differently. Because the assessment of personality involves a subtle mix of observation of behaviour, attribution of attitudes and beliefs, it can be assessed on several levels. The most common error is to over-simplify personality assessment, described by Vernon (1963) as the 'well known tendency to see people in blacks or whites, as goodies or baddies, to overestimate their unity and ignore their subtler variations'. This is seen in our tendency towards racial and national stereotypes. Thus, for example, we expect Italians to be volatile and pleasure loving, Germans to be dour and hard working, Swedes to be dull and depressed, and West Indians to be jolly and lazy. Once we have an over-simplified view of a person, we show selective perception, only seeing those characteristics that fit in with our stereotype and rejecting those that conflict with it. Similar stereotyping may also be present in the assessment of men and women. There is a tendency to regard women as having 'weaker' personalities, to be more emotional and less aggressive than men. This may explain why women are more often labelled as 'hysterical personalities' than men (Walton and Presly, 1973).

There is also a tendency to assess personality along subjective rather than objective lines. Thus, one of the first decisions that is often made when assessing personality is whether the observer likes or dislikes the person being rated. This may obviously affect the subsequent rating of characteristics and be responsible for some of the personality stereotypes already mentioned. This tendency

to use our own personal frameworks of interpretation was developed by Kelly as a new form of psychological assessment. Kelly noted that there was tremendous variation in an individual's views of others in society and that this could change over time. These *personal constructs* (Kelly, 1955) became formalized in the development of the Repertory Grid that has been used frequently in psychological testing and treatment. As each person has a different framework of interpretation it could account for a larger part of the differences between observer variation in personality assessment.

People also differ in the extent to which they study a person before making an assessment of personality. Those who are psychologically minded tend to go beyond superficial behaviour and try to interpret motives and attitudes, whereas others rely entirely on what is presented in the form of behaviour. This can also account for important differences in assessment of personality.

Contamination

The variations in a subject's behaviour and an assessor's perception are ones that disguise the underlying personality and therefore tend to misrepresent it. However, it is understood that the basic personality is unchanged and can be assessed adequately once the sources of confusion are removed. Contamination refers to the occasions when the personality does change through environmental circumstances or psychiatric illness. The change is not a permanent one and the personality reverts to its former state once the contaminating factors have been removed. However, during the contaminated state the personality is changed in a consistent fashion and both the subject and assessor can agree on the nature and extent of this change. It would be quite wrong to conclude on the basis of an assessment carried out during this time that the perceived personality is a permanent state.

Mention has already been made of the effect of environment on personality. People tend to adapt to a given environment and then change their behaviour when they move into a different environment. Just as a car changes its gear and speed depending on the nature of the road, people will change their behaviour and attitudes to suit a particular situation. This becomes a problem when an abnormal environment becomes long term or permanent. For example, offenders who are sent to prison or special hospitals for life at an early age will spend all their time in an abnormal environment which is nonetheless permanent. Their adjustment to that environment and their apparent personality structure will be different in that setting and cannot be described as normal. To take a less obvious example, people who grow up in economically deprived communities in which there is high unemployment are restricted to some extent in their personality development as well as in the more obvious aspects of occupation, housing and self-advancement. They have less opportunities to show their personality potential than those who are born into more favourable settings.

The effects of mental illness on personality are more tangible and have been studied extensively. It is well known that people's views of themselves change when they become mentally ill. The depressed patient may feel that he has always been inadequate and complaining and the schizophrenic may feel that he always had the power to influence events by magical thinking. It is, therefore, not surprising that assessments of personality based on the state of the patient at the time of assessment vary between times of mental illness and health. Thus, Coppen and Metcalfe (1965) found that scores on the Maudsley Personality Inventory changed after recovery from a depressive illness, with a decrease in scores for neuroticism and an increase in scores for extraversion. Similar findings were found by Knowles and Kreitman (1965) ex-

cept that extraversion scores did not change on recovery. Even when patients are asked to complete a questionnaire in terms of their normal personality they still score higher on neuroticism and lower on extraversion compared to their state when recovered (Kendell and DiScipio, 1968). The questionnaires that are often used for personality assessment are therefore inappropriate when testing people who are in long-term abnormal environments or who are mentally ill. Although attempts have been made to adjust for the effect of mental state on scores from personality inventories (e.g. Bianchi and Fergusson, 1977), these have not proved to be very satisfactory.

Specific studies of the reliability of the PAS

Reliability of the PAS (ICD-10 version)

The PAS has also been specifically adapted to make a diagnosis according to ICD-10 operational criteria for individual personality disorders. The full schedule is shown in Appendix 2 together with its scoring system for the different levels of severity of personality disorder. The ICD-10 version was piloted as part of the World Health Organization Field Trials programme, in which the inter-rater reliability was recorded using computer programs (Cicchetti *et al.*, 1977, 1978, 1984). The results showed excellent inter-rater reliability for each of the main personality disorder categories (*Table 4.6*) with all personality disorders achieving agreements of 0.75 or greater using the intra-class correlation coefficient (Merson *et al.*, 1994).

Table 4.6 Inter-rater reliability levels for the individual personality disorders in the PAS ICD-10 version

ICD-10 personality disorder	Inter-rater reliability (R_I)	F-ratio for inter-rater bias ($n = 29$) ns (not significant)	Level of agreement (after Cicchetti and Sparrow, 1981)
Paranoid	0.95	0.19	Excellent
Schizoid	0.90	0.03	Excellent
Dissocial	0.75	2.47	Excellent
Impulsive	0.96	0.24	Excellent
Borderline	0.97	0.68	Excellent
Histrionic	0.96	0.24	Excellent
Anankastic	0.88	2.40	Excellent
Anxious	0.96	0.46	Excellent
Dependent	0.97	0.97	Excellent

F-ratios for inter-raterbias non-significant at the 5% level

Quick Personality Assessment Schedule (PAS-Q)

The value of the PAS-Q as a screening measure was assessed in the course of a recent study of the value of different forms of case management in psychotic patients (the UK Case Management Trial) (Burns *et al.*, 1999; Creed *et al.*, 1999; for the UK700 Group). The PAS-Q was used to assess personality status for all patients entering the study and at one centre it was compared with the full PAS. In each case the PAS-Q was used to assess the patient first so that full information was not available from the full PAS when the PAS-Q was scored.

One hundred and fifty-four (76.6%) of 201 patients recruited at the centre (St Mary's and St Charles Hospital) had assessments of personality status using both the full PAS and the PAS-Q. The weighted kappa (κGr_w) statistic (Cohen, 1968) was used to gauge the agreement of the PAS-Q with the full PAS. The construct validity of PAS-Q was also indirectly evaluated through its relationship to psychopathology using the Comprehensive Psychopathological Rating Scale (CPRS) (Åsberg *et al.*, 1978).

Although the weighted kappa statistic for the four-point scale was 0.43, suggesting only moderate agreement between the full PAS and PAS-Q, much of the variation was due to dispute over the differentiation between no personality disorder and personality difficulty. However, much better agreement was found for the simple dichotomous separation of personality disorder versus no personality disorder ($\kappa_w = 0.83$). The CPRS scores at baseline supported the hypothesis that the PAS-Q was a valid identify of the four levels of personality pathology as the mean CPRS scores rose incrementally with each succeeding level of pathology (*Figure 4.3*).

Reliability of the full PAS

Several reliability studies have also been carried out with the PAS. In the first published study (Tyrer *et al.*, 1979), the intraclass correlation coefficient for ratings carried out with audio-tape interviews and separate interviews with two raters were only fair to good, ranging between 0.55 and 0.60 overall. Examination of individual attributes from the schedule showed that personality characteristics that were also clinical symptoms, such as pessimism, worthlessness and optimism, achieved lower levels of reliability whereas items such as conscientiousness, introspection, aloofness and childishness achieved much higher reliability. This suggested that raters had some difficulty in differentiating the present personality and clinical symptoms of patients from the premorbid personality that is formally rated by the PAS. This early study was carried out with a shorter version of the PAS and this was amplified to the present version (*see* Appendix 1) in later studies. A combination of inter-rater and cross-national reliability was carried out in West Haven, Connecticut and Nottingham, UK

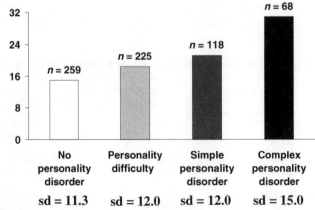

Figure 4.3 Baseline ratings of psychopathology from the Comprehensive Psychopathological Rating Scale in 670 patients assessed on the PAS-Q in the UK700 case management trial (reproduced by permission from the UK700 Group) [P < 0.001])

using videotaped interviews with informant and patient (Tyrer *et al.*, 1984a). The intraclass correlation coefficients between raters and between nationalities are shown (*Table 4.7*).

In general, satisfactorily high levels of agreement were achieved with both American and British raters (who included one from Ireland and one from Scotland), with little difference between the reliability for individual personality attributes. However, reliability levels for items of measured mood disturbance, particularly optimism, were lower than for other variables.

A combination of inter-rater and cross-national reliability was carried out in West Haven, Connecticut and Nottingham using videotaped interviews with informant and patient (Tyrer *et al.*, 1984). The intraclass correlation coefficients between raters and between nationalities are shown (*Table 4.7*).

In general, satisfactorily high levels of agreement were achieved with both American and British raters (who included one from Ireland and one from Scotland), with little difference between the reliability for individual personality attributes. However, reliability levels for items of measured mood disturbance, particularly optimism, were lower than for other variables.

In another study using a modified version of the PAS (M-PAS), in which 14 of the PAS items were included together with a further 4 new ones, particular attention was paid to the relationship between subject and informant ratings in which a 'best estimate' rating was used to get a consensus between the two sources of information (Piven *et al.*, 1994). This is similar to the method used in the PAS (Appendix 1) and was shown to produce intra-class correlations of >0.7 for all PAS traits apart from impulsive, with mean pairwise kappa ratings of 0.91.

Table 4.7 Cross-national inter-rater reliability ratings in Personality Assessment Schedule

Personality attribute	Informant as source information			Subject as source information		
	British raters	American raters	All raters	British raters	American raters	All raters
Pessimism	0.75	0.71	0.77	0.73	0.93	0.77
Worthlessness	0.92	0.19	0.11	1.90	0.19	0.91
Optimism	0.58	0.39	0.68	0.80	0.56	0.51
Lability	0.85	0.80	0.91	0.87	0.93	0.82
Anxiousness	0.79	0.85	0.87	0.83	0.91	0.82
Suspiciousness	0.81	0.79	0.78	0.77	0.80	0.80
Introspection	0.87	0.78	0.85	0.89	0.83	0.77
Shyness	0.88	0.92	0.94	0.94	0.93	0.90
Aloofness	0.76	0.71	0.68	0.66	0.76	0.74
Sensitivity	0.75	0.84	0.85	0.82	0.86	0.79
Vulnerability	0.77	0.77	0.75	0.72	0.90	0.77
Irritability	0.54	0.67	0.89	0.88	0.91	0.59
Impulsiveness	0.63	0.66	0.89	0.86	0.94	0.65
Aggression	0.74	0.87	0.86	0.87	0.85	0.76
Callousness	0.73	0.68	0.81	0.77	0.91	0.72
Irresponsibility	0.81	0.86	0.89	0.92	0.96	0.84
Childishness	0.68	0.69	0.81	0.79	0.87	0.66
Resourcelessness	0.75	0.77	0.86	0.84	0.95	0.73
Dependence	0.80	0.85	0.78	0.81	0.79	0.84
Submissiveness	0.76	0.76	0.79	0.76	0.78	0.76
Conscientiousness	0.84	0.80	0.85	0.83	0.91	0.82
Rigidity	0.82	0.78	0.83	0.81	0.87	0.74
Eccentricity	0.33	0.85	0.78	0.64	0.96	0.52
Hypochondriasis	0.86	0.87	0.66	0.78	0.59	0.85
Mean reliability across all items	0.75	0.77	0.82	0.81	0.86	0.75

In all assessments there were four English and three American evaluations. All correlations are of the intraclass correlation coefficient (R_I). The levels of statistical significant range between 0.01 and 0.0001. The levels of clinical significance, based upon the criteria of Cicchetti and Sparrow (1981), are poor ($R_I < 0.40$), fair ($R_I = 0.4$–0.59). Good ($R_I = 0.6$–0.74), and excellent ($R_I = 0.75$–1.00).

Despite these good levels of agreement comparison of the assessment of personality disorder by clinicians in a multidisciplinary team (using no measures apart from clinical impression), and by a research worker using the PAS, showed generally poor agreement for the presence or absence of a personality disorder (kappa = 0.23) but generally better agreement for flamboyant (kappa = 0.42) and odd/eccentric (kappa = 0.46) clusters (Hassiotis *et al.*, 1997). There was no agreement over the anxious/fearful group with kappa values of 0. This suggests that diagnoses of personality disorder diagnosed in ordinary clinical practice are not likely to be valid without better training of staff.

Temporal reliability of the PAS

Because of the contaminating effects of mental state the temporal reliability of personality disorder might be expected to be less good than inter-rater reliability and in general this view has been confirmed in clinical studies (e.g. Mann *et al.* 1981). This was also found to be true with the PAS in a formal study of temporal reliability (Tyrer *et al.*, 1983a) over 3 years. There was a reasonable agreement between the main four clusters of the PAS (κ_w = 0.64) but much less so for the individual traits in the PAS (*Table 4.8*). Those traits which have closer links to mental state (anxiety, pessimism, shyness, worthlessness and lability) have shown much less satisfactory reliability than those which are more independent (childishness, irresponsibility, impulsiveness, suspiciousness and conscientiousness).

Criticisms of the PAS

The PAS differs from all other instruments for assessing personality disorder in deriving the classification primarily from direct analy-

Table 4.8 Temporal reliability of the Personality Assessment Schedule in 28 patients (suffering from bipolar affective disorder (1), depressive episodes (8), schizophrenia (4), other neurotic disorders (8), primary personality disorder (4) and other diagnoses (3) at initial assessment) with reassessment after a mean of 2.9 years. (After Tyrer *et al.*, 1983a)

Personality attribute	Intraclass correlation coefficient (R_I)	Proportion of observed agreement (PO)	Weighted kappa (K_W)
Irritability	0.73**	0.91	0.47*
Submissiveness	0.68**	0.89	0.59*
Childishness	0.65**	0.85	0.43*
Irresponsibility	0.64**	0.88	0.44*
Impulsiveness	0.62**	0.87	0.40*
Resourcelessness	0.53*	0.87	0.33
Conscientiousness	0.51*	0.82	0.32
Suspiciousness	0.48*	0.82	0.28
Dependence	0.46*	0.80	0.33
Eccentricity	0.45*	0.90	0.30
Sensitivity	0.42*	0.79	0.31
Anxiety	0.35	0.83	0.31
Vulnerability	0.25	0.81	0.19
Optimism	0.24	0.88	0.25
Hypochondriasis	0.23	0.82	0.28
Worthlessness	0.22	0.75	0.24
Aloofness	0.15	0.71	0.14
Introspection	0.07	0.70	0.00
Lability	0.03	0.78	0.09
Pessimism	0.03	0.74	0.17
Shyness	0.01	0.70	0.00
Rigidity	−0.03	0.71	0.00
Callousness	−0.09	0.80	−0.10
Personality categories (after cluster analysis)	–	0.79	0.64**

(NB Reliability, following the criteria of Landis & Koch (1977a): * fair, ** good).

sis of traits using a computer program. In 1979 it was unusual in adopting a dimensional approach to diagnosis but now this has become much more popular, culminating in the development of the Dimensional Assessment of Personality Pathology-Basic Questionnaire (DAPP-BQ) (Schroeder *et al.*, 1992). Where it looks particularly strange to those familiar with the DSM-III classification is in its complete absence of operational criteria for diagnosis apart from the ICD-10 version. Each trait or characteristic is rated on the degree of social impairment it causes, not its intrinsic nature. This runs counter to the prototypical model which lies behind the DSM-III diagnostic system and which lies behind the operational criteria for the DSM-III personality disorders (Widiger and Frances, 1985). However, it is immediately understandable to trait psychologists, who have long argued for the superiority of this approach to personality assessment and have been in a bullish mood ever since the 'slaying of the dragon of situationism' (Matthews and Deary, 1998, p. 243).

Another obvious criticism is that the diagnostic categories of the PAS are not the same as the clinically derived categories of DSM and ICD. Because they are derived from a computer program, they could be regarded as arbitrary and of little clinical value. Only 24 personality characteristics are rated on the PAS and it could be argued that many others could be included which would alter the computer classification as well as reducing the overlap with other personality disorders. Indeed, Livesley (1987) identified 75 behavioural dimensions from DSM-III and has also shown that delineation of each dimension in the existing classification is not satisfactory, as several diagnoses use dimensions that are intrinsic parts of other personality disorders. The absence or presence of a computer-derived diagnosis is dependent on the questions in the schedule, and the assumption is made that these are representative of abnormalities found in the range of personality disorder.

The PAS differs from other classifications in employing a hierarchy of diagnosis so that the personality disorder producing the greatest social impairment becomes the primary disorder. Several personality disorders may be identified by the analysis but only one

becomes pre-eminent. This could be regarded as a procrustean decision that does not reflect clinical reality. However, the revised rating of severity (Tyrer and Johnson, 1996) allows the simultaneous presence of other disorders to be properly acknowledged if the disturbance extends beyond the initial cluster.

The PAS implicitly accepts a dimensional approach for personality disorder in rating all personality attributes on an eight-point scale. The cut-off points that divide normal from abnormal personality are not clear-cut and the clear separation that is achieved in DSM-III and DSM-IV is often considered superior by clinicians. Whether we like it or not, clinicians prefer a categorical to a dimensional classification (Kendell, 1975) and the PAS does not satisfy this requirement as much as other schedules. Those who prefer traits in place of categories also tend to use a much more detailed set of traits which are usually completed in the form of a questionnaire. We have always been concerned in clinical practice that the difficulties of separating mental state from personality, acknowledged by all but now often dismissed as an insoluble task, need to have clinical input and extra information wherever possible from informants. Getting information from many sources tends to lessen reliability but we are convinced it aids validity of assessment.

It could also be argued that the primary emphasis of PAS ratings is mistaken as it only refers to social adjustment. Both ICD and DSM definitions of personality disorder include the element of subjective distress. Indeed, DSM-IV specifically states that personality traits or behaviour can cause *either* impaired social functioning *or* subjective distress in order for the diagnosis of personality disorder to be satisfied. The PAS ratings suggest that those who have subjective distress as a consequence of their personality, but who are able to adjust to this so that it does not produce social impairment, do not therefore have a personality disorder.

Advantages of the PAS

Some of the criticisms made of the PAS can also be regarded as advantages. Although operational criteria have been of value in identifying mental state disorders, it is far from certain that they are equally appropriate for the personality disorders, which by definition are long-term and begin in adolescence or earlier. Many of the operational criteria for DSM-III personality disorders (e.g. the expression of 'constricted affect' in schizoid and schizotypal personality disorder, an 'impressionistic style of speech' – histrionic personality disorder) are likely to be influenced strongly by the subject's behaviour at interview and are not necessarily enduring features, particularly if there is concurrent mental state disorder. It would be ideal if we all had a consistent behavioural repertoire characterized by what Widiger and Frances (1985) term 'prototypic acts' to define personality. If certain of these acts would be representative of particular personality disorders then operational criteria would be in order. However, the repertoire of disturbance characteristically shown in personality disorder covers such a wide range of behaviour, that also varies greatly between cultures, that attempts at defining key behaviours may be doomed to failure. The prototypical model has been applied to personality disorder but the results suggest that, of several different disorders, there is considerable difficulty in achieving 'prototypicality' and only antisocial personality disorder is clear and distinct (Blashfield *et al.*, 1985).

Although the PAS diagnostic categories do not accord entirely with either ICD-10 or DSM-IV descriptions, there is a considerable degree of overlap between them (*see* Appendix 1) which is of interest in itself, as it suggests that the classification of personality disorders can be arrived at independently of clinical decision. A similar computer-derived diagnosis was used in the analysis of the Present State Examination (PSE; Wing *et al.*, 1974) using the Catego program.

There are also advantages in stability of diagnosis. It is not always wise for rating scales to be changed repeatedly, particularly with the long-term studies necessary in personality disorder. Our comment in the first edition of this book, 'unfortunately, those scales that are wedded to DSM have to follow their wayward bride wherever she chooses to take them, and at present she shows no sign of settling down', has proved to be true – and what horrors are round the corner when DSM-V is published. There is also a great deal

of evidence that the personality disorders of DSM-III overlap considerably and almost certainly there are far too many in the current classification. It is impossible to say which is the best classification, but where ICD-10, DSM-IV and other instruments such as the PAS and SAP all agree, it suggests that these are more likely to be enduring diagnostic categories. There are also some advantages in using a computer program to make the diagnosis as it helps to avoid stereotyping patients, a common fault in personality assessment (Vernon, 1963). If the ratings are made carefully for each item without expectation that the results will lead to a particular diagnosis of personality disorder, such bias is avoided.

The presence of a hierarchy in the diagnosis of personality disorder is obviously open to criticism. Nevertheless, the advantage of recording personality disorder in terms of the amount of social maladjustment created helps to provide a measure of severity that indicates which personality disorders are more serious than others. DSM-IV and ICD-10 do not allow this comparison to take place. Patients qualify for a diagnosis or they fail to do so and, if there are several personality disorder categories, there is no system for allocating their importance. This leads to confusion and difficulties in interpreting data.

The dimensional approach in scoring the PAS makes the diagnosis of personality disorder somewhat arbitrary, although the limits chosen by the computer program in reaching the cluster analysis have face validity and seem to separate groups of patients reasonably well. The advantage of having a dimensional approach with the recording of minor degrees of abnormality such as personality difficulty means that personality variation can also be recorded more satisfactorily. In most of the structured interviews for DSM and ICD diagnoses of personality disorder there is a rating equivalent to personality difficulty which describes characteristics that 'do not attain the level of severity required for personality disorder'. However, many of these characteristics are not defined in dimensional terms and are therefore difficult to rate. The scoring system of the PAS allows this to be recorded satisfactorily.

The criticism that the traits recorded in the PAS are somewhat arbitrary and limited may have some credence with two of the traits, submissiveness and optimism, which do not figure strongly in any of the cluster groupings, but most of the others are highly relevant. In *Table 4.9* there is a comparison between the 18 scale items of the Dimensional Assessment of Personality Pathology-Basic Questionnaire (DAPP-BQ) (Schroeder *et al.*, 1992) derived from 282 self-report items, and the 24 traits rated by the PAS. Despite the fact that they were derived from very different sources there is a surprising degree of com-

Table 4.9 Comparison between the 18 factors of the Dimensional Assessment of Personality Pathology-Basic Questionnaire (DAPP-BQ) (Schroeder *et al.*, 1992) and the 24 traits of the Personality Assessment Schedule (PAS)

DAPP-BQ dimension	PAS dimension	Comment
	Pessimism	No DAPP equivalent
	Worthlessness	No DAPP equivalent
	Optimism	No DAPP equivalent
Affective lability	Lability	Exact equivalent
Anxiousness	Anxiousness	Exact equivalent
Suspiciousness	Suspiciousness	Exact equivalent
Restricted expression	Introspection	Reasonable equivalent
Diffidence and social avoidance	Shyness	Reasonable equivalent
Intimacy problems	Aloofness	Reasonable equivalent
	Sensitivity	No DAPP equivalent
	Vulnerability	No DAPP equivalent
Rejection	Irritability	Rough equivalent
Stimulus seeking	Impulsiveness	Reasonable equivalent
Interpersonal disesteem	Aggression	Reasonable equivalent
Callousness	Callousness	Reasonable equivalent
Conduct problems	Irresponsibility	Rough equivalent
Narcissism	Childishness	Reasonable equivalent
Passive oppostionality	Resourcelessness	Reasonable equivalent
Insecure attachment	Dependence	Reasonable equivalent
	Submissiveness	No DAPP equivalent
Compulsivity	Conscientiousness	Reasonable equivalent
	Rigidity	Reasonable equivalent
Cognitive distortion	Eccentricity	Rough equivalent
	Hypochondriasis	No DAPP equivalent

Only two DAPP dimensions (identity problems and self-harm) have no equivalent in the Personality Assessment Schedule

Table 4.10 Reasons for selecting the Personality Assessment Schedule or other instruments in research studies

Purposes which may justify selection of PAS	Purposes which suggest the use of other instruments (preferred choice in brackets)
Need to assess premorbid personality	Need to assess current personality functioning (SCID-II)
A population that is unlikely to tolerate an assessment lasting longer than 30 minutes	Compliant population that is predominantly within normal or mildly abnormal range (SNAP or DAPP-BQ)
Significant Axis I comorbidity	Quick assessment for ICD-10 diagnosis (SAP)
Wish to record personality across severity range	Full assessment for ICD-10 and DSM-IV diagnoses (IPDE)
Longitudinal study requiring multiple assessments over a long time period	Forensic use with special attention to reoffending (PCL-R)
Studies in which either informant or patient may be required to complete assessment	Rapid screening instrument for DSM personality disorders (Iowa Personality Disorder Screen)

Glossary: SCID-II – Structured Clinical Interview for DSM-IV Axis II personality disorders
SNAP – Schedule for Nonadaptive and Adaptive Personality (Clark *et al.*, 1996)
DAPP-BQ (Dimensional Assessment of Personality Pathology-Basic Questionnaire (DAPP-BQ)(Schroeder *et al.*, 1992)
SAP – Standardized Assessment of Personality (Mann *et al.*, 1981; Hare Psychopathy Check-List – Revised (Hare, 1991)
Iowa Personality Disorder Screen (Langbehn *et al.*, 1999)

monality between the two systems that supports the notion that they are measuring the same basic constructs.

The rating of subjective distress and its contribution to the diagnosis of personality disorder is an important issue. However, it is generally accepted that most patients who are disturbed enough to qualify for the diagnosis of personality disorder do not have subjective distress alone and it is perfectly reasonable to postulate that those who only have subjective distress cannot usually be considered of sufficient severity as to qualify for the disorder label (although they may qualify for trait accentuation). By confining the rating to one of social dysfunction, then the confusion which might otherwise be engendered by scoring distress and social adjustment independently is avoided. The definition of personality disorder implied by the PAS ratings is somewhat different from DSM-IV and ICD-10 and has been expressed already as a persistent abnormality of personal and social functioning that is independent of mental integration. The implication of this is that those who have subjective distress as a consequence of personality abnormalities will automatically have impairment of personal and social functioning if the subjective distress is marked. If it is not marked, then the person comes within the range of normal personality function.

The effect of this position may be to raise the threshold of diagnosis of personality disorder and we do not know whether this is appropriate or not. Nevertheless, with the present criteria for diagnosis, a significant percentage of individuals, both in community samples and in psychiatric outpatient and inpatient groups, qualify for the diagnosis so it seems unlikely that the threshold is set at too high a level. In fact, the evidence from at least one study is that when the diagnostic criteria for an ICD-10 personality diagnosis are applied (in a consensus group meeting to formalize diagnosis) there is a tendency to overdiagnose personality disorder when the PAS records much of the same disturbance as personality difficulty (Merson *et al.*, 1994).

A much more important issue is whether the PAS is a reliable and valid instrument for recording abnormal personalities and this is discussed fully in the next chapter. However, there is nothing about its construction and internal consistency that suggests that it is intrinsically defective. In *Table 4.10* the research approaches that might justify, or militate against, using the PAS are listed. Most of these are clear from the information given in this chapter.

5

The epidemiology of personality disorder

Patricia Casey

Although the concept of personality disorder has been recognized since Hippocrates, the psychiatric profession has traditionally viewed it as a disturbance of inpatients and outpatients only. Among the lay-public, the phraseology of personality disorder has become commonplace, which can be judged by the widespread use of terms such as 'psychopathy' and 'introversion', and so it has been readily identified as a concept in non-clinical settings. Its relevance in these situations, however, has until recently been relatively unrecognized, dismissed or ignored by the psychiatric profession.

The main reason for this is an historical one and a reflection of attitudes to other psychiatric disturbances in non-institutional settings. With a few notable exceptions it is only in recent years that there has been any interest in or concern about psychiatric illness away from the traditional settings where psychiatrists practise. Now with the decarceration of the mentally ill, the shift to community-based service and the emphasis on prevention and early intervention, research has been stimulated in both general practice and the community as a whole. It is hardly surprising that an area such as personality disorder, with its uncertain aetiology, doubtful diagnostic status, and inadequate treatment, should receive such scant attention.

Its reality as an entity has been called into question by those who hold that it is a concept based on arbitrary criteria and value judgements, often used as a label for the un-conventional or eccentric (West, 1974). Philosophical uncertainties have arisen with regard to the most satisfactory approach to the measurement and labelling of personality disturbance. Many of these difficulties have been discussed fully in Chapter 2. In particular, those who advocate a nomothetic approach hold that general principles regarding personality can be developed from the study of large populations and can then be applied to individuals. By contrast those who advocate an idiographic approach argue that information based on population studies cannot be applied to the individual because of his uniqueness. Such treasuring of identity is even stronger in the domain of personality than for other mental disorders. Even among those who adopt a nomothetic approach, which probably includes most clinical psychiatrists and psychologists, there is argument as to whether one label or a profile (categories or dimensions) is more appropriate. We have argued earlier in this book for a dimensional approach, but the reluctance of clinicians to accept this despite overwhelming evidence to the contrary (Livesley *et al.*, 1998) has led many investigators to abandon the study of personality and concentrate on the less elusive formal psychiatric illness.

Traditionally, personality disorder and formal illness have been viewed as mutually exclusive. Psychiatric case conferences frequently find themselves impaled on the horns of an unnecessary dilemma: has the patient a real illness or just a personality disorder?

Professor Gunn has demonstrated the absurdity of this dichotomy in Chapter 3 but this division is still held strongly by many clinicians. In the past it has resulted in the prevalence of personality disorder being underestimated in clinical populations and has greatly hampered epidemiological studies. The advent of multiaxial systems of classification will improve the data available to future researchers in this field.

A further impediment to the study of personality disorder has been the paucity of adequate measures. These problems have been discussed in earlier chapters, but now that it is possible to separate the confounding influences of symptoms and traits in interview schedules (*see* Chapter 2), more valid assessments of personality disorder can be made. Such a separation now seems fundamental but, for many years, scepticism existed about the ability to assess personality in those who were ill. The additional use of informants to provide premorbid information has resulted in an improvement in the validity of such assessments. Nevertheless, epidemiological studies in this field are still in their infancy and much needs to be done.

Personality disorder in the community

One of the earliest epidemiological studies which concerned itself with measuring the prevalence of personality disorder was that by Essen-Möller (1956). He interviewed 2550 people to determine the prevalence of abnormal personalities in the community using predetermined criteria. He identified 29% of males and 19% of females as having evident or probable personality disorder. In addition, 13% of the men and 38% of the women had asthenic states and 14% of the men and 2% of the women had asociality and alcohol abuse. Although this study was one of the first major studies of its kind incorporating both illness and personality disorder within the definition of psychiatric disturbance, the vagueness of the terminology and absence of full description makes it difficult to comprehend fully the author's meaning. Moreover, some of the categories of personality disorder (e.g. indo-

lent, ixioid) are now rarely used and difficult to equate with current personality disorders.

Srole *et al.* (1962) in the midtown Manhattan study also attempted to assess personality using the Minnesota Multiphasic Personality Inventory (MMPI) on the 1660 adults who were interviewed. Ten per cent were judged to have probable personality disorder. Leighton *et al.* (1963), in Stirling County, interviewed 1010 heads of households and independent assessors decided on the presence or absence of 'significant psychiatric symptoms'. Sociopathy and personality disorder were differentiated from each other: 11% of men and 5% of women met the criteria for sociopathy while 7% of men and 6% of women had personality disorder. Sociopathic disturbances were three times more common in *disintegrated than integrated* areas. It is important to note that neither of these studies used clinicians to assess the respondents and it is likely that the prevalence figures are therefore overestimated.

More recently Weissman *et al.* (1978) in New Haven systematically interviewed 938 adults over the age of 18 and followed up 511 of these 8–9 years later. Information was collected using the Schedule for Affective Disorders and Schizophrenia (SADS) (Spitzer and Endicott, 1983). The information was operationalized using the Research Diagnostic Criteria and a lifetime diagnosis given to those with personality disorder, together with a current diagnosis for all the other psychiatric illnesses: 4.5% were found to have depressive personalities, 0.2% each had cyclothymic and antisocial personalities and a further 0.4% had a probable diagnosis of abnormal personality. Although SADS does not regard personality and illness as being mutually exclusive, no attempt was made to investigate the relationship of one to the other. DSM-III notes that antisocial personality is present in 3% of males and 1% of females in the USA. It does not provide epidemiological information on the other categories of abnormal personality described in it.

A large-scale study by Myers *et al.* (1984) as part of the Epidemiological Catchment Area (ECA) study was conducted in three urban centres (Baltimore, St Louis and New Haven) to investigate the 6-month prevalence of psychiatric disturbance including personality disorder in the community. The Diagnostic

Interview Schedule (DIS) was used to generate diagnosis based on DSM-III. It does not, however, cover all Axis I diagnoses and only identifies antisocial personality among the personality disorders. The 6-month prevalence for this was 0.8–2.1% in men and 0.3–0.5% in women. Abnormal personality was not found in women over the age of 45. The lifetime prevalence of personality disorder (Robins *et al.*, 1984) in the same three sites and using the same methodology was between 2.1 and 3.3% and, as with the 6-month figure, was significantly more common in men than women. The highest rate was in the 24–44 age group. The rate in those over 65 was less than 0.8% in all three sites and there were no significant racial or educational differences. As in other studies (Dohrenwend and Dohrenwend, 1969), personality disorder was significantly more common in the inner city areas. In contrast to this, Blazer *et al.* (1985) failed to find any urban–rural differences in the prevalence of antisocial personality disorder. When this team investigated five separate areas of the USA as part of the ECA study, personality disorder decreased with increasing age, was higher in men than in women and highest in those subjects with less than a high school education. None of the studies in the ECA series investigated the relationship between Axis I and Axis II diagnoses.

More recent studies from the USA include those of Reich (1989) and Zimmerman and Coryell (1990). Using the Personality Diagnostic Questionnaire (PDQ) Reich assessed 235 adults drawn from the general population and 11.1% were diagnosed as having any personality disorder with compulsive (6.4%), dependent (5.1%) and schizotypal (5.1%) the most common. Zimmerman and Coryell interviewed 697 relatives of psychiatric patients and healthy controls using SIDP (semi-structured interview) and the PDQ (self-report questionnaire). Personality disorder was somewhat more common using the SIDP (13.5% vs 10.3%). Regrettably there was no agreement on the most common categories and this depended on the interview schedule used. Schizotypal, histrionic, antisocial and passive–aggressive were the most frequent diagnoses with SIDP whilst dependent personality disorder was the most common category using the PDQ. Multiple categories were more frequent with the PDQ. Findings in this study point to the poor concordance between questionnaire and interview measures for personality disorder.

Several European studies are also worthy of consideration. Casey and Tyrer (1986) recorded the personality status of 200 subjects chosen at random from a population registered with a general practitioner. As almost all people are registered with general practitioners in the UK this can be regarded as a true epidemiological sample. The Personality Assessment Schedule (PAS) was used to assess personality status and, in the original report, a simplified classification was used which was then converted to the equivalent categories of the *International Classification of Disease* (ICD-9). Explosive personality disorder was the most common (6%), followed by anankastic (3%), asthenic (2.5%), schizoid (1%) and hysterical (0.5%). The asthenic category was significantly more common in women and the explosive type predominated in men. The personality status of these 200 subjects using the revised classification of the PAS is illustrated (*Table 5.1*).

A significant relationship was found between personality disorder and PSE caseness, but there was no association between personality and specific Catego classes. Not surprisingly, the numbers with psychoses were so low that investigation of their relationship to personality was precluded. This study also examined the relationship of personality to social functioning. This was significantly worse in those with personality disorder than in those with normal personalities, but did not differ between specific categories of personality disorder. It was found that there was broad overlap in the areas of functioning affected by personality and PSE caseness.

Maier *et al.* (1992) interviewed 109 German families in order to measure the presence of lifetime Axis I and Axis II diagnoses. Using SCID-II for personality disorders they found a prevalence of 10.3% for all personality disorders, a figure similar to that obtained by Casey and Tyrer (1986), Reich (1989), Zimmerman and Coryell (1990). Significant associations were found between the Axis I diagnoses of anxiety disorders and affective disorders and the Axis II diagnoses of avoidant and borderline personality disorders, respectively. The rates of personality disorder

Table 5.1 Personality classification of 200 randomly selected subjects using revised PAS diagnosis

Personality type (PAS)	Sex M	Sex F	Personality difficulty	Personality disorder	Combined personality disorder	Severe personality disorder	Gross personality disorder	Total*	
Normal	74	90						164	(82.0)
Sociopathic	1	4	2	3				5	(2.5)
Explosive	2	2	1	1		2		4	(2.0)
Sensitive–aggressive	2	4	2			3	1	6	(3.0)
Passive–dependent	0	3	1	1	1			3	(1.5)
Histrionic	0	1	1					1	(0.5)
Asthenic	0	2			2			2	(1.0)
Anankastic	1	0		1				1	(0.5)
Anxious	2	3	3		1	1		5	(2.5)
Hypochondriacal	0	0							
Dysthymic	1	2	1	1	1			3	(1.5)
Schizoid	1	0	1					1	(0.5)
Avoidant	1	0	1					1	(0.5)
Paranoid	0	4	1	1	1	1		4	(2.0)
Total*	164		14	8	6	7	1	200	
(Percentage)	(82.0)		(7.0)	(4.0)	(3.0)	(3.5)	(0.5)	(2.0)	

* The percentages of the total are given in parentheses.

were non-significantly higher among females than males and schizoid and compulsive were the most common categories.

In summary, the epidemiology of personality disorder has not been investigated with the same vigour as have other psychiatric disturbances. A lifetime prevalence of between 2.1 and 18% has been found depending on the population and criteria used. Personality disorder is associated with youth and the association with gender is uncertain.

Personality disorder in primary care

Although some work has been done in assessing the prevalence and natural history of formal psychiatric illness in general practice, such attention has not generally been accorded to the study of abnormal personality in this setting. Kessel (1960), on examining the prevalence of conspicuous psychiatric morbidity in a single general practice, noted that 5% of patients were considered on clinical grounds by their general practitioner to have abnormalities of personality independent of their presenting illness. In a larger study, Shepherd *et al.* (1966) found a similar

prevalence and noted the excess in males. Cooper (1965) identified a group of chronic psychiatric patients in general practice and found that the psychiatrist identified 8% as having a primary diagnosis of personality disorder while the GP identified 3%. Both of these studies viewed formal psychiatric illness and personality disorder as mutually exclusive. In a primary care study in which 87 patients were diagnosed by their general practitioners as having a non-psychotic disorder, Mann *et al.* (1981) identified 31 of these as having a personality disorder using the Standard Assessment of Personality as the measure. Personality was assessed independent of any other Axis I disorder.

A similar approach was used by Casey *et al.* (1984) who assessed the personality of every patient with conspicuous psychiatric morbidity in urban general practice. The general practitioner and psychiatrist both diagnosed personality disorder as the primary diagnosis in 8.9% and 6.4% of the study population, respectively. However, when each patient was formally assessed using a structured interview, 33.9% were identified as having personality disorder. Diagnostically, 17% had explosive personalities followed by anankastic (4.7%), asthenic (4.1%), schizoid (3.5%) and hysterical (2.3%). Explosive personality was especially common (50%) in those patients showing alcohol abuse. The relationship between personality and PSE caseness was explored and there was no relationship to caseness; overall personality disorder was significantly more common in patients with a Catego class of anxiety states. There was no association with the diagnosis of depressive neurosis. The difference in proportion with personality disorder when a clinical diagnosis as compared to a research diagnosis is used is not surprising. In the former, only the primary diagnosis was considered whereas the latter refers to the personality assessment of each patient irrespective of the primary diagnosis. This may also explain the seemingly higher proportion with the personality disorder in the present study when compared with the other studies described earlier. Further information concerning the features of those with personality disorder was obtained by extending the above study into rural practice (Casey, 1985). A similar discrepancy was noted when clinical and research diagnoses were used. The diagnostic trends were similar to those in the urban study. When both urban and rural practices were compared, personality disorder was significantly more common in the urban than in the rural sample. For specific types, explosive personality was more common in the urban, and anankastic personality in the rural sample. The only sex difference was for explosive personality which was more common in men than in women. The traditional view that hysterical and asthenic personality disorder is associated with being female was not upheld. When social functioning was assessed using a structured interview, there was no difference between the diagnostic categories of personality disorder; all produced roughly equal impairment. Much lower levels of personality abnormality were found in the Upper Bavarian studies (Dilling *et al.*, 1989) when 9.4% of a sample of identified psychiatric patients attending 18 general practitioners were so diagnosed using the Clinical Interview Schedule and rates were somewhat higher among men than women.

More recently, Moran *et al.* (1999) have examined the prevalence of personality disorders attending primary care by studying 303 consecutive attenders. This approach is likely to overestimate the true prevalence because those with personality disorder attend more frequently than others (*see* Chapter 9) and so in any short specified period more would be likely to attend. They found a prevalence of 29%, covering the range of personality categories from paranoid (8–10%) down to 2–4% for dissocial and antisocial personality disorders. Those with personality disorder had greater psychiatric morbidity, particularly in the cluster B group.

Comparative studies from the USA are uncommon because of the different pattern of primary care provision. Hoeper *et al.* (1979), using primary care attenders rather than those with conspicuous psychiatric morbidity, found that 2.7% of clinic attenders met RDC (Research Diagnostic Criteria) for labile personality and 2% for cyclothymic personality. This study did not attempt to investigate the relationship between personality and diagnosis. Even though the proportion with abnormal personality is smaller than in other studies, it must be realized that this study used a population base which was different from that of the British studies described above.

In summary, abnormalities of personality are the primary diagnosis in 5–8% of patients with conspicuous psychiatric morbidity in primary care and are more common in men than women. When the assessment is made independent of the primary diagnosis this rises several-fold. Recent studies have thrown new light on the links between personality disorder and neurosis and helped to explain the alleged sex differences in relation to personality. The likely reasons for this are the separation of symptoms and traits and the use of structured techniques to assess personality rather than just relying on clinical judgement.

Hospital populations

The wealth of data on the prevalence of personality disorder in hospital populations through case registers and government sources must be counterbalanced by the lack of descriptive precision and the inadequacy of definitions. Moreover, the view that disturbances of personality and illness are mutually exclusive has resulted in the former being obscured from hospital and case register data, because these utilize only the primary diagnosis as identified by the clinician. The arbitrary use of terms such as 'immature', 'hysterical' and the acknowledged pejorative and prejudicial use of many labels make this information less useful than might initially be apparent.

Dilling and Weyerer (1980) gathered data on those receiving in- and outpatient treatment over a 6-month period and extrapolated to the community. In all the psychiatric hospitals and clinics in three counties of Upper Bavaria, 0.4 per thousand were treated for personality disorders and these were twice as common in men as in women.

In England and Wales, 7.6% of all admissions and 8.5% of first admissions were diagnosed clinically as having disorders of personality as the primary diagnosis. This is equivalent to a rate of 32.3/100 000 and for first admissions the rate is 9.8/100 000 (Department of Health and Social Security, 1985). In Ireland the rates of personality disorder among all admissions (34.7/100 000) and among first admissions only (11.1/100 000) are similar to the British figures (O'Hare and Walsh, 1986). In hospital settings, abnormalities of personality are slightly more common in men than in women and rates peak in the 20–44 age group and in unskilled workers. These official statistics suggest that personality disorder is much less common than do studies designed to investigate their prevalence specifically – probably due to the failure of this data to separate Axis I from Axis II disorders and only including those where personality disorder is the primary diagnosis. Evidence to support this comes from the study of Loranger (1990) who compared the last 5 years of the DSM-II era (1975–1980) with the first 5 years of the DSM-III era and showed that the move from a single axis to a multiaxial classification did indeed impact upon the rate of personality disorder diagnoses which rose from 19% to 49% with no change in admission policies in the unit under investigation.

A study of consecutive admissions to an urban psychiatric unit, selected because they suffered from one of the functional psychoses, attempted to assess the prevalence of personality disorder in this population and investigate the link between the primary diagnosis and personality (Cutting *et al.*, 1986). Using a semi-structured interview, 44% were found to have abnormalities of personality and a further 6% had lesser degrees of personality disorder. The proportions with abnormalities of personality were similar in all diagnostic categories, but patients suffering from affective disorder had an excess of personality disturbance accounted for by cyclothymic and anxious premorbid traits. There was no association between schizoid personality and a clinical diagnosis of schizophrenia. In a more severely ill population of recurrent psychotic patients, the UK700 case management trial, 186 (28%) of 670 patients assessed using the Quick Personality Assessment Schedule (PAS-Q) had a personality disorder but 34% had personality difficulty (see *Figure 4.3*, p. 64). A similar rate of personality disturbance in psychiatric inpatients has been noted in one American study (Stangl *et al.*, 1985). Among depressed inpatients Zimmerman *et al.* (1988) diagnosed personality disorder in 57% according to informant reports and in 36.4% based on subject interviews with borderline predominating among the informant data group and histrionic being the most common on the basis of subject interviews. Although this study used the SIDP interview schedule it points to some worrying discrepancies between subjects and informants particularly for specific categories. More recent studies have confirmed the high prevalence of personality disorders among various diagnostic inpatient groups. Casey and Butler (1995) found that among inpatients with major depression receiving electroconvulsive therapy (ECT), 45% met the criteria for personality disorder when the assessment was made, using a structured interview (Personality Assessment Schedule) with patients, after recovery and with their relatives providing collateral information. The single most common categories were anankastic (10%) and avoidant (7.5%). Among a consecutive series of first ever admissions to two acute psychiatric units in Ireland, one private, one public, 26% met the criteria for an Axis II diagnosis using the Standardized Assessment of Personality (SAP; Cooney *et al.*, 1996). There were no significant differences in the rates of personality disorder between the two institutions.

The anxious, anankastic and dependent and paranoid categories predominated and gender differences were also observed with females dominating these categories with the exception of the paranoid group. Numbers however were small.

Among new outpatients in the USA, 11% were diagnosed as having a personality disorder (National Institutes for Mental Health, 1971) as the primary diagnosis. In an outpatient sample selected for study because they suffered from one of the neuroses, Tyrer *et al.* (1983c) found that 39% had an underlying personality disorder when assessed using structured interviews and independent clinical diagnosis. Anankastic and passive–dependent types predominated. By contrast, 60% of those assessed had normal personalities: a finding at variance with much of the impressionistic thinking common in clinical practice. Studying 298 Norwegian outpatients, of whom 97% had an Axis I disorder, Alnaes and Torgensen (1988) found that 81% had an Axis II diagnosis using SIDP to make the assessment. A much lower prevalence of 12.9% was obtained by Fabrega *et al.* (1993) when 18 179 outpatients were assessed using DSM-III criteria. As in the Norwegian study the most common diagnoses were affective disorders and antisocial and borderline personality disorder predominated. The latter were associated with being male and under the age of 36. In this study the diagnosis was made at intake and appropriate reluctance to make a diagnosis of personality disorder after a single assessment may partly explain the low prevalence. Recent studies from outpatient populations in the USA have confirmed the trend of personality disorder being very common in that population with Kass *et al.* (1995) obtaining a figure of 51% and Jackson *et al.* (1991) a figure of 67%.

Other studies in hospital settings have concentrated on emergency clinics for assessing acute emotional problems. A comparative study of five different clinics found that 7.4–17.1% of those assessed received a clinical diagnosis of personality disorder (Muller *et al.*, 1967). Bowman and Sturgeon (1977) obtained a much higher figure of 31% for abnormal personality in a similar clinic.

In summary, estimates of the prevalence of personality disorder based on hospital populations are underestimates because of the single axis of classification used by most case registers and hospital records. The introduction of multiaxial classification, pioneered by DSM-III, has led to an increase in the apparent prevalence of personality disorder in psychiatric patients, so that between 30 and 40% of outpatients and between 40 and 50% of inpatients are now recognized as having a personality disorder. The prevalence of personality disorder in a university hospital (Cornell) in New York rose from 15% in 1979 to over 50% after the introduction of DSM-III in 1980 (A. W. Loranger, 1987, personal communication). This dramatic increase reflects the higher detection rate personality disorder in a multiaxial classification. It is, therefore, likely that prevalence rates in studies carried out before 1980 are far too low.

Personality disorder in other populations

In no other population is the problem of assessing personality more obvious than in the forensic one. There are close associations between crime and personality disorder, although the link is not a direct one-to-one relationship. Also the issue may be confounded by circularity, i.e. inferring personality disorder from antisocial behaviour and then explaining this behaviour by abnormal personality. There is general assent to the need for vigilance in assessing personality in offenders and in separating specific behavioural abnormalities, e.g. criminal behaviour, from underlying personality traits such as callousness and irresponsibility. Between 39 and 76% of prisoners have been found to have antisocial personality disorder in various studies (Bluglass, 1977; Gunn *et al.*, 1978; Bland *et al.*, 1990; Cote and Hodgins, 1990). A comprehensive randomly selected population of one in six prisoners in English prisons (Singleton *et al.*, 1998) using SCID-II revealed more than three-quarters of the population were personality disordered, with antisocial personality disorder found in 63% of male remand prisoners, 49% of sentenced prisoners, and 31% female prisoners. Paranoid personality disorder was the second most prevalent condition in 29% of male remand prisoners, 20% of male sentenced, and 16% of female prisoners, but borderline personality disorder was more common in female prisoners. The variation is most probably a reflection of differences in the concentration of hardened criminals in various prisons. Patients detained in psychiatric units and hospitals under the terms of the Mental Health Act comprise 0.24% of the general population and up to 25% of the population in special hospitals (Coid, 1993). Not surprisingly, other types of abnormal personality are rarely described in the offender population.

A quasipsychiatric group seen in general hospitals is the parasuicide population. It is acknowledged clinically that personality disorder abounds although the belief in a specific suicidal personality is no longer held. Very high prevalences ranging from 48 to 65% have been reported by Ovenstone (1973), Casey (1989) and Ennis *et al.* (1989) with the antisocial type predominating in all three studies in spite of diverse methods of assessment. Surprisingly, Jacobson and Tribe (1972) found abnormalities of personality in only 14% of men and 9% of female parasuicides, and Urwin and Gibbons (1979) obtained figures of 26 and 16%, respectively, for men and women with a personality disorder. Disorders of personality are especially common in those who make non-serious attempts (Pallis and Birtchnell, 1977). An association between serious attempts and obsessional traits of personality was found by Murthy but other studies by Pierce (1977) and Casey (1989) failed to find such a link. Both studies recognize that personality is important in the genesis of parasuicide but not as a determinant of its seriousness. The mechanisms by which personality factors generate this self-destructive behaviour or interact with social variables have yet to be elucidated.

Borderline personality

Recent years have seen a mushrooming of studies of the borderline personality, also variously known as ambulatory schizophrenia, borderline schizophrenia and pseudo-neurotic schizophrenia in the past. It is now probably one of the most studied categories. These investigations have invariably emanated from the USA where the disorder is formally recognized in DSM-IV. Although borderline personality was not incorporated in the European classification until the publication of ICD-10, there were sufficient similarities between some of the ICD categories in previous editions and the concept as defined in DSM (*see* Chapter 2) to have general application.

There is little information available on the epidemiology of this disorder and most of the work has consisted of describing the socio-demographic profile of patients and identifying distinguishing features from other disorders. In one study, Spitzer *et al.* (1979) used data obtained from members of the American Psychiatric Association whom they selected at random. Each member was asked to identify two patients with a clinical diagnosis of borderline personality and compare them with two other patients who acted as controls. Patients were rated on a number of symptoms and these combined to achieve the best discrimination between the two groups. The borderlines were more often female and under 25. Approximately one in 10 was an inpatient, the remainder being private psychiatric outpatients.

An epidemiological study by Weissman and Myers (1980) using SADS found a point prevalence of 0.2% among 511 adults in New Haven. Somewhat higher rates have been obtained by Reich *et al.* (1989) who reported a prevalence of 1.3% in the general population using the PDQ and Zimmerman and Coryell (1990) who found disparate rates when using the PDQ (4.5%) and SIDP (1.7%). A study derived from the ECA study found that among 1541 adults from one of the sites 1.8% met the DIS criteria (Swartz *et al.*, 1990). A even lower rate of 1.1% was described by Maier *et al.* (1992) using SCID in a German population.

Castaneda and Franco (1985) obtained information on the sex and ethnic distribution for this disorder by studying those patients who were discharged from a New York psychiatric teaching hospital. There were no significant differences between blacks, whites and Hispanics but there were variations in the sex distribution across the ethnic groups. The male–female ratio varied from 1:1 to 4:1. Overall, 6.4% of the population under study met DSM criteria for borderline personality disorder. A study by Sheehy *et al.* (1980), using a psychiatric outpatient sample, expanded the findings of Spitzer in discovering that most borderlines were female, were more likely to be divorced or separated, and also younger than the non-borderline controls. Features distinguishing the two groups were difficulties in impulse control, in tolerating unpleasant affect and in emotional control. Social withdrawal, periodic substance abuse, promiscuity, bizarre sexual fantasies and projection were also features which discriminated borderlines from other patients. Although the community-based study by Swartz *et al.* (1990) conformed the clinical impression that borderline personality disorder was a female attribute, other large-scale studies have not replicated this finding (Kass *et al.*, 1985).

In a British psychiatric population, an interesting study by Kroll *et al.* (1982) attempted to establish whether patients seen by British psychiatrists met the criteria for borderline personality disorder, to identify the ICD-9 category to which such patients belonged and to compare British and American borderline patients. All those seen were inpatients on two acute psychiatric wards. Four per cent met DSM criteria for borderline personality disorder, while Gunderson's criteria yielded a prevalence of 14.9%. The condition was four times more common in women than in men. The diagnosis was not made in any patient over the age of 40 and all had been given ICD diagnosis of abnormal personality (hysterical,

explosive, 'inadequate' and immature). Some of the borderlines had also received an additional DSM-III diagnosis of major depressive episode and the authors concluded that current depressive symptoms were confounding the presentation of personality traits.

Conclusion

It is apparent that the widely differing prevalence rates for personality disorder in different settings are a reflection of both historical changes in attitudes to personality assessment, the conflict between different measures of personality assessment and of the confusion surrounding its relationship to other disorders. It is only when the rigour that has been applied to the study of other disorders such as depressive illness can be applied in this area, that the epidemiology of personality disorder will provide firm figures that will be of public health significance. This should be facilitated by recent advances in techniques for assessing personality and by the development of a multiaxial classification of psychiatric disorders in ICD-10 as well as changes in the DSM concepts. This would augur the end of judgemental and restrictive views that have governed this aspect of psychiatric research and clinical practice in the recent past.

6

Comorbidity of personality and mental state disorders

Peter Tyrer

Comorbidity is one of the necessary evils of current psychiatric practice and is really an indictment of our present system of psychiatric classification. It is a relatively recent import into psychiatric terminology but is now used so widely that some marvel how we managed to do without it for so long. Its significance and meaning is far from clear as it is a confusing word that covers many different types of association ranging from complete independence of two or more disorders to such close association that the conditions can be thought of as identical and the association therefore consists of 'consanguinity' (Barsky *et al.*, 1994; Tyrer, 1996; Lyons *et al.*, 1997). This deviates greatly from the original definition of comorbidity described by Feinstein as 'any distinct additional clinical entity that has existed or that may occur during the clinical course of a patient who has the index disease under study' (Feinstein, 1970).

In describing comorbidity of personality disorders it is important to mention that the commonest form of comorbidity of personality disorder, that with other personality disorder, is not being discussed here. It is described elsewhere in Chapter 2 and is argued there to be largely an artefact of incorrect classification. In this chapter the nature and extent of the relationship between personality disorders and those of mental state are described together with their implications and consequences. It is first necessary to describe the association before trying to interpret it.

Comorbidity identified in research studies

The main elements of comorbidity between personality and mental state disorder are shown in *Tables 6.1* and *6.2*. To avoid making the table too large both the mental state and personality disorders are described in general terms in most cases, with classification of mental disorders using the main categories of ICD-10 and personality disorders in the three (sometimes four) major clusters of both DSM-IV and ICD-10 classifications. However, there is occasionally some merit in identifying a specific relationship between a single personality disorder and a single Axis I diagnosis, particularly when the association is abnormally strong, and some examples of these are also included in *Table 6.1*.

There are five areas in which there is a strong relationship between personality and mental state disorders. In this context, we define a strong relationship in which over 50% of all patients with a specific mental state disorder also have an associated personality disorder from the appropriate cluster, so the association is an intimate one. The strong associations are the relationship between:

1. Substance use and the flamboyant cluster of personality disorders (cluster B);

2. Somatization disorders, and to a slightly lesser extent, eating disorders and both flamboyant (cluster B) and anxious/fearful personality disorders (cluster C);

Table 6.1 Strong associations between mental state (Axis I in DSM) and personality disorders (Axis II)

Axis I disorder	Axis II disorder	Degree of association	Source
Alcohol abuse and dependence	Antisocial and other disorders in cluster B	Strong, most marked for antisocial personality disorder but extends cross the range	Helzer and Pryzbeck, 1988; Morgenstern *et al.*, 1997; Johnson *et al.*, 1998;
Opioid abuse	Antisocial and borderline disorder	Strong, with a mixed group of abusers having links to cluster C also	Brooner *et al.*, 1993, 1997; Darke *et al*, 1994; Links *et al.*, 1995; Rutherford *et al.*, 1997;
All substance use	Many comorbid personality disorders, but association with antisocial personality disorder very strong	Very strong, particularly in polydrug abusers	Dejong *et al.*, 1993; Eronen *et al.*, 1998; Rounsaville *et al.*, 1998
Obsessive-compulsive disorder	Obsessive–compulsive (anankastic) personality disorder	Strong, but not as great as between social phobia and avoidant personality disorder	Tyrer et al, 1983b; Diaferia *et al.*, 1997; Bejerot *et al.*, 1998
Social phobia	Cluster C (specifically avoidant personality disorder) C	Very strong indeed so only a minority of people with one disorder (1 in 5) do not have the other	Dahl, 1996; Alpert *et al.*, 1997; Stein *et al.*, 1998
Neurotic disorders	C	Strong	Tyrer, 1985; Flick *et al.*, 1993; Rees *et al.*, 1997
Bulimia nervosa	Cluster B	Moderate	Dowson, 1992a; Yates *et al.*, 1989
Bulimia nervosa	Cluster C (particularly obsessive–compulsive personality disorder)	Moderate	Fahy *et al.*, 1993; Lilenfeld *et al.*, 1998
Post-traumatic stress disorder	Cluster B	Strong	O'Toole *et al.*, 1998; Zanarini *et al.*, 1998, 1999
Pathological gambling	All clusters	Strong	Black and Moyer, 1998; Crockford and el-Guabaly, 1998; Cunningham-Williams *et al.*, 1998
Somatization disorder	Cluster C and (to a lesser extent) B	Very strong	Stern *et al.*, 1993; Fink, 1995; Hudziak *et al.*, 1996

The degree of association for each of these disorders is so high (over 10 times greater than would be expected by chance) that it is possible to argue that the association represents a co-axial syndrome, or a diagnosis that has both mental state and personality elements. (Chance association is determined by the base rates of each disorder. Thus if a study found that alcohol dependence was present in 40% of a population and cluster B personality disorder in 40% the chance association would be 16%.)

3. Neurotic disorders and the anxious/fearful personality disorders (cluster C);
4. Post-traumatic stress disorder and flamboyant personality disorders (particularly borderline) (cluster B);
5. Habit and impulse disorders (F63 in ICD-10) and cluster B personality disorders.

Difficulties in separating personality disorder from mental state

Before discussing individual examples of comorbidity it is important to acknowledge that the separate identification of personality disorders from those with mental state (Axis I) disorders is relatively new and still far from easy. Prevalence figures from a number of sources have established from population-based epidemiological studies (Chapter 5) that approximately one in 10 of all individuals suffers from a personality disorder (de Girolamo and Reich, 1993) and that the rates climb progressively with each rung negotiated in the ladder of care, with rates rising from 15% in primary care to over 50% in in-patient samples. However, in general clinical practice the identification of personality disorder is often missed unless it is obvious, and Oldham and Skodol (1991) have noted that many patients seen in the public sector almost certainly have personality disorders that are currently unrecognized (*see* also Chapter 5). For example, there appears to be a high rate of comorbidity between schizo-affective and abnormal personality in clinical practice but this has not been studied much by researchers. There may be, therefore, some significant examples of comorbidity between Axis I and Axis II disorders that are currently uninvestigated but of considerable clinical importance.

It also needs to be admitted that it is very difficult to measure personality disorder if it exists in the presence of a mental state disorder. There is now abundant evidence that most mental illness distorts premorbid personality and makes it appear more abnormal (Coppen and Metcalfe, 1965; Hirschfeld *et al.*, 1983) and this impairs reliability of measurement (Tyrer *et al.*, 1983a), although with newer, more structured and better defined instruments such as the International Personality Disorder Examination (Loranger *et al.*, 1994) the degree of contamination is much less (Loranger *et al.*, 1991). Assessments of personality status are usually carried out by interviewing the subject and cannot be accurate in patients with many severe mental illnesses who have an impaired grasp of reality. Unless assessment is made from other sources, and this leads to other possible sources of error, the presence or absence of a personality disorder may be impossible to determine. This problem is particularly prominent in the schizophrenic group of disorders, not least because the schizophrenic illness commonly changes personality because of its pervasive intrusion into all aspects of functioning. Because of these methodological difficulties researchers have generally avoided studies of personality comorbidity in schizophrenia which probably has more important associations than many of the other less serious mental state disorders.

Strong associations

Relationship between avoidant personality disorder and generalized social phobia

Almost the strongest comorbidity relationship in psychiatry is between social phobia, particularly the generalized form of the condition, and avoidant personality disorder. There are strong reasons for believing that the two conditions cannot be usefully separated (Herbert *et al.*, 1992; Sanderson *et al.*, 1994) and when it is found that those with avoidant personality disorder respond equally well to psychopharmacological treatment as those with social phobia (Deltito and Stam, 1989), it is reasonable to question whether there is any real justification for maintaining the Axis I–II distinction (Livesley *et al.*, 1994). To clarify whether avoidant personality disorder reflects a personality variant of generalized social phobia research is needed to show that the avoidant disorder precedes generalized social phobia and that they have a shared form of familial, presumably genetic, transmission. As recent evidence from community epidemiological studies suggests social phobia begins early in adolescence (at the same time as personality disorders) (Burke *et al.*, 1990) it becomes even more difficult to separate the two, and if the two terms were regarded as equivalent many would be satisfied (Dahl, 1996).

Substance use in cluster B personality disorders

Alcohol and the reasons for addiction to it have long been studied by psychiatric research workers and personality aspects are high on the list of these. For many years it has been debated if those who became addicted to alcohol have 'addictive personalities' (Barnes, 1979), or whether the main reason for dependence is just a consequence of persistent increased consumption of alcohol. We now know the latter to be much the most important but the reasons why people turn to alcohol and drugs for pleasure and comfort is related to personality factors, and Kendler and his colleagues have shown that once alcohol and other drugs of addiction have been sought as a refuge for coping with the problems of life genetic factors play a major part in leading the individual to addiction or just occasional recreational use (Kendler and Prescott, 1998; Prescott and Kendler, 1999). As in all studies of associated disorders, longitudinal enquiries involving one condition before the second has developed are preferable to cross-sectional ones, but, unfortunately, there are very few of these in the study of the relationship between personality and mental state. However, the evidence from the cross-sectional studies is compelling and consistent; there is a very strong link between all forms of substance use and cluster B personality disorders, particularly with antisocial and borderline personality disorder (*Table 6.1*). However, the link with cluster B personality is not a universal one. In many patients with multiple or polydrug abuse there are many other personality disorders present as well as the cluster B group and this association of many mixed personality disorders and substance use may constitute a separate group (Brooner *et al.*, 1993). In one study of polydrug abusers 91% of all patients had a personality disorder as well as their substance use but the categorization of these was extremely difficult because of the extensive comorbidity of personality disorder (DeJong *et al.*, 1993). However, this may reflect the 'ripple effect' of greater severity of personality disorder affecting more and more categories as severity increases (Tyrer and Johnson, 1996).

A major problem in drawing conclusions from these studies is the absence of studies recording personality status before substance abuse developed. Once abuse has become established it is not surprising that antisocial and borderline features may develop; the crucial question is whether they are present in the premorbid state. Despite this gap in enquiry there is indirect evidence that these personality features are present at an early stage in those prone to alcohol abuse (Mulder *et al.*, 1994).

Eating disorders and cluster B and C personality disorders

It has long been claimed that anorexia nervosa was associated with personality abnormality, with histrionic and personality features lying behind the excessive self-absorption that is so characteristic of the condition, and the obsessional ones with the steely determination to continue dieting to excessive thinness (Dally and Gomez, 1979). Since formal assessments have been made in patients having both anorexia and bulimia nervosa, this association has been confirmed. In general, bulimia nervosa tends to be associated more strongly with cluster B personality disorder (Herzog *et al.*, 1992; Fahy *et al.*, 1993; Skodol

et al., 1993) but the association with anorexia nervosa is less strong with a more heterogeneous group, including not only cluster B personality but also obsessive–compulsive and avoidant personality disorder (Gillberg *et al.*, 1995; Thornton and Russell, 1997). The presence of self-induced vomiting is strongly correlated with cluster B personality disorders (Dowson, 1992a) and might almost be regarded as a key core symptom of bulimia nervosa even though it is present in anorexia nervosa also.

Neurotic disorders and cluster C personality disorders

This association is perhaps the best known form of all relationships between mental state and personality and stems back to the early days of psychoanalysis (Freud, 1916). Anxious, dependent and 'oral' personality features are commonly associated with anxiety disorders and could be part of the overlapping comorbidity model described by Lyons *et al.* (1997) in which the Axis I and Axis II conditions could be perceived as all part of the same syndrome. The presence of a personality disorder in the anxious/fearful cluster and any anxiety or non-psychotic depressive diagnosis is common but by no means universal, and it has been suggested that those with this type of comorbidity have a separate disorder formulated as the general neurotic syndrome (Tyrer, 1985; Andrews *et al.*, 1990; Tyrer *et al.*, 1992).

Examining the merits of the arguments for and against the general neurotic syndrome depends on whether you are a 'splitter' or a 'lumper' when it comes to psychiatric classification. This difference is often felt to be one that depends on a fundamental philosophical dichotomy between the two approaches but it is really one of timing. Splitters see tremendous potential in separating disorders early in their investigation whereas lumpers do not want to separate them until they have been demonstrated to be distinct syndromes.

The general neurotic syndrome is not just a collection of diagnoses which have been lumped together. Several issues are intrinsic to it beyond the simple co-occurrence of neurotic disorders and personality abnormality. The general neurotic syndrome was described as a core disorder in which 'two or more of the common neurotic disorders (agoraphobia, social phobia, panic disorder, non-psychotic depression, generalized anxiety and hypochondriasis) have been present together, there are abnormal dependent or anankastic personality features (*now subsumed under cluster C personality disorder*), at least one episode has developed in the absence of major stress, and there is a history of a similar syndrome in a first degree relative' (Tyrer, 1985). The latter two requirements are necessary to separate the general neurotic syndrome from adjustment disorders and to emphasize the genetic component of the condition, a suggestion that has been supported strongly by twin data (Andrews *et al.*, 1990; Kendler *et al.*, 1995). Examination of the literature on the subject to June 1999 shows that of 14 articles devoted to the subject 10 are broadly in favour of the concept and find it valuable both as a practical and theoretical notion (Tyrer, 1985, 1989; Tyrer *et al.*, 1987, 1992; Andrews *et al.*, 1990; Larkin *et al.*, 1992; Rey *et al.*, 1994; Manicavasagar *et al.*, 1997; Langs *et al.*, 1998; Seivewright *et al.*, 1998) and only one, a study of the stability of panic disorder over 5 years, directly contradicts it (O'Rourke *et al.*, 1996).

Many studies have also been carried out into the relationship between individual Axis I neurotic disorders and Axis II conditions. Many of these have been stimulated by the desire to find better criteria to separate the Axis I disorders but have not always been successful. The results are not consistent. Patients with generalized anxiety disorder have been found to have a higher association with antisocial personality disorder in one study (Blashfield *et al.*, 1994), whereas in another the association was strongest with avoidant personality disorder (Noyes *et al.*, 1995). Panic disorder is more commonly associated with cluster C personalities (Sanderson *et al.*, 1994), particularly with dependent personality disorder (Noyes *et al.*, 1995). Agoraphobic patients also have links with dependent personality disorder and those without panic are more likely to have avoidant personality disorder (Hoffart *et al.*, 1995).

Although these studies of comorbidity occasionally have some value, as for example elucidating the difference between agoraphobia with and without panic disorder, most of them have been relatively pointless. There are

many suggestions that the comorbidity identified justifies even further division of the Axis I disorders depending on their comorbidity relationships, but there is insufficient evidence that these conditions constitute a group of disorders that enjoys clinical validity with respect to other criteria. The anxiety disorder–cluster C association is by far the most robust association apart from the somatization disorders discussed later in this article.

There are several other instances of comorbidity of neurotic disorders and personality disorder and these too need to be taken into account. Obsessive–compulsive personality disorder has criteria which are closely linked to those of obsessive–compulsive disorder in the Axis I classification and one might expect that there would be extensive comorbidity between these two conditions. The results are equivocal, with some finding such a close relationship (Tyrer *et al.*, 1983b; Aubuchon and Malatesta, 1994; Baer, 1994) and others showing no particular association with obsessive–compulsive personality (Black *et al.*, 1993; Kolada *et al.*, 1994). The latter study found an association between obsessive–compulsive disorder and antisocial personality disorder and as this was an epidemiological study, there may be some differences between those who present for treatment and those in the community with these conditions.

Somatoform and personality disorders

Many of the somatoform disorders, particularly somatization disorder, are associated with major personality disorder comorbidity. In almost all published studies more patients with somatization have comorbidity with personality disorder than do not (Fink, 1991; Rost *et al.*, 1992; Stern *et al.*, 1993). The association is roughly equal between clusters B and C personality disorders and in this respect differs from hypochondriasis which shows more association with the cluster C group (Barsky *et al.*, 1992). An argument has also been made for hypochondriacal personality disorder being regarded as a condition in its own right and this is discussed further in Chapter 4.

Somatization disorder is the most common of the somatoform disorders to be associated with personality disorder. This condition has developed from careful definition of the characteristics of what used to be labelled hysteria (Perley and Guze, 1962) and follow-up studies reveal it to be a remarkably consistent diagnosis over periods as long as 25 years (Guze *et al.*, 1986). The same characteristics are characteristically found to the same extent in personality disorder and it has been argued that, like social phobia and avoidant personality disorder, somatization disorder is indistinguishable from personality disorder (Stern *et al.*, 1993). This may be true, but the chronicity and temporal stability of somatization disorder might be quite independent of personality and the high incidence of co-occurrence may reflect independent causation (Lyons *et al.*, 1997).

Habit and impulse disorders and cluster B personality disorders

These conditions, particularly pathological gambling, might be expected to occur frequently in the presence of the flamboyant cluster of personality disorders and certainly reflect the need of this group to act in such a way that they generate potentially adverse life events. Published reviews (Crockford and el-Guebaly, 1998; Cunningham-Williams *et al.*, 1998) have also shown (predictable) morbidity with other risk-taking activities including drug abuse, nicotine dependence and alcohol dependence.

Post-traumatic stress disorder and borderline personality disorder

This association is somewhat of an embarrassment to the legal profession. The fundamental notion behind the diagnosis of post-traumatic stress disorder is that it, in the words of ICD-10, although individual vulnerability may predispose to occurrence 'the condition would not have arisen without the stressor' (World Health Organization, 1992). Thus once responsibility has been established any suffering caused by the stress is a direct responsibility of the source of the stressor.

However, this implies that stressful events are entirely independent of the apparent consequences of the stress. This is a very dubious conclusion. There is now good evidence that the cluster B group of personality disorders create, or at least predispose to, an increased

rate of life events in patients with neurotic disorder and adjustment disorders (Seivewright, 1987, 1988, 1999; Tyrer *et al.*, 1988c) and therefore such personality disorders might be expected to be associated with more stress disorders. This immediately throws doubt on the common assumption that conditions such as borderline personality disorder are caused, or at least triggered, by serious negative life events such as physical or sexual assault (McFarlane, 1988; Herman *et al.*, 1989; Zanarini *et al.*, 1989). It is plausible to test the notion that these individuals are already prone to experience such events because their personalities are already formed and associated with greater rates of life events.

Weaker associations and spectrum disorders

The less prominent examples of comorbidity are summarized in *Table 6.2*. Again it is worth while emphasizing that these are associations only and causal connections cannot be inferred except by speculation.

Relationship between schizotypal personality disorder and schizophrenia

There are many more types of association that could be equally relevant to the strong ones mentioned above and the concept of spectrum disorders has been introduced to explain the range of pathologies that can be covered, with personality disorder at one extreme and mental illness at the other. The best known of these is the schizophrenia/schizotypy spectrum, developed from the Danish adoption studies published over 20 years ago (Kety *et al.*, 1975), in which first degree relatives of schizophrenic patients were found to have a high proportion of people for whom the diagnosis of schizophrenia could not be sustained but who were nonetheless odd and had curious beliefs and behaviours. For many, this is where the concept of schizotypal personality disorder was born. Spectrum relationships exist between disorders when the separate descriptive syndromes represent phenotypic variations of the same basic underlying psychopathology, usually indicating common heritable dispositions. Apart from

Table 6.2 Weak or diffuse associations between mental state (Axis I in DSM) and personality disorders (Axis II)

Axis I disorder	Axis II disorder	Degree of association	Source
Schizophrenia	cluster B (including association with sexual offending)	Moderate	Phillips *et al.*, 1999
Schizophrenia	cluster A	Weak	Cutting *et al.*, 1986
Schizophrenia	cluster A	Moderate	Peralta *et al.*, 1991
Bipolar disorder	no clear associations with any specific cluster or single personality disorder	Weak	Barbato and Hafner, 1998
Depressive episode	B and C	Moderate	Alnaes and Torgersen, 1988; Gunderson and Phillips, 1991
Anxiety disorders	B and C	Moderate	Zanarini et al, 1998
Adjustment disorders	B and C	Moderate	Tyrer *et al.*, 1988c; Strain *et al.*, 1998
Anorexia nervosa	Cluster C	Moderate	Gillberg *et al.*, 1995
Eating disorders	B and C	Moderate	Dowson, 1992a; Fahy *et al.*, 1993

In these conditions there are no clear links between the Axis I and II conditions although some form of association is likely to be present

the relationship having been thought to exist between schizophrenia and the odd or eccentric group of personality disorders (cluster A), other postulated spectra are between borderline and depressive personality disorder and depression, between dependent personality and mixed anxiety/depressive disorders and between social phobia and avoidant personality disorder. These are given added weight by genetic evidence and that derived from family studies, although the failure of so many of these to address personality status is a cause for regret.

The relationship between schizotypal personality disorder and schizophrenia is described in more detail in Chapter 2. However, the notion of a heritable spectrum of disorders with the milder expression as personality disorder and more severe expression as a mental state disorder is best supported by the evidence for the 'schizophrenia spectrum' which is reinforced now by a considerable body of evidence from clinical and family studies (Peralta *et al.*, 1991; Siever and Davis, 1991; Kendler *et al.*, 1993).

Although it has long been assumed that there is a close relationship between schizoid, and more particularly, schizotypal, personality disorder and schizophrenia, this has rarely been shown in practice. This is partly because personality disorder assessments, particularly in the USA, are normally carried out with subjects and in the case of major psychoses

such as schizophrenia, which in many cases began many years ago and distort personality during the course of their development, adequate assessments of premorbid personality have not been made. Most of the evidence that schizophrenia is linked to the schizoid and schizotypal personality disorders comes from family studies only (Kendler *et al.*, 1993; Silverman *et al.*, 1993) and a review of studies carried out before personality assessment became more formalized (Cutting, 1985) revealed that only around one in five of schizophrenic patients has premorbid schizoid personality disorder. More recently there has been limited evidence of this association in actual probands with schizophrenia but this is based on retrospective report (Peralta *et al.*, 1991). Despite these reservations, it is clear that the relationship between cluster A personality disorders and schizophrenia is not just a chance finding and gives support to the spectrum concept of personality and mental state being on the same continuum (Siever and Davis, 1991).

Relationship between personality disorder and depression

The operational criteria for borderline personality disorder include 'unstable (or marked reactivity) of mood', 'chronic feelings of emptiness' and 'recurrent suicidal behaviour' (World Health Organization, 1993; American Psychiatric Association, 1994), so obviously a relationship with depressive illness is likely. However, the extent of comorbidity between these disorders is not nearly as great as might have been expected. Studies from many different sources have concluded that the association is only a vague and indeterminate one whose significance is also uncertain as both these disorders are common (Soloff *et al.*, 1987, 1991; Gunderson and Phillips, 1991; Southwick *et al.*, 1995). There are qualitative differences; the depression in borderline personality disorder differs from that in major depressive episodes in showing greater evidence of personal emptiness without hopelessness together with a strong element of self-destructiveness and self-criticism (Westen *et al.*, 1992; Rogers *et al.*, 1995). Of particular interest is the evidence that those with borderline personality disorder do not have a higher frequency of depressed relatives (after controlling for comorbidity), do not change their diagnoses over time into depressive or other mood disorders, and do not respond particularly well to antidepressants (although there is some recent evidence that contradicts this (*see* Chapter 8). Although there may be a heritable component that is common to both mood disorders and borderline personality disorder it does not fit into a straightforward spectrum relationship in the same way as schizotypal personality disorder and schizophrenia.

Relationship between depressive personality disorder and depression

Depressive personality disorder and dysthymia possess high comorbidity (19–60%) and overlap between them is shown by family studies (Klein and Miller, 1993: Hirschfeld and Holzer, 1994). Depressive personality disorder may be included in the next American classification (DSM-V) and whether it deserves such status depends on whether it represents a syndromal variant or basic disposition to dysthymia and depression. Phillips and colleagues (1998) support the notion of depressive personality disorder (which has nosological logic if anxious personality disorder is included) and found that of 54 patients with long-standing mild depressive features 30 satisfied the proposed criteria for depressive personality disorder. Nearly two-thirds of these did not have dysthymia or a current

major depressive episode and 40% had no other comorbid personality disorder. After reassessment 1 year later those with depressive personality disorder had changed little. Similar findings have been reported by Klein and Shih (1998), who concluded that the associations with other mood disorders were sufficiently low to conclude that depressive personality disorder 'contributed unique information beyond that available from the two emotional superfactors'.

It should also be noted that there is still a close relationship between the mental state diagnosis of dysthymia and personality disorder of all sorts (Seivewright and Tyrer, 1990; Klein *et al.*, 1995; Pepper *et al.*, 1995). However, as the association is not seen particularly within the borderline group, this is one of the arguments for the inclusion of depressive personality disorder as a condition that is completely independent of borderline personality disorder (Tyrer *et al.*, 1990b; Gunderson and Phillips, 1991; Klein *et al.*, 1995). The presence of personality disorder, particularly borderline pathology, in depressed patients leads to greater morbidity. Such patients are more prone to suicide attempts and could also be responsible for greater mortality (Lepine *et al.*, 1993; Runeson and Beskow, 1991).

Personality diathesis and mental state disorder

One way of relating the comorbidity of Axis I and II disorders is to regard the personality disorder as an Achilles heel that makes the individual more likely to suffer from a specific mental disorder when exposed to certain stressful events. In this model the personality characteristics represent a diathesis that increases vulnerability to the disorders concerned and therefore is part of an aetiological model (Lyons *et al.*, 1997). Thus the association between substance misuse and cluster B personality disorder could be regarded as a likely consequence of high risk-taking and the need for constant stimulation that is part of the personality structure of the flamboyant group. The notion that people with personality disorder could create their own life events that might to others appear to be independent might seem odd but is now supported from many quarters (Seivewright, 1987, 1988, 1999; Samuels *et al.*, 1994; Heikkinen *et al.*, 1997;

Seivewright and Daly, 1997). The findings support the four-cluster model of classifying personality disorder with both cluster B and C showing an increase in life events compared with others and those with the obsessive–compulsive (inhibited) group (now able to be called cluster D) showing fewer life events. In particular, the evidence from epidemiological studies is crucial in testing this hypothesis as this avoids the confounding factors of health-seeking behaviour found in clinical studies. One recent epidemiological study of 2000 randomly selected people in Oslo (Torgersen, Cramer and Kringlen, to be published) showed that both those with antisocial and borderline personality disorder had experienced a mean of 3.4 life events in the previous 6 months but that those with avoidant personality disorder (the most prevalent individual personality disorder in the study) had only experienced a mean of 1.5 life events. It is clear from these figures that people with personality disorders to some extent control their lives so that their experience of life events is far from random.

The greater vulnerability of obsessional personalities to life events may be the sole explanation necessary for the restricted life-

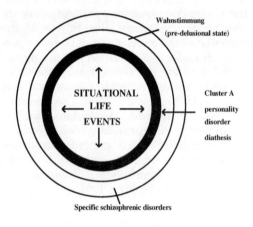

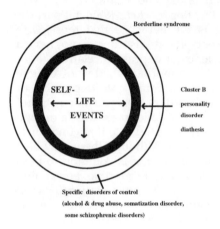

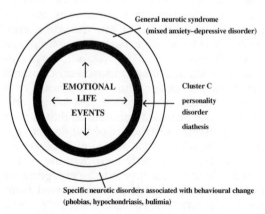

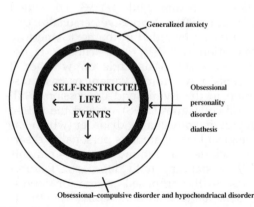

Figure 6.1 How personality disorder might predispose to Axis I disorders

styles these people lead and the high levels of anxiety created by minor stresses and the subsequent development of other conditions, particularly obsessive–compulsive personality disorder. Similarly, but perhaps less convincingly, the isolation and loss of social norms created by the schizoid (and schizotypal) personality disorder might provoke vulnerability to schizophrenia (provided there is underlying susceptibility), and the anxious/fearful cluster of personalities lead to an excessive response to threat and loss with the development of neurotic symptoms as postulated in the general neurotic syndrome (*Figure 6.1*).

The difficulties in investigating this hypothesis are considerable. Nevertheless, the subject can be investigated using strategies of both secondary and tertiary prevention, as by limiting the extent and impact of life events it would be possible to test whether Axis I disorders could be made less frequent and increase the time to relapse after successful treatment of an acute episode. There is sup-port for this notion from studies in obsessive–compulsive disorder (McKeon *et al.*, 1984) and post-traumatic stress disorder (Reich *et al.*, 1996).

In evaluating theories such as these the importance of getting an accurate descriptive classification cannot be over-stressed. For example, it would be very easy to explain the high degree of association between avoidant personality disorder and social phobia as the personality disorder creating the milieu in which social phobia could germinate and develop to a full-blown disorder. This has obvious face validity but is almost certainly wrong; the diagnostic descriptions of generalized social phobia and avoidant personality disorder are too close to argue convincingly for any view other than the two conditions represent one described in different ways. The association of many disorders simultaneously or consecutively is a much reported observation best summarized in Shakespeare's words, 'when sorrows come, they come not single spies, but in battalions'.

7

Psychosocial treatment in personality disorder

Kate M. Davidson and Peter Tyrer

The treatment of personality disorders appears to have been neglected by cognitive and behavioural therapists but with the introduction of DSM-III (American Psychiatric Association, 1980) which separated Axis I (mental state) from Axis II disorders (disorders of personality), there has been growing acknowledgement that patients may suffer from personality disorder and comorbid conditions and that personality disorder may influence treatment outcome in those with Axis I disorders. Almost 20 years on, this radical change in diagnostic practice has resulted in the development of cognitive and behavioural therapies of personality disorder and clinical research in the outcome of treatment of patients who have personality disorders. These developments have arisen partly in response to the recognition that the presence of personality disorder does not necessarily have a negative impact on the treatment outcome of a range of Axis I disorders such as depression (Shea *et al.*, 1990), panic disorder, agoraphobia, obsessive–compulsive disorder (Dreesen *et al.*, 1997), social phobia and eating disorders (*see* van Velzen and Emmelkamp (1996)). From the clinician's perspective, there is a pressing need to develop treatment approaches which are explicitly aimed at helping patients who fail to respond to traditional brief psychotherapies and who remain impaired in several domains. In addition, treatments which may improve the problematic behaviours of those with a diagnosis of personality disorder such

as self-harm and improve social functioning and interpersonal relationships are to be welcomed but also require thorough evaluation.

Beck *et al.* (1990) and Young (1990, 1994) have suggested that certain clinical signs and difficulties which arise in therapy may be indicative of the presence of a personality disorder or problem:

• The patient or significant others report that the problems are long-standing.

• The patient is persistently non-compliant with therapy.

• Progress in therapy comes to a halt and further change seems blocked.

• The patient seems unaware of the effect their behaviour has upon others.

• Interpersonal problems are more obvious during the interview and from the patient's history.

• The patient has difficulty reporting specific feelings, thought or problems.

• The therapist suspects patient of lacking motivation for change.

• The problems are reported as seeming natural to the patient (e.g. 'That's the way I am').

• The patient's problems may appear ill-defined, less severe and less acute.

Recently, attention has particularly focused on borderline personality disorder. This appears to be due to the nature of this disorder which has as one of its main features intentional self-injurious behaviour. The challenge of treating these patients has been taken up by several branches of psychotherapy including psychodynamically orientated therapists, cognitive therapists, behavioural therapists and more recently, cognitive analytical therapists (Ryle, 1997a). Each of these separate schools of psychotherapy have developed different models to explain the features of personality disorder and from these, different treatment approaches have developed. Some authors have suggested that lack of a clear identity is the central problem in borderline patients (Millon, 1987; Ryle, 1997b) whereas Linehan regards borderline patients as primarily suffering from a dysfunction in emotional regulation (Linehan, 1992). Beck *et al.* (1990) conceptualize borderline patients as primarily suffering from a dysfunction in the cognitive domain. An individual's beliefs and assumptions 'play a central role in influencing the perception and interpretation of events and in shaping both behavioural and emotional responses' (Beck *et al.*, 1990, p. 186).

Dynamic model of personality disorder

There are many different dynamic models for understanding personality disorder and they have been studied in borderline personality disorder for over 60 years (Stern, 1938). In addition to the original Freudian explanations of development being held up at the oral, anal and genital phases of development to explain dependent, obsessional and histrionic personality types there have been continued attempts to link childhood development with personality disturbance in adult life. Bowlby's theory of attachment behaviour (Bowlby, 1973) comprised the hypothesis that unresolved separation anxiety would lead to anger and subsequent antisocial personality disorder but this has not been supported by any empirical studies. Lorna Benjamin (1993) has developed an interpersonal theory of development which is operationalized as a structural analysis of social behaviour (SASB) in which early experiences are thought to be of major importance in forming adult personality characteristics and, by direct development, personality disorder. The dynamic forces of identification, internalization and introjection are established early and tend to replicate themselves in adult personality development.

Kernberg (1984) has been a major influence in describing the personality organization of people with borderline personality disorder. Whereas others have relatively clear 'layers' within their personality structure those with borderline personality disorder have a diffuse and unfiltered reaction to experience that prevents them from putting adversity into perspective and thereby creating crisis. It is not clear to what extent this 'borderline personality organization' is found in other personality disorders; but the impression given is that it is specific to borderline personality disorder or others within the cluster B grouping, particularly narcissistic personality disorder.

Therapeutic community treatment

Although there was a dramatic growth in mental hospitals between the early years of the nineteenth century and the middle years of the twentieth, this did not necessarily indicate satisfaction with this model of care. Although the concept of 'institutionalization' may appear to be a relatively recent one (Barton, 1959), concern about the damaging effects of mental hospitals on patients had been recognized for much longer. In particular, the hierarchical and dehumanizing elements of mental hospitals has been recognized since the early years of the twentieth century (Manning, 1989).

There has also been some confusion of the term therapeutic community. In this chapter we are referring only to an intensive form of treatment in which every aspect of the environment is part of the treatment setting in which behaviour can be challenged and modified, essentially through the mechanism of education and inquiry. Rapoport (1960) identified four principles of this type of therapeutic community; democratization, permissiveness, communalism and reality confrontation. These principles were maintained through the functioning of many different types of interaction between patients and staff, both in groups and individually, and in particular during the daily community meeting, which all staff members and patients are required to attend. Haigh (1999) has developed these further into the Big Five principles of the therapeutic community (ACCIA) (our acronym); Attachment or the feeling of belonging, Containment and the feeling of safety, Communication and the culture of openness, Involvement and participation, and Agency and the development of empowerment. These also have parallels in human development. These can only be achieved fully in an inpatient setting in which confidentiality is respected as fundamentally as 'aseptic technique is to surgery' (Campling, 1999). These all-embracing and ambitious aims are very different from other approaches in which attempts have been made to prevent dehumanization of mental hospitals by creating a general therapeutic and democratic atmosphere (Clark, 1965). Perhaps the best definition of a therapeutic community in the setting of the treatment of personality disorders is 'a consciously-designed social environment and program within a residential or day unit in which the social and group process is harnessed with therapeutic intent' (Roberts, 1997).

Cognitive models of personality disorder

Beck *et al.* (1990) regard personality traits as reflecting strategies which are described as forms of programmed behaviours designed to serve the biological goals of survival and reproduction. These programmes involve cognitive, affective, motivational and arousal processes and result in patterns of stereotyped behaviours which have developed through an interaction between genetically determined structures and experience. Natural selection is assumed to have brought about a fit between programmed behaviour and the environment and as a result programmed patterns will be either adaptive or maladaptive depending on the circumstances. In a rapidly changing environment there may a mismatch between these automatic strategies and the social and organizational structure of the environment. Beck *et al.* (1990) suggest that a bad fit may be a factor in the development of cognitive, affective, motivational and overt behavioural patterns which we diagnose as personality disorder.

Beck *et al.* (1990) place central importance on the concept of schemata (which we will also refer to as schemas). Schemas are stable knowledge structures which represent specific rules that affect the processing of information. Schemas not only determine the way in which an individual will attend to and process information from the environment but they will also determine the product of the operation of schemas through overt behaviour. As well as cognitive schemata, Beck *et al.* (1990) propose that affective, motivational, action and control schemas interact with one another to produce specific patterns of thinking, emotion and behaviour thought to be characteristic of personality disorder. The example below of the way in which an antisocial personality disordered individual obtained agreement of colleagues at work illustrates how these schemas interact. (*Table 7.1*). As these separate schemas are interrelated, it follows that in personality disorder, certain patterns of behaviour are overdeveloped and other patterns underdeveloped. For example, antisocial personality disorder is characterized, on the one hand, by a tendency to behave as a predator through exploiting others and behaving aggressively

Table 7.1 Interrelated schemas in a person with antisocial personality disorder

Schema	Example
Cognitive *self/others*	I am better and stronger than other people
Affective	Anger (if thwarted), pleasure (if goal attained)
Action	Seeks to meet own goals by intimidating others
Control	(Appraises situation as low risk, so no inhibitory process becomes operational)
Motivational	I can get what I want from others

and, on the other, a relative deficiency in behaviour which could be described as socially sensitive, considerate and reciprocal.

Beck and Freeman's cognitive model of personality disorder (1990)

Cognitive therapy with personality disordered patients focuses on changing maladaptive schemas and behaviours. Patients with personality disorder (particularly in cluster B) are often found to hold three predominant maladaptive beliefs which are seen as central to the disorder: These are 'I am inherently unacceptable', 'I am powerless and vulnerable' and 'the world is dangerous and malevolent'. These beliefs are assumed to account for the borderline patient's inherent sense that the world is threatening and their feelings of insecurity and powerlessness which leads to a vacillation between dependence on others and autonomy with neither strategy being entirely effective or reliable. A second cognitive factor thought to be important is the borderline patient's tendency to think dichotomously. Experiences are evaluated in mutually exclusive categories such as bad or good and trustworthy or untrustworthy. This type of cognitive distortion, or error, then forces extreme interpretations on events that would otherwise be regarded as lying on a continuum. This black and white interpretation of experience results in extreme emotional and behavioural responses to events.

Compared to cognitive therapy with patients with Axis I disorders, cognitive therapy for patients with personality disorders places more importance on working with patient's dysfunctional schemata. A distinction is made between core beliefs or schema which are expressed as unconditional statements such as 'I am bad', and dysfunctional assumptions, expressed as conditional statements such as 'if my children are not successful, I will have failed as a mother'. For example, a depressed patient may hold a dysfunctional assumption such as 'unless I am liked by others, I am worthless' whereas in personality disorder, these attitudes take the form of fundamental beliefs including unconditional rules such as 'I am worthless' and 'everyone is out for themselves'. In personality disorder these maladaptive core schemas are thought to be 'hypervalent' and evoked across many situations. This leads to the schemas being overgeneralized, inflexible and resistant to change. It is this exaggeration of the content of schemas and from the associated strategies arising in association with the core beliefs that is thought to be a major difference between normal and disordered personality. Cognitive therapy aims to address these unconditional and rigid core beliefs.

The early maladaptive schema model of Young (1990)

Some differences in emphasis have arisen between cognitive models of personality disorder. Young (1990) has introduced a fourth level of cognition, early maladaptive schemas, in his schema focused therapy. He regards early maladaptive schemas as stable and enduring themes that develop during childhood and are elaborated throughout an individual's lifetime. These early maladaptive schemas concern themes relating to the self and the world and others such as over-vigilance and inhibition. Beck *et al.* (1990) describe schemas in personality disorder as core beliefs which are thought to arise from an interaction between childhood experience and pre-programmed patterns of behaviour and environmental responses. The schemas control the processing of information and the bias in the operation of the schema leads to differences in behavioural action. Beck *et al.* (1990) suggest that personality disordered individuals may also suffer from a dysfunction in self-control strategies which leads to either impulsivity or over-inhibition.

Young (1990) has suggested that early maladaptive schemas are reinforced by three different types of processes. These are schema maintenance, avoidance and compensation. In schema maintenance, information is distorted to fit the schema by information processing errors such as arbitrary inference and minimization. Schema avoidance is used to describe the process whereby unpleasant thoughts and emotions that might allow full access to negative schemata are avoided through behavioural, cognitive and emotional manoeuvres. This prevents an individual from experiencing the schema and therefore any opportunity for modifying the content of the schema through disconfirming experiences. Schema compensation is depicted as the process of adopting the opposite cognitive and behavioural stances predicted from underlying content of schemas. As this then functions to maintain the schema, no modification in the content of the schema can take place.

Linehan's dialectical model of borderline personality disorder (1993)

Linehan (1993) regards borderline personality disorder as primarily a dysfunction of emotional regulation which is assumed to have resulted from biological irregularities combined with certain dysfunctional environments. Significant others are thought to reinforce this dysfunction by discounting or invalidating their emotional experiences. Borderline patients are regarded as emotionally vulnerable and as having difficulty in regulating patterns of responses associated with emotional states. The maladaptive behaviours which form part of the borderline syndrome are thought of as either the product of emotional dysregulation or as attempts by the individual at regulating intense emotional states by maladaptive problem solving strategies. Dialectical behaviour therapy (DBT), as its name suggests, contains within it the notion of opposites: common themes that emerge in therapy with borderline patients, such as acceptance of things as they are and change, may appear incompatible but are brought together in the therapy.

Ryle's cognitive analytical therapy for borderline personality disorder (1997b)

This recent extension of cognitive analytic therapy suggests that borderline personality disordered patients suffer from the subjective experience of a range of partially dissociated 'self states' which account for the clinical features of this disorder (Ryle, 1997a). Such patients for example may describe switching from one state of mind to another, experiencing states of intense uncontrollable emotions or alternatively feelings muddled or emotionally cut off. Dissociative states are thought to initially occur in response to unmanageable external threats and to be maintained by repetitions of threat and internal cues such as memories or situations which are similar to

the original source of threat. Borderline patients are thought to have experienced abusive and neglectful relationships in childhood and the internalization of harsh parental attitudes leads to intrapsychic conflict in which the emotions of guilt and anxiety are repressed or result in symptomatic behaviours. Borderline patients are regarded as having deficits in self-reflection resulting from an underdeveloped emotional vocabulary and a narrowing of focus of attention and to experience disruptions in self-reflection such that a coherent sense of self and others is impaired.

Psychosocial treatments for personality disorder

Dynamic psychotherapy

Classical psychotherapy since the time of Freud and Jung has long regarded the treatment of personality disorders to be a fundamental component of therapy. However, from classical descriptions it is clear that psychoanalysts were mainly treating neurotic disorder with associated personality pathology (from the cluster C group) when ostensibly treating personality disorder. No evidence of efficacy of treatment of personality disorder *per se* has been claimed for this approach until recently, and even now the view of Andrews (1991) that dynamic psychotherapy 'has not been demonstrated to be superior to placebo in the treatment of the neuroses and personality disorders' is probably the consensus one.

However, there has been considerable interest in the dynamic psychotherapy of borderline personality disorder in the last 20 years. As mentioned elsewhere in this book, borderline personality disorder is not typical of other personality disorders and patients often seek treatment for it repeatedly. Because it is associated with intense anger and emotion the normal processes of psychoanalysis, involving interpretation, transference and countertransference, are not considered suitable for this group and more subtle approaches are needed (Adler, 1979; Higgitt and Fonagy, 1992).

Kernberg and his colleagues at the Menninger Clinic (Kernberg *et al.*, 1972; Kernberg, 1984) provided evidence that a dynamic approach that was neither supportive nor openly confrontational but which aimed to tackle patients' core psychopathology, considered to be inchoate and confused and which quickly can be converted to aggression. This approach, expressive psychotherapy, has been developed further by Masterson (1976) as confrontative psychotherapy which anticipates the difficulties often found when therapy ceases. Kohut (1975) adopts an approach that identifies the inner functioning of borderline and narcissistic personalities and how they have developed in response to trauma in childhood and adolescence. None of these approaches have been formally evaluated with a control group.

The only formal evaluation of two forms of dynamic psychotherapy, short-term dynamic psychotherapy and brief adaptational psychotherapy, was carried out by Winston and colleagues (1991) but specifically excluded patients with borderline and narcissistic pathology. The results essentially showed no differences between treatments and as they were both better than a waiting list control group it suggests that these approaches have some value. Group psychotherapies are also being evaluated using similar approaches at the Cassel Hospital in the UK by Chiesa and his colleagues.

Cognitive analytical therapy

Cognitive analytical therapy is concerned with describing different self states and helping patients to identify 'reciprocal role procedures' which are patterns of relationships which are learned in early childhood and are relatively resistant to change (Ryle, 1997b). The patient is taught to observe and try to change damaging patterns of thinking and behaviour which relate to these self states and to become more self-aware. The therapist's role is to gather information about the patient's experience of relationships and the different states the patient experiences. Any countertransference reactions experienced by the therapist are considered as useful data as they may represent identification with the patient or some reciprocating response to the patient's overt or covert behaviour and having identified and labelled these appropriately, the latter is assumed to help maintain a working alliance with the patient. Having identified the pa-

tient's various self states, the therapist's task is to help the patient reliably recognize these and to encourage the patient to become aware of these separate states without dissociating.

Although the application of CAT for borderline personality disordered patients has not been compared with other psychotherapies and no published studies are available at this time, Ryle (1997a) suggests from experience of treating over 30 patients that this form of psychotherapy shows promise.

Dialectical behaviour therapy

Dialectical behaviour therapy (DBT) is a manualized treatment programme for borderline personality disordered patients which involves weekly individual psychotherapy and group psychoeducational behavioural skills training. In addition, patients receive telephone consultation with their therapist. The treatment consists of a variety of problem-solving techniques including teaching the patient skills to help regulate emotions, tolerate distress, methods for validating the patient's perceptions, and behavioural and psychological versions of meditation skills. Therapists are also trained in case management. Linehan describes core mindfulness skills which are aimed at teaching the patient to observe, describe and 'participate' in events and responses to events without separating oneself or dissociating from what is happening. DBT encourages patients to take a non-judgemental approach to events and interactions and to do what is effective in situations rather than what the patient may feel is the 'right' thing to do.

Schema-focused cognitive therapy

This cognitive therapy consists of identifying and modifying early maladaptive schemas and schema driven behaviours. Young recommends a thorough and detailed assessment of the patient's history of problems and symptoms and the use of questionnaires such as his own Schema Questionnaire (Young, 1990) and the Lazarus Multimodal Life History Questionnaire (Lazarus and Lazarus, 1991) to assess dominant maladaptive schemas and long-standing behavioural problems. Schema-focused therapy involves educating patients about schemas and raises the expectation in patients that their schemas will be difficult to change and that they will resist by systematically distorting information to maintain their beliefs about themselves and the world. He differentiates between primary and secondary schemas and suggests that it is important to concentrate on changing one or two primary schemas initially in therapy. Primary schemas are identified clinically as those which are associated with high levels of affect, are linked to enduring and pervasive problems and closely associated with the patient's developmental problems with significant others. His stance in therapy is described as one of 'empathic confrontation'. He uses terms such as fighting and battling with schemas to describe the degree of challenge and persistence required to produce change in the rigidly held unconditional beliefs about self-worth and the world. As well as educating patients about schemas and confronting schema avoidance and compensation, Young's therapy focuses on identifying and changing schema-driven behaviours. Interpersonal schemas concerned with issues such as dependence or mistrust which may arise within the therapeutic relationship are assessed and considered legitimate targets of treatment. It is in the treatment of personality disorder that cognitive therapy has had to take into account the concept of transference within therapy and although the therapeutic relationship has always been considered an important aspect of therapy, it is now given much more attention and this is likely to lead to increasing acknowledgement of the factors which impede and enhance collaboration and alliances in therapy.

Cognitive therapy for personality disorders

Although several important differences exist between cognitive therapy for Axis I and Axis II disorders, there are many common features. As in cognitive therapy for Axis I disorders, cognitive therapy for personality disorders is a goal-directed, problem-solving therapy which aims to teach the patient specific cognitive and behavioural skills which are also thought to be helpful in preventing relapse. The focus in therapy is on defining the patient's presenting problems, goal setting, and modification of dysfunctional thinking and problematic behaviour which

interfere and impede with adaptive functioning. The clinician teaches the patient to identify and modify dysfunctional thoughts and beliefs through the use of specific cognitive techniques such as Socratic questioning.

Several differences in cognitive therapy between Axis I disorders and personality disorders have been emphasized by cognitive therapists (Beck *et al.*, 1990; Young, 1990; Beck, 1996; Davidson, 1998). One of these differences is on the emphasis and attention paid to the therapeutic relationship. In cognitive therapy for personality disorder, more emphasis is placed on establishing and maintaining a therapeutic alliance as interpersonal difficulties which arise in the patient's life outside of therapy are also likely to arise within therapy. Interpersonal difficulties are thought to arise from the patient's maladaptive beliefs about themselves and others. One of the goals of cognitive therapy with personality disordered patients is to utilize these interpersonal difficulties in treatment by assessing and modifying the underlying beliefs about others and relationships *per se*. The therapist encourages the patient to test out their beliefs and assumptions about others by using the therapeutic relationship as a relationship laboratory and to learn new more adaptive strategies in relating to others. In comparison to the treatment of Axis I disorders, cognitive therapy with personality disordered individuals is assumed to take more sessions and to span a longer time-frame due to the long-standing nature of the patient's difficulties and the possible inflexibility and rigidity of the patient's beliefs and behavioural responses. Although most personality disordered patients can recognize difficulties, they experience the problems as being ego-syntonic and 'just the way I am'. As a result, new alternative and more adaptive beliefs about self, others and the world need to be explicitly identified and evaluated for their adaptiveness. These alternative, more adaptive beliefs require to be systematically reviewed and reinforced and new behaviours and ways of relating to others need to be practised repeatedly if changes are to be consolidated (Davidson and Tyrer, 1996). In order for these changes to take place, the therapist is likely to have to be more directive at times and will be more concerned with identifying and overcoming cognitive, emotional and behavioural avoidance which acts to suppress or maintain core beliefs. As these maladaptive patterns of behaviour and beliefs are likely to have their origin in childhood experience, cognitive therapy for personality disorders will be more concerned with historical data than cognitive therapy for Axis I disorders. Also apparent in cognitive therapy for personality disorders is the need for the therapist to be inventive in developing behavioural and cognitive interventions to test out the validity of the patient's maladaptive core beliefs. Patients are requested to keep logbooks to record new ways of behaving as they attempt to change their schema-driven behaviours, and to keep records of evidence which support more adaptive beliefs about themselves and others (Padesky and Greenberger, 1995). Although most of the techniques utilized to change beliefs are focused in the here and now, historical and developmental perspectives have been developed to aid in re-examination of core beliefs and attached emotion. Young's historical review of schema traces the development and reinforcement of schema through recall of memories which are perceived by the patient to be relevant to their core belief (Young, 1990) and restructuring of the meaning of earlier memories using psychodrama (Edwards, 1990) have been described as being useful in that the emotional impact of the schema can be evoked and this is assumed to allow changes in, or re-assessment of, the core belief to occur more readily.

Both Beck *et al.*'s (1990) and Linehan's (1993) clinical model of personality disorder have in common an attempt to integrate biological and psychosocial factors. All models of treatment recognize the importance of building a secure therapeutic relationship but transference and countertransference issues in therapy are perhaps not yet dealt with adequately by current treatment strategies, except for Ryle's (1997b) cognitive analytical therapy. Cognitive therapists have yet to develop a cognitive model of these reactions which may interfere with the aim of developing a collaborative working relationship. Cognitive therapy for personality disorder is experimental in approach. Although the patient's overt problems are the initial focus of treatment, the therapist utilizes hypotheses about underlying mechanisms which drive these problems to aid under-

standing (Persons and Bertagnolli, 1994). This formulation allows therapy to proceed with a coherent strategy rather than following a piece-meal approach to symptoms and problems. The development of cognitive models of personality disorder does however aid the therapist in understanding this group of often diverse patients and provides a framework in which to formulate problems and intervene.

Is there evidence that psychosocial interventions are effective?

So far, very few studies have been published which attest to the efficacy of psychosocial treatment in personality disorder. Where studies have been published, the target of treatment has usually been behaviours or acts which are indicative of personality disorder rather than change in personality traits.

The efficacy of the therapeutic community

Therapeutic communities have operated as tertiary referral systems in health care since their introduction many years ago (Jones, 1952, 1956). Patients are referred to other units in their area as first and second lines of treatment but some cases prove particularly difficult (and usually incur a great deal of expense) and the therapeutic community is turned to, often as a last, rather than a first, resource. Those who are referred are accepted primarily on the basis of their behaviour and acceptance by the democratic therapeutic community, not as a consequence of any pre-defined diagnostic criteria. Despite this, most therapeutic communities regard themselves as specialists in the treatment of people with severe personality disorders. In this context it is important to note that the definition of severe personality disorder is not formalized. Studies at the Henderson Hospital have used instruments that record personality disorder according to the standard diagnostic systems (mainly the *Diagnostic and Statistical Manual of Mental Disorders* (DSM)) with the Personality Disorder Questionnaire (PDQ-IV) (Hyler, 1994) used to record personality category.

Although this has no category for severe personality disorder the fact that the mean number of personality disorder diagnoses in those accepted by the Henderson Hospital is greater than four (Norton and Hinshelwood, 1996) suggests that those who are referred do have severe disorder (*see* Chapter 2 and Tyrer and Johnson, 1996).

The treatment given is almost entirely confined within the description of group psychotherapy. Because there are so many different groups going on throughout the day and interactions are being monitored closely it could be said that the patients are in a state of permanent group therapy while at the hospital. In general there is no individual psychotherapy given because this undermines the group approaches. The length of stay is variable but typically lasts for around 7 months.

Evidence of efficacy

There have been no randomized controlled trials of therapeutic community intervention in personality disorder. There is no fundamental reason why such trials could not be used in such settings and four major difficulties – ethical problems, a lack of objective outcome measures, resistance from the field, or a reluctance to compare treatments – identified by McPherson (1994) are not really present in these settings. Indeed, one of the more positive aspects of therapeutic communities in recent years has been their willingness to embrace a wide range of research methodologies in evaluating the success of treatment.* The major difficulties are over the random allocation of patients to treatment programmes (bearing in mind that the democratic views of the residents in selecting individuals are a key part of the programme), the high rate of attrition with treatment (which makes the case for a pragmatic rather than an explanatory trial), and some difficulties in selecting the right outcome measures.

All the studies have included cohort studies in which patients have been followed up and in some cases compared with those patients

*Since this book went to press a randomized controlled trial has been initiated by the National Programme of Forensic Mental Health in the UK.

who are referred to treatment but are not taken on for care, mainly because funding has not been provided from their relevant health authorities. The findings of such studies were impressive, with savings (cost offsets) of over £12 500 per patient because so many of the patients not taken on by the hospital remain as inpatients for prolonged periods (Dolan *et al.*, 1996). However, it should be noted that the comparison group is not likely to be comparable with those selected for care at the therapeutic community. The democratic process could preferentially select patients who are more likely to do well (or at least could be postulated at carrying out this function) and until a pragmatic trial investigates this and includes all randomized patients such comparisons have limited viability.

There is sufficient circumstantial evidence to suggest that the therapeutic community might well be effective in at least some patients with severe personality disorder. Whether this group would fare equally well with different treatments cannot be decided on the basis of present evidence. However, the evidence to date certainly suggests that there are some important therapeutic elements present within these systems and that they deserve to be evaluated more closely.

Dialectical behaviour therapy (DBT) for parasuicidal patients with borderline personality disorder has been compared with treatment as usual in a randomized controlled trial and found to be superior to treatment as usual in reducing the number of parasuicidal acts and number of medically treated episodes in the year of treatment (Linehan *et al.*, 1991). In addition, DBT was found to be superior to treatment as usual during the 6 months after treatment had ended but no differences were found between the two groups in the number of parasuicidal episodes after 6 months post-treatment (Linehan *et al.*, 1993). Furthermore, no differences were found between treatment as usual and DBT in reported levels of depression, suicidal ideation, hopelessness and reasons for living during the treatment phase of the study but those women who received DBT did report less anger and better social adjustment compared with those who had received treatment as usual. The numbers in this study were relatively small ($n = 44$), the treatment intensive, the therapists highly trained, and all the participants in this study were women, which may limit the generalizability of the study. Nonetheless, this important and innovative study has led to growing interest in psychological treatment for this group of parasuicidal patients who are known to have a relatively high suicide rate compared with other psychiatric patients and the general population (Stone, 1993).

A related study in this area has evaluated a manualized brief cognitive treatment for patients with personality disturbance who epeatedly self-harm (Evans *et al.*, 1999). Patients were randomly assigned to treatment as usual or manualized cognitive therapy, which was extremely brief compared with Linehan's standard treatment (patients received a package of a set of self-help and training booklets and between two and six sessions of treatment). The booklets comprised six short chapters which contained information and examples of problem solving and cognitive strategies aimed at reducing problems, emotional disturbance and the risk of further self-harm. The results of this study demonstrated promise in brief manualized cognitive treatment in parasuicidal patients in that there was a trend in favour of the cognitive treatment reducing the rate of self-harm episodes compared with treatment as usual ($P = 0.11$) and there were significant reductions in self-rated depressive symptoms after 6 months and more positive future thinking (MacLeod *et al.*, 1998). However, because of the small numbers in the study ($n = 34$), no clear conclusions can be drawn at this stage about the general value of this treatment.

One difficulty in the evaluation of psychosocial treatment or indeed any treatment for personality disorder is reaching a consensus about exactly what is expected to change with treatment. Both the above randomized controlled trials had as the primary outcome measure a reduction in the number of parasuicidal acts, and other measures such as affective symptomatology, social functioning and cost of care as secondary outcome measures. Case studies provide some evidence that psychological treatment can be helpful in reducing dysfunctional behaviour and improving relationships (e.g. Turkat and Maisto, 1985; Ryle, 1997b) but without any standardized way of assessing outcome, whether this be in terms of personality traits, symptom-related acts such as self-harm or general measures of social functioning, studies are hard to compare and evaluate. In a consecutive series of patients, we used single case experimental methodology to assess the impact of cognitive therapy on baseline measures of patients' problems. We demonstrated that cognitive therapy can produce clinical, and to a lesser extent, statistically significant change in a wide range of domains, including interpersonal relationships, self-harm and affective symptoms in borderline and antisocial personality disorder (Davidson and Tyrer, 1996). Given the increasing awareness of personality disorder at a clinical level, the development of clinical models of personality disorder and the availability of treatment manuals for personality disorder, further larger-scale studies using randomized controlled trials of treatments for personality disorder are needed.

8

Drug treatment of personality disorders

Peter Tyrer

Drugs are often used for treating personality disorders although it is important to note that none of them are yet licensed for the treatment of these conditions. As with all areas of medicine in which there is no clear treatment there are many competing drugs that have been tried in the treatment of these disorders, and a full and comprehensive account of these good review articles are available (Stein, 1992; Soloff, 1994). However, because so many of the drugs used in treatment have not been evaluated in a way that could even remotely allow a view on their efficacy, many will not be discussed. As with other forms of treatment, borderline personality disorder constitutes the biggest group in which drug treatment is being used and is therefore worth examining separately. However, again it is important to note that borderline personality disorder is one of the most heterogeneous of all groups within the personality classification and includes extensive comorbidity with other personality disorders as well as mental state disorders, particularly mood disorders and stress-related ones.

To establish the efficacy of personality disorder it is really necessary to satisfy four strict conditions (Tyrer, 1998a):

1. The treatment should be effective in the pure form of the personality disorder (i.e. independent of comorbidity).
2. Efficacy needs to be established using the classical methodology of the randomized controlled trial (despite inherent difficulties in

using this methodology for personality disorders).
3. Because there are no established drug treatments for personality disorder any treatment tested has to be superior in efficacy to a placebo pill using the methodology described in point 2.
4. The treatment should show evidence of its efficacy over a period of at least 6 months in view of the long duration of personality disorder.

A fifth criterion concerns the outcome measure for personality disorder. Benjamin (1997) has criticized the tendency for researchers to look at changes in symptoms or behaviours rather than the underlying attitudes and proclivities that lie behind all personalities and which would have to change if personality altered significantly.

Borderline personality disorder

Antipsychotic drugs

The antipsychotic drugs have been tested in the treatment of borderline personality disorder using more rigorous methodology than any other treatments. Despite this, the results are equivocal, even though the subject has been a focus of study for over 20 years (Brinkley et al., 1979). Two studies published in 1986 (Goldberg et al., 1986; Soloff et al., 1986) suggested in randomized placebo-controlled trials that low doses of haloperidol and thiothixene, respectively, were effective in reducing typical borderline behaviour and associated symptoms. These symptoms included depression, and as in one of these studies (Soloff *et al.*, 1986) amitriptyline was one of the comparison drugs it is of particular interest that haloperidol was superior to this drug in reducing depressive symptoms. However, since these impressively clear-cut findings were published further studies have failed to show the same level of efficacy. When treatment is extended over many weeks the gains of antipsychotic drugs over placebo are lost by the time of the fourth month. One of the major problems of antipsychotic drugs is their tendency for poor compliance leading to relapse (Kemp *et al.*, 1996) and even in low dosage used to treat borderline personality disorder (e.g. haloperidol up to 7 mg daily) they can create adverse effects. Whilst in a secure penitentiary it may be possible to ensure that all patients take their drugs at the appropriate times, in most other settings it is necessary to allow the patient to maintain their own motivation to take treatment. The possibility of giving antipsychotic drugs in low dose depot injections is an option in the treatment of these disorders but because it is unlikely to appeal to most it will probably never be a major plank of treatment.

Antidepressants

Tricyclic antidepressants, mainly in the form of amitriptyline, have been compared with other treatments, including placebo in the treatment of borderline personality disorder (and the results are difficult to interpret). Some patients show extremely good response to this treatment whereas others show no benefit whatsoever and there are suggestions that more than one type of borderline personality disorder exists which respond differently to therapy (Soloff *et al.*, 1991). The monoamine oxidase inhibitor, phenelzine, also seems to help patients with borderline personality disorder, possibly to a greater degree than other antidepressants in the short and medium term (Cornelius *et al.*, 1993).

There are now clear suggestions that selective serotonin re-uptake inhibitors (SSRIs) are effective with one randomized controlled trial showing superiority over placebo using fluoxetine (Salzman *et al.*, 1995) and another suggesting that SSRIs reduce impulsiveness and deliberate self-harm (Verkes *et al.*, 1998a,b). This is of particular interest because of the apparent differences between SSRIs and tricyclic antidepressants, although neither of these studies involved a tricyclic antidepressant comparison. In one of the early controlled studies the monoamine oxidase inhibitor, tranylcypromine, was compared with alprazolam, carbamazepine and trifluoperazine (Cowdry and Gardner, 1988). The results were equivocal which is not surprising considering that the sample only included 45 patients, and some gains from all treatments were judged to be present. However, since no placebo control was included this could only be speculative.

The results of these studies are very difficult to interpret because of the unsatisfactory diagnostic status of borderline personality disorder, its heterogeneity and extensive co-morbidity. The evidence of efficacy in the short term, disappearing in the longer term, suggests that improvement is more likely to be a consequence of successful treatment of a mental state disorder rather than the personality component, although the opposite has been argued by Ekselius and von Knorring (1998) in another study with SSRIs.

Other personality disorders

Flamboyant group

Low dosage of antipsychotic drugs has been recommended for the treatment of antisocial (now called dissocial) personality disorder for many years (Bennie and Kinnell, 1975) and these recommendations have included treatment by depot injection. Most of these reports are anecdotal and no control comparisons have been made. Mood stabilizers have also been considered for the treatment of personality disorder. Carbamazepine was one of the comparison drugs used in the study by Cowdry and Gardner (1988) and lithium has been claimed to reduce anger and impulsiveness in those with antisocial personality disorder (Tupin *et al.*, 1973b; Sheard *et al.*, 1976) but although the second of these was a randomized trial it has never been replicated. There are similar benefits argued for treatment with lithium in the treatment of alcohol dependence as this condition is often associated with personality disorder (although personality was not mentioned in the study (Merry *et al.*, 1976) and so it is impossible to judge whether personality status was a key issue in the response). Similar antiaggressive action of lithium has been demonstrated in learning disability (Dale, 1980; Tyrer, S. *et al.*, 1984).

Odd and eccentric group (cluster A)

There is limited evidence that antipsychotic drugs may also be effective in the odd or eccentric cluster of personality disorders (schizoid, schizotypal and paranoid). This is generally unsatisfactory evidence and the only controlled trial (Goldberg *et al.*, 1986) included both borderline and schizotypal personality disorder in its selection criteria. No studies have been published of drug treatment in paranoid personality disorder and, indeed, perhaps predictably – it might even meet the requirements for a diagnostic criterion – this condition seems to escape formal assessment of all therapeutic interventions. Adherence to drug treatment is also likely to be a major problem with all forms of treatment for this group and makes one gloomy about the prospects for further advances in management except in institutional settings.

Anxious fearful cluster (cluster C)

There is a strong association between neurotic disorder and what is commonly known as cluster C group of personality disorders, comprising dependent, obsessive–compulsive and anxious (avoidant) personality disorders (Rees *et al.*, 1997) (*see* Chapter 6). There is considerable overlap between the criteria for many neurotic disorders and these disorders within the cluster C group and, as noted in Chapter 6, is particularly prominent with social phobia and avoidant personality disorder. In view of this the evidence that antidepressants are effective in avoidant personality disorder (Deltito and Stam, 1989) should be taken with a degree of scepticism; it is more likely that the antidepressants have been effective in treating social phobia or other anxiety symptoms.

A retrospective study of patients who had

received both tricyclic antidepressants and monoamine oxidase inhibitors (Shawcross and Tyrer, 1985) compared the outcome of the treatment of depression. Assessment was made with the Personality Assessment Schedule (PAS) and showed that those who had dual diagnosis of personality disorder and depressive illness found that tricyclic antidepressants were in general superior. In one long-term study, the Nottingham Study of Neurotic Disorder, in which drug treatment, mainly in the form of tricyclic antidepressants, was compared with cognitive and behaviour therapy, and self-help, in patients with neurotic disorder over 2 years, it was found that although there was no difference in outcome between the three treatments overall (Tyrer *et al.*, 1993) there was a significant difference in outcome when patients were separated by personality status (*Figure 9.3*). These data show that outcome, as measured by mean scores on the Comprehensive Psychopathological Rating Scale (CPRS) (Åsberg *et al.*, 1978), was much better in patients with complex personality disorder treated with drug treatment (predominantly the antidepressant, dothiepin) after the first 10 weeks of treatment (Tyrer *et al.*, 1988a) than by the two psychological treatments. This suggests that the notion of personality disorder should be treated more appropriately by psychological than by drug treatment could be challenged, but more evidence is required, particularly as this finding was not one of the original hypotheses tested in the study.

In a study of antidepressant drug treatment with fluvoxamine in obsessive–compulsive disorder it was found that those with concurrent obsessive–compulsive personality disorder had a better outcome (Ansseau *et al.*, 1991). It is difficult to know if this was a consequence of better response or better adherence to treatment in those who were personality disordered, and although it might be assumed that those with obsessive–compulsive personality disorder might adhere to treatment more closely than others this also needs to be compared.

In the treatment of apparent benzodiazepine dependence the role of personality disorder in selection of treatment is important. People who take benzodiazepines long-term are more likely to have a personality disorder than those with no personality disorder

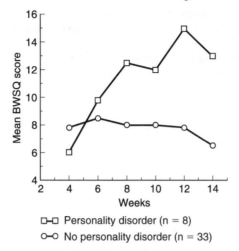

Figure 8.1 Changes in withdrawal symptoms in 41 patients who had taken benzodiazepines regularly for 6 months or more and who were switched to one of three benzodiazepines, lorazepam, diazepam or bromazepam and had these drugs withdrawn gradually after 4 weeks of treatment, so that on the 10th week after withdrawal they were taking no drugs. Withdrawal symptoms were recorded using the Benzodiazepine Withdrawal Symptom Questionnaire (BWSQ) (Tyrer *et al.* 1990c). (Figure reproduced by permission of the *British Journal of Psychiatry* and Dr Siobhan Murphy.)

(Seivewright *et al.*, 1991) but many who have taken them long-term (at least in the more distant past) have done so for other reasons. The assumption that all those who take benzodiazepines long-term are likely to become dependent is a myth. In *Figure 8.1* the outcome of a group of patients with putative benzodiazepine dependence (i.e. they thought they were dependent because they had been on their drugs for over 6 months in regular dosage) is shown. Personality disorder was assessed before withdrawal using the PAS and the 41 patients completing treatment switched to one of three benzodiazepines, lorazepam, diazepam or bromazepam in equivalent dosage before being gradually withdrawn after 4 weeks in 25% proportions at 2-week intervals so that all had withdrawn by 10 weeks. Those with premorbid personality disorder had an increase in benzodiazepine withdrawal symptoms whereas those with no personality disorder showed no change during withdrawal (Murphy and Tyrer, 1991) (*Figure 8.1*). Similar results were found in an earlier study (Tyrer *et al.*, 1983c). It is therefore reasonable to conclude that gradual withdrawal of benzodiazepines is all that is necessary to help people stop benzodiazepines if they have been taking them regularly for many weeks or months.

Conclusion

Despite the fact that there have been several controlled trials involving psychotropic drugs and placebo in the treatment of personality disorder none of them satisfy the full requirements for establishment of efficacy set out at the beginning of this chapter and it seems unlikely that this will change in the immediate future. This does not mean that drugs are ineffective in personality disorder but there is no satisfactory evidence that allows specific recommendations to be made. Bearing in mind that most patients receiving drug treatment have a mental state disorder independent of their personality status further studies such as those of Ansseau *et al.* in which patients with mental state disorders undergoing drug treatment also have their personality status assessed would be helpful in elucidating the role of personality in treatment response.

It is also necessary to carry out more investigations in which personality status itself is the main outcome being measured, along the lines that Benjamin (1997) has suggested. Changes in symptoms, which we know are likely to be created by successful drug treatment for mental state disorders, should not be regarded as the main prerogative for the treatment of personality disorders. Ideally, in randomized trials the outcome of personality disorder should be carried out directly by measuring personality status before and after treatment (and also after long-term follow-up). This is not a pipe dream, but it needs will and enterprise to succeed.

9

Outcome of personality disorder

Peter Tyrer and Helen Seivewright

Outcome is a straightforward word and seems to be unequivocal in what it describes. Unfortunately it is an ambiguous term and has been interpreted in different ways by research workers evaluating what happens to psychiatric disorders. Reviews attempting to compare studies of outcome tend to become handicapped by these different interpretations (e.g. Puccinelli and Wilkinson, 1994) and, if there are difficulties in understanding outcome studies with mental state conditions such as schizophrenia and depression, the problems become much greater when personality disorders are studied. A major difference of opinion involves the time-scale of disorder. Does outcome refer to the measurement of personality disorder (or any other measure) at a certain point in time or does it refer to progress made ever since the initial treatment was completed? If a longitudinal perspective is taken, what is the position of a patient who, for example, is considerably handicapped for 2 years after initial treatment but then spends the rest of the time well? Similarly, what is the position of the patient who pursues an episodic course and is either completely well or severely ill at the time of follow-up? These questions have clear answers, but until there is universal agreement over scoring them there will continue to be different interpretations and attempts to combine data, such as meta-analysis, will be fraught with difficulty (Emmanuel *et al.*, 1998).

Another important source of difficulty is the choice of primary outcome measure. The natural one is a global measure which is a synthesis of all the aspects of outcome relevant to clinical practice – symptoms, social functioning and disability, use of services, satisfaction of needs – but often these have to be derived from scratch and are therefore *ad hoc* measures that cannot be combined. The best measures are dichotomous ones (e.g. dead/alive, no diagnosis/diagnosis) but these conflict with the longitudinal approach mentioned above. In the case of personality disorder the obvious measure is absence or presence of personality disorder at follow-up but this can be misleading. In *Figure 9.1* the outcome of two populations, one with a more severe personality disorder at initial assessment compared with the second, is illustrated. Each group improves equally but because the first is more handicapped at the outset, it will wrongly appear to have a worse outcome at follow-up. Despite the criticisms of dichotomous measures, it must be appreciated that patients have to be categorized for purposes of treatment and management; 0.4 of a patient cannot be transferred to a special hospital.

In the case of personality disorder the problems are compounded by the unwelcome complication of comorbidity. If two or more conditions exist in the same person, even if they might be part of the same disorder and therefore consanguineous rather than comorbid (Tyrer, 1996), it is difficult to know how to separate those elements of outcome that are due to one disorder and those which are a

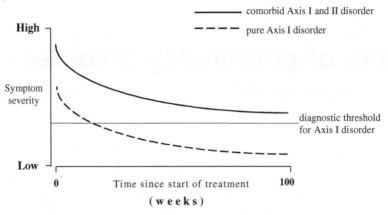

Figure 9.1 Explanation of apparently poor outcome in comorbid bi-axial disorders

consequence of the other. The much better outcome of borderline personality disorder compared with others may be nothing to do with any fundamental property of the personality disorder but to the fact that the condition is almost invariably associated with affective symptoms (Fyer *et al.*, 1988). As depression generally has a fair to good outcome in follow-up studies (Puccinelli and Wilkinson, 1994; Emmanuel *et al.*, 1998) it is therefore not surprising that borderline personality disorder would do better than other personality disorders not associated with affective disturbance.

Methodological problems in assessing outcome of personality disorder

The problems mentioned in the previous chapter about interpreting response to treatment in personality disorders apply with even greater force when examined in the context of outcome studies. A longer time-scale is necessary for all outcome studies and, in the case of personality disorders, this should ideally be measured in decades rather than just a few years. However, there are few prospective studies that have employed this time-scale and almost all studies of outcome have been retrospective ones. Because most of these have not employed any formal assessment of personality disorder at time of initial

contact, the diagnosis of personality disorder has, to some extent at least, been retrospective also.

The main aspects of outcome that have been examined in studies of patients with personality disorder are (a) the personality status of patients at follow-up, (b) their general level of functioning, (c) the psychiatric services they have received or are currently receiving, and (d) the impact on the symptoms and other measures of outcome of psychiatric disorder other than personality disturbance. Because most of the studies have not recorded the outcome of different categories of personality disorder individually, outcome can only be discussed in general terms. This is obviously unsatisfactory, and so separate discussion of the outcome of individual personality disorders is discussed where data exist.

Prevalence of personality disorder in different age groups

One way of studying the possible relationship between the time course of different personality disorders is to examine the relationship between age and personality disorder in a cross-sectional study. This is no substitute for close follow-up studies but, if some personality disorders or subtypes are more commonly represented in some age groups than others, some tentative conclusions can be made about the natural history of each personality disorder. We therefore studied the relationship between age and the key trait scores for a population of 928 patients on our main database. Their key trait scores allow for the range of personality disturbance to be studied even though most patients do not qualify for the formal diagnosis of a personality disorder.

The key trait scores for each of the personality categories in the PAS were calculated and their relationship with age studied by means of regression analysis. All the categories showed a negative slope, so that the older the patient the lower were the key trait scores. Although only a relatively small percentage of the variance could be explained by the age factor, the findings showed that the flamboyant group of personality disorders (cluster B) were less common in older people suggesting a favourable outcome in this group (*Table 9.1*), and although other categories contributed some of the variance they were dwarfed by the flamboyant group.

As almost all the patients had a mental state disorder as well as a personality one, these findings might be regarded as secondary to factors other than personality. We therefore examined the key trait scores for the PAS personality categories in the randomly selected sample (200) of the population (of Nottinghamshire) described by Professor Casey in Chapter 5. The results showed a similar pattern. Personality disorders in cluster B,

most marked for histrionic personality disorder, were much less frequent in the older age groups (*Table 9.2*). The withdrawn group (cluster D) showed very little change with increasing age. Examination of the individual PAS variables showed that lability was most dependent on the age factor and rigidity the least. Indeed, there was a small positive slope for rigidity, indicating that older subjects had rather higher scores for this variable than younger ones (*Table 9.3*). These results are consistent with other epidemiological findings that antisocial disorders in particular are less prevalent in older age groups (Myers *et al.*, 1984; Robins *et al.*, 1984). However, there could be several factors that could falsify these conclusions. Those with flamboyant personality disorders may die at a younger age or have higher refusal rates in research studies than other groups, and longitudinal examination of personality change is necessary to be more certain what is happening to personality over time.

Change in personality disorder over time

Descriptions of personality disorder since the term was introduced over 100 years ago have always been accompanied by the adjectives *enduring* and *persistent*. To qualify for the diagnosis, it is assumed that the condition

Table 9.1 Regression analysis to study relationship between age and PAS diagnostic categories in 928 psychiatric patients

Diagnostic group	Main cluster link (DSM-IV)	Significance of age relationship (P)	Direction of slope*	Percentage variance explained by age factor (R^2)
Schizoid	A	<0.0001	N	3.9
Paranoid	A	<0.0001	N	4.3
Avoidant	A&B	<0.0001	N	3.4
Sociopathic	B	<0.0001	N	10.7
Sensitive–aggressive	B	<0.0001	N	8.1
Impulsive	B	<0.0001	N	11.0
Histrionic	B&C	<0.0001	N	7.6
Passive–dependent	C	<0.0001	N	5.6
Asthenic (dependent)	C	<0.0001	N	2.4
Anankastic	C (D)	<0.025	N	0.7
Dysthymic	C (D)	<0.001	N	1.2
Anxious	C (D)	NS	N	0.2
Hypochondriacal	C (D)	<0.025	N	0.6

*N = negative, P = positive
A negative slope indicates lessening of severity of the personality characteristic with increasing age

Table 9.2 Regression analysis to study relationship between age and personality disorder categories in 200 randomly selected subjects

Diagnostic group	Main cluster link (DSM-IV)	Significance of age relationship (P)	Direction of slope*	Percentage variance explained by age factor (R^2)
Schizoid	A	NS	N	1.4
Paranoid	A	<0.05	N	2.2
Avoidant	A&B	<0.005	N	4.1
Sociopathic	B	<0.0001	N	8.6
Sensitive–aggressive	B	<0.01	N	3.4
Impulsive	B	<0.0001	N	7.9
Histrionic	B&C	<0.0001	N	10.0
Passive–dependent	C	<0.01	N	3.7
Asthenic (dependent)	C	NS	N	0.7
Anankastic	C (D)	<0.05	N	2.4
Dysthymic	C (D)	NS	N	1.0
Anxious	C (D)	NS	N	1.3
Hypochondriacal	C (D)	<0.01	N	3.7

*N = negative, P = positive
A negative slope indicates lessening of severity of the personality characteristic with increasing age

Table 9.3 Regression analysis to study relationship between age and PAS scores in 200 randomly selected subjects

Diagnostic group	Main cluster link (DSM-IV)	Significance of age relationship (P)	Direction of slope*	Percentage variance explained by age factor (R^2)
Pessimism	C	NS	N	0.9
Worthlessness	C	<0.02	N	3.1
Optimism	C	<0.05	N	1.8
Lability	B	<0.0001	N	9.4
Anxiousness	C	NS	N	1.1
Suspiciousness	A	NS	N	0.2
Introspection	A	<0.05	N	2.3
Shyness	C	NS	N	0.8
Aloofness	A	NS	N	0.7
Sensitivity	A	NS	N	0.6
Vulnerability	C	<0.025	N	2.7
Irritability	B	<0.01	N	3.3
Impulsiveness	B	<0.001	N	6.5
Aggressiveness	B	<0.005	N	4.1
Callousness	B	<0.01	N	3.5
Irresponsibility	B	<0.005	N	4.2
Childishness	B	<0.005	N	4.4
Resourcelessness	C	<0.02	N	2.7
Dependence	C	NS	N	1.6
Submissiveness	C	NS	N	0.9
Conscientiousness	C	NS	Level	0.1
Rigidity	C	NS	N	0.4
Eccentricity	A	<0.02	N	3.1
Hypochondriasis	C	<0.01	N	3.5

*N = negative, P = positive
A negative slope indicates lessening of severity of the personality characteristic with increasing age

begins in adolescence or even earlier and continues throughout most of adult life (World Health Organization, 1992). This is a presupposition that has now been tested and shown to be not always correct (see later in this chapter). There has long been reason to doubt it from clinical experience, as many personality disorders seen in early adult life do not present in anything like the same degree when identified in the elderly. When we mellow as we get older this seems to describe changes in our personalities as well as other characteristics.

One of the longest periods of observation in any outcome study is the 30-year follow-up study of Lee Robins (1966) which has become a famous landmark in studies of outcome of psychiatric disorders. She showed unequivocally that children referred to a child guidance clinic for delinquent behaviour, particularly thieving and aggressive conduct, were significantly more likely to show all the features of sociopathic (now antisocial) personality disorder than those children referred for other reasons. Twenty-eight per cent of delinquent children developed such personality disorder whereas only 4% of other referrals did so. This does not, however, tell us that antisocial personality disorder is a permanent state as at follow-up this population had not reached the age of 50. The fifth decade of life is the one which many past clinicians regard as the turning point for patients with personality disorder; if they are protected from society until this time it was suggested they can be released with safety because they had matured (Sargant and Slater, 1962; Curran and Partridge, 1963; Davis, 1972). However, it should not be assumed that all personality disorders achieve this pleasant state of resolution, and indeed, the striking nature of such improvement when it occurs may lead to the conviction that what is uncommon is really the norm. Certainly there are many in the criminal justice system seen by forensic psychiatrists, who find that a significant proportion (probably at least a third) have sufficient disorder to require treatment and cannot be left with time as their only therapy (Gunn *et al.*, 1978). Nevertheless, it is extremely important to know if personality disorders do improve or indeed deteriorate over time, not least because the natural history of each condition needs to be known to determine the value of specific treatments and length of management policies before review.

Early studies were small with selected groups and had several methodological deficiencies. Maddocks (1970) followed up a group of psychopathic patients (probably regarded mainly as antisocial personality disorder in DSM-IV) and found that, of 52 patients, three had committed suicide and only 10 had improved sufficiently to be regarded as having 'settled down'. The ages of the patients were not given in his report. Rather better results were reported by Whiteley (1970) who found a 40% improvement in a similar group of difficult sociopathic individuals. However, the improvement rate was measured only in terms of criminal convictions or psychiatric admissions and many personality disordered patients can avoid these events but still remain disordered.

In Robins' study (1966) a poor outcome was also found with girls who presented to a child guidance clinic with conduct disorder. Of the 76 girls followed up 30 years later, 20 had developed what would probably be labelled as histrionic or borderline personality disorder in DSM-IV, but in her book was described as hysteria. This gender difference in personality diagnosis with somewhat similar personality disturbance being diagnosed as histrionic in women and antisocial in men has been noted many times in the American literature (Cloninger *et al.*, 1975; Lilienfeld *et al.*, 1986) and so it is not surprising that the outcome of histrionic personality disorder should be somewhat similar to that of the antisocial one (and incidentally supports the argument that gender bias is involved in diagnosing these two conditions).

The member of the flamboyant personality cluster (cluster B) studied most closely with regard to outcome is borderline personality disorder. Pope *et al.* (1983) examined closely the outcome of 33 patients with borderline personality disorder 4–7 years after initial contact. All patients were seen in a psychiatric hospital (McLean Hospital, Belmont, Massachusetts) and diagnosed as borderline personality disorder using the Diagnostic Interview for Borderlines (DIB) (Gunderson *et al.*, 1981). Of the 33 patients, two had committed suicide and 27 of the remaining 31 were seen or interviewed by telephone. Thirteen of these had *pure* borderline personality disorder at initial assessment and 14 had mixed borderline personality disorder and a major affective disorder (depression). Of the *pure* group, 10 had possible or definite personality disorder at follow-up, but six of these had a diagnosis of histrionic, narcissistic or antisocial personality disorder. Of the 14 patients with borderline personality disorder and depression, three patients were well and had no psychiatric diagnosis, three others had no personality disorder, and eight had definite or possible borderline personality disorder. However, six of these had other personality disorders also, mainly the histrionic category. The authors concluded naturally that borderline personality disorder did not appear to be a stable condition.

Another major study of outcome in personality disorder has been the Chestnut Lodge follow-up study reported in a series of papers by McGlashan (1984a,b, 1986a,b). Chestnut Lodge is a private psychiatric hospital in Rockville, Maryland, USA, which specializes in the long-term residential treatment of severely ill patients. Most of these are described as suffering from schizophrenia, affective disorder or borderline personality disorder. An additional group was also felt in retrospect to be suffering from schizotypal personality disorder. The patients were followed up between 5 and 20 years after their admission to hospital and most interviews were carried out by telephone except for those patients who lived close to the hospital. As a formal personality disorder diagnosis was not made at initial assessment, McGlashan used a standardized retrospective technique to record the original personality status in DSM-III terms (McGlashan, 1984a). The initial comparisons between the Chestnut Lodge diagnoses and DSM-III ones for personality disorder were not good, but after application of this standardized method of assessment they improved significantly.

McGlashan found that the borderline personality disordered patients generally had a better outcome than the schizophrenic patients and those with affective disorder (McGlashan, 1983, 1984b). Of 81 patients followed up a mean of 169 months after discharge, 87% were alive and had an average age of 47. Of these 44% were still diagnosed as suffering from borderline personality disorder and 24% were diagnosed as having schizophrenia. The follow-up revealed an interesting time course in symptomatology and functions. Up to 9 years after admission there was some improvement but this was not marked. Follow-up carried out between 10 and 19 years after admission showed a much greater level of improvement with many pa-

tients having few or no symptoms of personality difficulties. Follow-up carried out after a period of 20 years or longer, however, suggested that improvement was less marked after this longer time interval. McGlashan concluded that borderline personality disorder was more closely linked to affective disorders than any other mental state diagnoses and, unlike Pope and his colleagues, considered that the diagnosis of borderline personality disorder was a stable one. However, it is important to emphasize that his original diagnoses were retrospective ones, whereas those of Pope and his colleagues were prospective.

McGlashan (1986b) has also studied the outcome of retrospectively diagnosed schizotypal personality disorder. Of 119 patients followed up, only 10 had the pure syndrome without any other diagnosis and 18 had both borderline and schizotypal personality disorders. An additional 91 had schizotypal personality disorder in association with schizophrenia, including 30 who also had borderline personality disorder. Schizotypal personality disorder had a poorer outcome than the borderline group and many developed schizophrenia subsequently. This accords with McGlashan's earlier findings in which 55% of patients with schizotypal personality disorder developed schizophrenia at follow-up (McGlashan, 1983). The group which had both schizotypal and borderline personality disorder showed a similar pattern of improvement to the borderline group and so McGlashan concluded that the mixed syndrome was more likely to be a variant of borderline personality disorder and the schizotypal component was relatively less important. Schizotypal personality disorder therefore appeared to be a much less stable diagnosis than that of borderline personality disorder. McGlashan (1986b) concluded that 'ironically, our results indicate that schizotypal personality disorder, rather than borderline personality disorder, can most legitimately lay claim to the label borderline, in the sense of existing on a midground between health and schizophrenia'.

Michael Stone and his colleagues (Stone *et al.*, 1987; Stone, 1993) have examined the outcome of borderline personality disorder over periods ranging up to 20 years. He has found tremendous variation in his population, ranging from some who have achieved commanding positions in government and major companies and others who committed suicide or continued on a path of continued disruption in relationships and behaviour. Rather paradoxically, those who had more comorbid Axis I and II disorders fared better in the second decade of follow-up than the first.

Most of these studies have been carried out in specially selected populations with the more severe personality disorders, mainly in the flamboyant DSM-III cluster, in patients who were in hospital at the time of first contact. In personal work we have followed up a much less seriously ill group, those with neurotic disorders and comorbid personality disorders. In the Nottingham Study of Neurotic Disorder a cohort of patients referred to general practice psychiatric clinics with generalized anxiety disorder (GAD), panic disorder and dysthymic disorder had their clinical and personality status assessed at baselines. Of 198 with personality assessments, 72 (36%) had a personality disorder using the PAS, 39 (20%) had personality difficulty and 87 (44%) had no personality disorder classification (Tyrer *et al.*, 1990b). Of those with personality disorder or difficulty 22 (20%) had a diagnosis within cluster A, 43 (39%) in cluster B and 46 (41%) in the cluster C groups.

After 12 years the same patients were assessed again using the same instruments, including personality status with the PAS, by one of us (HS). The data were collected over a 4-year period between 1995 and 1999 (to match the timing of the original data collection so that all assessments were exactly 12 years after baseline ones). Whilst the full data have not yet been analysed at the time of writing, it was felt appropriate to examine changes in each of the 24 personality traits of the PAS to test whether the age findings shown in the cross-sectional comparison were replicated in this prospective study.

The results are shown in *Table 9.4*. The results of 150 patients (78F : 72M) are shown and at the time of follow-up their mean age was 50 years. Although these in general support the findings of the cross-sectional study, there are some important differences. The cluster B attributes of impulsiveness, childishness, aggression and irresponsibility showed significant reduction over the 12-year period but lability showed no change. Most

of the cluster C traits (pessimism, worthlessness, hypochondriasis, dependence and resourcelessness) showed no change but some showed an increase (anxiousness, vulnerability and conscientiousness). In addition, several of the cluster A elements (suspiciousness, introspection, eccentricity, shyness and aloofness) showed an increase (albeit from a low baseline). A separate analysis was also carried out to determine if there was an interaction between age and outcome in the population studied (this would, for example, detect groups who improved over 12 years if they presented early in life but got worse over this period if they presented with the same characteristics later). These findings suggest that the traits of anxiousness and obsessionality do not improve over time (at least in this original group who all had a neurotic diagnosis initially) and so what constitutes 'mellowing' in old age refers more to impulsiveness and aggression than anxiety and nervous preoccupation.

In the first edition of this book we suggested that the findings from the studies till that time indicated that personality disorders could be divided into mature and immature groups, with the immature ones developing early and improving over the medium term whereas the mature ones persisted (Tyrer and Seivewright, 1988). With our later findings the hypothesis still holds up but there is a caveat that allows the possibility of at least some personality characteristics getting more pronounced with increasing age.

The McLean Hospital and Chestnut Lodge studies suggest that borderline personality disorders have a better functional outcome than the schizotypal ones, at least in the medium term, and the evidence from other studies uniformly confirm that borderline personality disorder has the best outcome overall. However, even this conclusion has to be qualified as it is such a heterogeneous group and one outcome, death, cheats maturation by putting a stop to time. The outcome of antisocial personality disorders suggests continued conflict with society when taken from childhood onwards, but is more optimistic when adult patients are studied (Maddocks, 1970; Whiteley, 1970). There are a number of studies that indicate a relationship between antisocial personality and bodily complaints of illness (Cloninger *et al.*, 1975;

Table 9.4 Change in PAS scores in 150 patients with neurotic disorder (generalized anxiety disorder, dysthymic disorder and panic disorder) seen at baseline and after 12 years

Diagnostic group	Main cluster link (DSM-IV)	Significance of age relationship (P)	Implication of findings
Pessimism	C	NS	no change over time
Worthlessness	C	NS	no change over time
Optimism	C	NS	no change over time
Lability	B	NS	no change over time
Anxiousness	C	increase ($P < 0.01$) no interaction	increase in anxiety with increasing age
Suspiciousness	A	increase ($P < 0.001$) no interaction	increase in suspiciousness with increasing age
Introspection	A	increase ($P < 0.001$) significant interaction	increase in introspection with increasing age but less in middle age
Shyness	C	increase ($P = 0.02$) no interaction	some increase in shyness with increasing age
Aloofness	A	increase ($P < 0.001$) no interaction	increase in aloofness with increasing age
Sensitivity	A	NS	no change over time
Vulnerability	C	increase ($P < 0.01$) no interaction	increase in vulnerability with increasing age
Irritability	B	decrease ($P < 0.02$) interaction with increase up to middle age and then reduction	decrease in irritability after middle age
Impulsiveness	B	small decrease ($P < 0.05$)	decrease in impulsiveness with increasing age
Aggressiveness	B	decrease ($P < 0.02$)	decrease in aggression with increasing age
Callousness	B	NS	
Irresponsibility	B	decrease ($P < 0.0001$) no interaction	decrease in irresponsibility with increasing age
Childishness	B	decrease ($P < 0.0001$) no interaction	decrease in childishness with increasing age
Resourcelessness	C	NS	no change over time
Dependence	C	NS	ditto
Submissiveness	C	NS	ditto
Conscientiousness	C	increase ($P < 0.001$) no interaction	increase in conscientiousness with increasing age
Rigidity	C	NS	no change over time
Eccentricity	A	increase ($P < 0.001$) no interaction	increase in eccentricity with increasing age
Hypochondriasis	C	NS	no change over time

Lilienfeld *et al.*, 1986) and also with affective illness (Winokur, 1972; Reich and Vasile, 1993). These relationships have been established in cross-sectional and family studies and receive some support from the examination of outcome of patients with antisocial personality disorders. Maddocks (1970) found that a substantial minority of the patients with psychopathic personality disorder at follow-up had developed hypochondriacal symptoms and frequent co-occurrence of depressive disorder and borderline personality disorder in follow-up studies has already been noted (McGlashan, 1983; Pope *et al.*, 1983).

This might seem somewhat paradoxical, the idea of amoral, unfeeling people developing symptoms that are more typical of those shown by inhibited people with neurotic disorders who show no antisocial tendencies. However, it would be wrong to equate the two because the characteristic feature of affective disturbance in antisocial personality is its instability and unpredictability. Intense feelings of depression may be just as quickly followed by sudden optimism and energy that is quite separate from the mood disturbance of manic depressive disorder and the physical complaints have a flamboyant quality about them that differs from the symptoms of hypochondriasis. This is one of the major reasons for the separation of somatization disorder from hypochondriasis in current psychiatric classifications. Nevertheless, a great deal more needs to be done in classifying the phenomenon of somatization in psychiatric illness. The implication that somatization is somehow linked to antisocial and other personality disturbance, which is suggested by the studies of the St Louis group, is not necessarily justified. Somatic presentation of symptoms is extremely common and the current criteria for somatization disorder only account for a small part of its spectrum (Bridges and Goldberg, 1985). There is also a strong case for regarding classical somatization disorder as a personality disorder in its own right, as its comorbidity with personality disorder is so marked (up to 80%) that it is more likely that they are consanguineous than comorbid conditions (Stern *et al.*, 1993).

The high incidence of affective disturbance, almost exclusively depression, in the outcome studies of personality disorder suggests that suicide might be a more common outcome in personality disordered patients than in others. Because mortality is more often (and reliably) reported than any other measure of outcome, there are a number of studies that examine this hypothesis. In general, the results showed that patients with personality disorder have greater mortality than other psychiatric diagnoses and that a significant part of this increased mortality is due to suicide (Innes and Millar, 1970; Sims and Prior, 1978; Black *et al.*, 1985). Suicide is commoner in the early follow-up period, usually within 5 years of initial assessment. The differences between personality disordered and other psychiatric populations tend to disappear after this period.

This finding again suggests that the maturation hypothesis is supported by study of the antisocial personality disorders; with increasing age impulsiveness lessens and suicide is therefore less likely. It might also be argued that the improvement is due to a lower incidence of depressive episodes with increasing age. However, the increased mortality in personality disorders is considerably greater than that for affective disorders. For example, the standardized mortality ratio (SMR), the ratio of observed to expected deaths, is 4.6 for men and 17.8 for women for

unnatural deaths (principally suicide) and personality disorder, and 3.1 for men and 13.0 for women in patients with affective disorders from one recent study (Black *et al.*, 1985). Most studies have been carried out with inpatients, but similar findings have also been noted in an outpatient population (Martin *et al.*, 1985). The SMR for patients with antisocial personality disorder was 8.57 by comparison with 0.84 and 0.62 for unipolar and bipolar affective disorder.

It seems, therefore, as though the combination of personality disorder and affective symptoms is a powder keg that can easily explode into successful suicide. The increased risk taking of antisocial personality disorders and their ability to generate more threatening life events (Seivewright, 1999; Seivewright *et al.*, 2000) probably accounts for the higher mortality from accidents (Schuckit and Gunderson, 1977) and the co-occurrence of depression leads to self-directed aggression. Indeed, the high risk of early mortality in personality disorders represents one of the major challenges for preventative psychiatry. If such unnatural deaths can be prevented in, say, the first 5 years after identification of the disorder, the high-risk period is over and subsequent mortality is not excessive.

Outcome of personality disorders in primary care

All the studies reported so far in this chapter have been concerned with highly selected groups of patients. Most studies have been carried out with inpatients, as much more information is available about this group at the time of initial assessment than in others. However, we have already established that a significant proportion of patients with personality disorders have little or no contact with the psychiatric services and it is important to know how they fare.

An opportunity to study this came about when carrying out a follow-up survey of the outcome of the patients with conspicuous psychiatric morbidity in primary care described in Chapter 5 (Casey *et al.*, 1984; Casey, 1985). Exactly three calendar years after Dr Casey's assessments in urban and rural general practice, the patients' medical (and, where relevant, psychiatric) notes were examined by one of us (HS) and all forms of medical and psychiatric contact recorded using a standardized form. Where there was doubt about data, the general practitioner was seen for clarification. A detailed record was obtained of all psychotropic drug treatment, frequency of contact with the general practitioner, information about all psychiatric admissions and other forms of psychiatric treatment (day hospital, outpatients, community nurse support, psychological treatment and social work). HS was unaware of the clinical and personality status of each patient at initial contact with Dr Casey and so her results could not be biased by this knowledge.

Of 357 patients seen by Dr Casey, 318 (93.8%) had follow-up information available. However, for 17 of these patients, full follow-up data for the 3 years were not available; 15 of these had died, one by suicide, and two had emigrated. Full follow-up data therefore concerned 301 patients, which represents 84.3% of the original sample. The notes were not available for 39 of the patients because they could not be traced. In the UK, all individuals are registered with a general practitioner and details of this are co-ordinated through Family Practitioner Committees. However, a small number of patients forget or refuse to register unless they become ill and others change their address so frequently that further information is difficult to trace. Thirty-nine patients fell into this category and examination of their initial diagnoses showed that 18 had normal personalities but 21 had a personality disorder, including nine in the antisocial group and five in the schizoid one. This represents a significant excess of personality disorders in those patients who were not traced ($\chi^2 = 13.1$, d.f. = 1, $P < 0.001$), a significant statistic that should be noted by those involved in follow-up studies of personality disorder. Of the 15 patients who had died, 12 had a diagnosis of normal personality, three had personality disorders.

It therefore seems likely that those patients not followed up in studies of this nature are more likely to contain an excess of personality disorders. Nevertheless, 72 of the patients (24%) who had their notes studied also had a personality disorder. We wished to study the difference in the service patterns of those with

and without personality disorder (taking all groups of personality disorder together) over the 3-year period. We were interested in knowing whether patients with personality disorder received less or more treatment from their general practitioners and psychiatric services, both outpatient and inpatient. It is possible to argue that patients with personality disorder receive more treatment from each of the services because their social difficulties make them more likely to come to the attention of the caring services, but it is also possible to argue that they receive less treatment because they are not inclined to seek help. It is important to know if patients with personality disorder in hospital are representative of personality disorders in the community; from experience with other mental disorders it is unlikely that they are equivalent.

Overall, there were no differences between the personality disordered and normal patients as far as rate of contact with the general practitioner was concerned in the 3-year period. Eleven (15.3%) of the personality disordered patients had no contact with their general practitioner as opposed to 24 (10.5%) of those with normal personality but 18 (25%) consulted their general practitioner at least 11 times during the 3 years compared with 63 (28.2%) of the normal group. However, patients with neurotic disorders had significantly more appointments with the general practitioner if they also had a personality disorder (mean appointments 11.9) than those patients with neurotic disorder and normal personality (mean appointments 8.9). By contrast, the rates of contact for schizophrenia were higher in those with normal personality (7.3 vs 4.8), as were the appointment rates for affective psychosis (11.4 in those of normal personality and 7.0 in those with personality disorder).

Patients with personality disorder were significantly more likely to be referred to psychiatrists, community psychiatric nurses, social workers or psychologists ($\chi^2 = 23.8$, $P < 0.001$), with 190 (83%) of those with no personality disorder having no contact with psychiatric services compared with only 42 (58%) of those with a personality disorder. This also applied across all diagnostic groups but was particularly marked for neurotic disorders. Only four of the 102 patients with a neurotic disorder who had a normal personality were seen by other psychiatric personnel, whereas nine out of the 29 patients who had a combined neurotic diagnosis and personality disorder were so referred ($\chi^2 = 23.3$, d.f. = 3; $P < 0.001$). Patients with personality disorder also tended to have more day care, with a mean of 1.6 weeks in treatment for each patient with no personality disorder and 5.2 weeks for those with personality disorder (Mann–Whitney U-test ($z = 2.09$), $P < 0.04$). There were 81 psychiatric admissions in the 301 patients during the 3-year study. Four of these were compulsory ones, three of these were diagnosed as having a schizophrenic illness at initial contact and the fourth had no psychiatric abnormality when seen by Dr Casey. Two of the four patients had a personality disorder, one schizoid and one anankastic personality disorder.

Of the other 77 admissions, 30 were personality disordered. This rate of admission was over twice that of the patients with normal personality and was highly significant ($\chi^2 = 11.8$; d.f. = 1, $P < 0.001$). The mean duration of admission was nearly three times as long in patients with personality disorder (3.7 weeks) compared with normal personalities (1.3 weeks) (Mann–Whitney U-test ($z = 2.38$), $P < 0.02$).

The personality disordered patients therefore had more psychiatric admissions and spent longer in hospital than those with normal personality, but this did not apply to hospital admissions for non-psychiatric reasons. There were 82 admissions for non-psychiatric reasons in the normal personality group and 36 in the personality disordered one. These admissions were for short periods in the main. The group with normal personality had a mean admission duration of 4 days and those with disordered personality of 5 days in the whole 3-year period.

The results indicate that psychiatric patients with personality disorder identified in primary care have significantly greater rates of contact with all forms of the psychiatric service than those of normal personality. This indicates that one of the major factors leading the general practitioner to refer a patient for psychiatric care is the presence of a personality disorder, although in many, if not most, instances referral is made without personality status being mentioned. The results also go a long way towards explaining the higher incidence of personality disorder in psychiatric patients described in Chapter 5 in comparison with the prevalence of personality disorders in primary care. These findings show that the diagnosis of personality disorder, notwithstanding its poor reliability, overlap with other mental disorders and difficulty in measurement, needs to be recorded if only for its public health implications, as it suggests that those with personality disorder will make significantly more demands on the services and thereby cost significantly more than patients of identical mental state diagnoses with no personality disorder. Indeed, we go so far as to predict that in the future the recording of personality status will be mandatory in diagnostic coding within psychiatric services precisely for this reason. The results also go some way towards validating the computer-coded separation of personality disorder from non-personality disorder in the PAS. The threshold may be determined by a statistical manoeuvre rather than by clinical judgement, but it nonetheless helps to separate patients in a way that makes clinical sense and has service implications.

Outcome of comorbid personality and mental state disorders

The combination of a mental state disorder and a personality disorder is almost always associated with a less good outcome than the mental state disorder alone. The subject has recently been comprehensively reviewed by a group of colleagues who met at the National Institute of Mental Health in Maryland (Tyrer et al., 1997) and the following major associations were described and their impact on outcome reached:

1. Borderline personality disorder and major depressive disorder are not closely related even though they often occur together (Gunderson and Phillips, 1991).
2. There is a close relationship between the new diagnosis of depressive personality disorder (likely to appear in DSM-V), dysthymia and depressive episodes that may indicate a spectrum of disturbance.
3. Schizotypal disorder and schizophrenia are also closely linked and represent excellent

evidence of a spectrum from mild expression (personality disorder) to severe expression (schizophrenia).

4. Comorbidity of personality disorder with either neurotic disorders of any kind, depressive disorders, eating disorders, schizophrenia, those with affective disorder undergoing day hospital treatment, adolescent emotional and conduct disorders, and most substance misuse disorders, leads to a significantly worse outcome.

However, although in general the influence of personality disorder is like a particularly unwanted guest at a wedding who behaves abominably and upsets almost everybody, there are some variations on this general negative theme and so the outcome for each mental state (Axis I) disorder is worth discussing separately.

Impact of personality disorder on the outcome of neurotic disorders

A number of reviews have established that personality disorder in any form has a negative effect on the outcome of neurotic disorder (Reich and Green, 1991; de Girolamo and Reich, 1993). This is important in practice, as between 20 and 50% of neurotic disorders have a significant degree of personality disturbance and so might be expected to have a major impact on outcome generally. One of the earliest studies of the impact of personality disorder on neurotic disorder was by Greer and Cawley (1966). They followed up 175 patients 4–6 years after admission to hospital with a neurotic disorder. Premorbid personality was assessed from the case notes at the time of admission. Although, in general, this is an unsatisfactory method of collecting data, all the patients concerned were admitted to the Professorial Unit at the Maudsley Hospital which is noted for its zeal in documentation and assessment and the findings were probably more valid than those achieved by a structured clinical interview administered by a junior researcher. Patients were classified into normal or abnormal personalities after examination of the case notes; 77 (44%) had normal and 98 (56%) had abnormal personalities and as these figures reflect

those of inpatients with personality disorder (de Girolamo and Reich, 1993) it is reasonable to regard abnormal personality and personality disorder as equivalent.

The results showed that abnormal personality, defined from the case notes using the general descriptions of the *International Classification of Disease* (ICD), was associated with a significantly worse outcome than in similar patients of normal personality (*Figure 9.2*). Although both the assessments of personality disorder and of outcome had some methodological deficiencies the magnitude of the differences in outcome between the two groups is too great to be ignored and the study is a pioneering one whose conclusions have been abundantly confirmed during the 35 years following completion of the study. Greer and Cawley's conclusion that personality status is one of the 'outstanding correlates of a good prognosis in neurotic disorder' can hardly be bettered.

Sims (1975) came to similar conclusions after examining the outcome of 146 patients admitted to a psychiatric hospital or day hospital with a diagnosis of neurotic disorder (ICD category 300). Sims' studies are remarkable in that he has been able to get a much higher follow-up rate than most other investigators, and in this group 97% of the patients were interviewed at a mean of 4 years later. The initial assessment of personality disorder was not particularly satisfactory, but it was found that using their particular criteria, 'pathological and immature personality' led to a significantly less satisfactory outcome than patients of normal personality. However, this difference was only significant at the 5% level of probability.

Other studies have come to broadly similar conclusions. The outcome of hysteria in patients with hysterical personality (Ciompi, 1969), anxiety and depressive neurosis in the presence of personality disorder (Kerr *et al.*, 1974), and of agoraphobia and social phobia in dependent personalities (Mullaney and Trippett, 1979) are uniformly worse in the presence of personality abnormality or disorder. No study has provided any evidence that personality disorder confers any advantage on the outcome of any neurotic condition.

However, this does not mean that personality disorder has a uniform effect on outcome irrespective of treatment. We examined

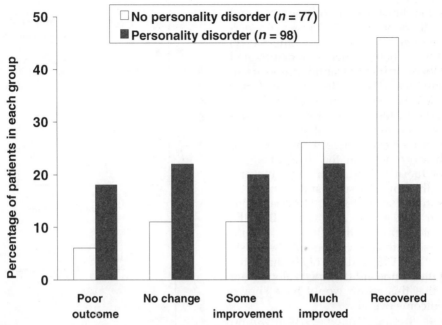

Figure 9.2 Outcome of 175 patients with neurotic disorder followed up after a mean of 5 years (after Greer and Cawley, 1966)

the influence of treatment in our long-term cohort study linked to a randomized controlled trial of treatment, the Nottingham Study of Neurotic Disorder. This involved the recruitment of 210 patients with generalized anxiety, dysthymic and panic disorder who were referred to general practice psychiatric clinics in Nottingham, England between 1983 and 1987. The patients were assigned randomly to drug therapy, cognitive behaviour and self-help and treated for 10 weeks under double-blind conditions. After 10 weeks patients continued to be treated in the same mode as that originally allocated as much as possible (with all those allocated to drug therapy originally being asked to continue antidepressants in the first instance) and patients were followed up for 5 years. After 2 years nearly three out of four patients had stayed within the same treatment 'mode' as that originally allocated (Tyrer *et al.*, 1993) (most of the 'deviations' involved similar prescriptions for benzodiazepines in all three treatment groups) and so the effects of treatment could still be judged as essentially similar to those of a randomized trial. Assessments of clinical symptomatology were made before treatment and at regular intervals for 2

years using the Comprehensive Psychopathological Rating Scale (CPRS) (Åsberg *et al.*, 1978) and associated scales for depression, Montgomery and Åsberg Depression Rating Scale (MADRS) (Montgomery and Åsberg, 1979) and the Brief Anxiety Scale (BAS) (Tyrer *et al.*, 1984b). Diagnostic status using the Structured Clinical Interview for DSM-III (SCID) was used initially to define the diagnostic status of each patient and also record it serially on four occasions throughout the 2 years. After 5 years the patients were assessed again using a five-point outcome scale based on their service contact at that time (*Table 9.5*). At both 2 and 5 years the PAS diagnoses of personality disorder were converted into the four-point scale of severity (Tyrer and Johnson, 1996) so that additional information could be obtained beyond that available from simple dichotomous separation of normal personality from personality disorder.

After 2 years the results showed an interesting interaction between personality disorder and treatment (Tyrer *et al.*, 1993) that is worth reporting in full because of its potential implications. People with one of the three neurotic disorders alone (unimorbidity) had an excellent outcome if they were treated by self-help and, to a lesser extent, by cognitive and behaviour therapy, whereas those with personality and neurotic disorders (comorbidity) had a relatively better outcome when treated by drug therapy (mainly antidepressants in the first instance). This is illustrated in *Figure 9.3*, in which the outcome is recorded by the scores on the CPRS. The most noticeable difference between the treatment groups is the much wider disparity between the scores for the self-help group than the drug one. The results for those treated with cognitive and behaviour therapy may suggest that this is no more effective than self-help. However, it is fair to add that it was also found that the outcome of cognitive therapy was significantly worse with less competent therapists (Kingdon *et al.*, 1996) and it is likely that if the results of the competent therapists alone were included that this group would have shown the best outcome overall.

The most striking differences were found with the complex (diffuse) personality disorders, in which the outcome with drug treatment was little different from those with normal personality. The main drug used in the treatment was the tricyclic drug, dothiepin, and it is possible that the same findings might not have been shown with other antidepressant drugs. The monoamine oxidase inhibitors have been found to have a much less satisfactory response to treatment in those with personality disorders (Tyrer *et al.*, 1983b) and this response is less than with tricyclic antidepressants (Shawcross and Tyrer, 1985).

It is also important not to interpret too much about the effect of personality disorder on treatment in the long term from the findings. The differences between the treatment groups were only marked between 16 weeks and 1 year and by 2 years were getting much less. Although this could reflect greater overlap between treatments later in the time period it might also indicate that personality disorder only has a delaying rather than an absolute effect on the outcome of psychological treatments and self-help.

This suggestion is to some extent supported by the analysis of the data at 5 years. After this length of time the adverse influence of personality disorder on outcome is even more marked and is one of the most important clinical predictors (Seivewright *et al.*, 1998).

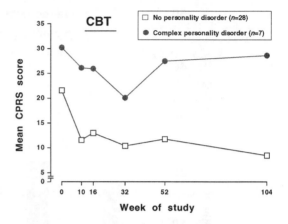

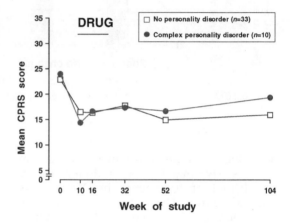

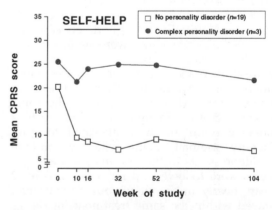

Figure 9.3 Influence of personality status in determining response to treatment (measured by change in symptoms on the Comprehensive Psychopathological Rating Scale (CPRS)) in patients with generalized anxiety disorder, dysthymic disorder or panic disorder randomized to drug treatment (mainly antidepressants after initial 10 weeks), cognitive and behaviour therapy (CBT) and self-help over 2 years. (For illustrative purposes the findings for personality difficulty and simple personality disorder are omitted in these figures.)

Outcome at this time was recorded from the information derived from both general practice and hospital notes and scored on a five-point scale (*Table 9.5*). The results showed that those with diffuse personality disorder had the worst outcome (*Figure 9.4*) and that neither treatment nor original diagnosis contributed anything of importance. The worst outcome was found in those who qualified for the diagnosis of hypochondriacal personality disorder at baseline assessment (*Figure 9.5*). Although there will continue to be dispute over the status of this condition as a personality disorder, as there is overlap with the hypochondriacal syndrome, its nearest neighbour in the classification (Tyrer *et al.*, 1999), the worse outcome of hypochondriacal personality disorder compared with other personality disorders is an empirical finding partly supporting the validity of the diagnosis.

Table 9.5 Outcome scale used to record good or poor outcome in neurotic disorder (after 5 years)

Code	Description	Number of patients (%)
Good	Very good: no psychiatric contact with either general practice or psychiatric services since initial period of care (up to 9 months)	50 (27)
Good	Good: some contact for psychiatric problems in general practice or psychiatric clinics but at least half time well	57 (31)
Poor	Fair: frequent contact with services for psychiatric problems for more than half of time of follow-up but intensity of care not great (e.g. short period of day-care, many outpatient contacts but no inpatient care)	38 (21)
Poor	Poor: little or no time in follow-up period well. Intermittent contact as outpatient or day-patient	28 (15)
Poor	Very poor: continuously ill with frequent contact with all parts of psychiatric services or death from deliberate self-harm	9 (5)
	Total	182

(Data from Seivewright *et al.*, 1998, reproduced with permission of *Psychological Medicine*)

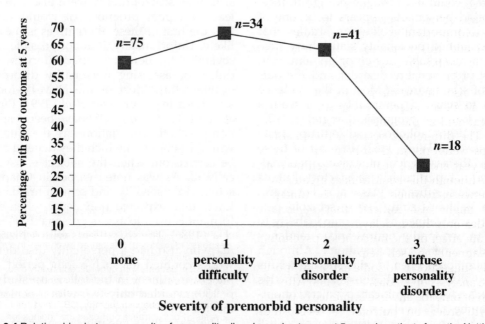

Figure 9.4 Relationships between severity of personality disorder and outcome at 5 years in patients from the Nottingham Study of Neurotic Disorder

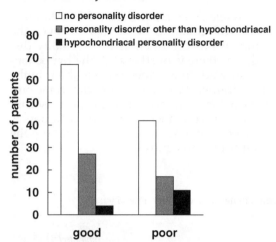

Figure 9.5 Five-year outcome in 168 patients with one of three neurotic disorders (generalized anxiety disorder, dysthymic disorder and panic disorder) separated by personality status on entry to the study. $\chi^2 = 6.8$; d.f. 2; $P < 0.05$. (Reproduced from Tyrer *et al.* 1999 with permission of the *Journal of Psychosomatic Research*.)

Outcome of schizophrenia in the presence of personality disorder

Schizophrenia has been subjected to more studies of outcome than almost any other psychiatric disorder. Among the many variables that could have prognostic significance, premorbid personality appears to be one of the most important. Follow-up studies that have examined personality status have produced a remarkable degree of unanimity in respect of personality disorder and the outcome of schizophrenia. Most of the evidence points to schizoid personality as a feature leading to a bad prognosis (Langfeldt, 1937; Rennie, 1939; Holmboe and Astrup, 1957; Vaillant, 1964; Wing, 1982). In most of these studies, the assessment of schizoid personality was not particularly satisfactory but its prognostic significance was major. For example, in Vaillant's study (1964), schizoid personality was defined as 'a chronic inability to relate to non-family figures and a tendency towards autistic preoccupation'. Although this definition is open to criticism, the results showed that clinical diagnosis made in this way was a highly significant predictor of outcome at the 0.1% level of significance. Thus 31 (24%) of 128 patients who did not achieve full remission from schizophrenia at follow-up

had a non-schizoid premorbid personality, whereas 29 (66%) of 44 patients who achieved full remission had a personality status that was non-schizoid.

These data are less impressive than they appear. All these studies employ unsatisfactory measures of personality assessment, but, more particularly, the natural history of schizophrenia makes it difficult to establish the difference between schizoid premorbid personality and an insidious onset (the prodrome) of schizophrenia. It is well established that an insidious onset of the condition also leads to a poor prognosis (Wing, 1982) and so it is possible that apparent schizoid personality traits are confused with the early symptoms of schizophrenia. The status of schizoid personality as a predisposing factor and prognostic indicator in schizophrenia is therefore open to some doubt. As Cutting (1985) puts it: 'it [schizoid personality] is a cause of schizophrenia in that the florid psychosis may supervene in someone with this personality when they encounter an event to which they cannot adapt', but 'in another sense it is not a cause because the personality and florid psychosis share a similar pattern of psychological dysfunction' (p. 124).

If other types of personality disorder that did not share the same psychological constructs as schizophrenia were also shown to lead to a poor prognosis, it would suggest that the first of these alternatives is the more likely. Unfortunately, it is not possible to use several of the new structured interview schedules for assessing personality disorder to evaluate this. Most of the DSM-IV–focused schedules (e.g. Loranger *et al.*, 1994; Pfohl *et al.*, 1994; First *et al.*, 1995) have been tested on non-psychotic populations as the interview with the subject on which they depend cannot be carried out when the subject is psychotically ill. As was noted earlier in Chapter 8, schizoid personality and schizophrenia has a lower than expected prevalence when an informant is used to assess personality (Cutting *et al.*, 1986). The six patients with schizophrenia who also had a personality disorder and who accounted for such a long period of inpatient treatment in the follow-up study (*see* p. 130) included only two with a personality disorder in the schizoid group.

There are also some indications from American studies that premorbid antisocial personality characteristics are associated with a poorer outcome in schizophrenia (e.g. Robins, 1966). These findings show that studies of outcome of established schizophrenia in the presence of personality disorder are difficult to carry out. In addition to the problem that most of the instruments available for assessing personality disorder rely so much on self-report, there is also the significant problem of personality change associated with schizophrenia, a phenomenon colloquially known as 'burn-out' which represents the trend towards a negative, anergic personality with little drive and motivation in the latter stages of the illness.

It is worth describing one recent study with which we have been involved in some detail. This is the UK700 case management trial, a randomized controlled trial in which 708 patients with recurrent psychosis were recruited in four centres and randomly allocated to intensive case management, with an average case load of 10–15 patients per worker, or to standard case management, with an average case load of 30–40 per worker (UK700 Group (Burns *et al.*), 1999).

A total of 708 patients was recruited from the four centres, three in London and one in Manchester. Fifty-six per cent were male, 41% were inpatients at the time of recruitment and the average age of the sample was 38 years. Although the project was concerned with recurrent psychosis it was essentially a sample of people with schizophrenic pathology. Diagnosis was made according to the OP-CRIT system (based on operational criteria for ICD and DSM classifications) (McGuffin *et al.*, 1991) and 345 (49%) of the sample had schizo-affective psychosis and 270 (38%) had schizophrenia, together with a further 6% with associated conditions within the schizophrenia group. It was therefore felt appropriate to include all the diagnoses in the analysis since only a fraction (7%) were not related to schizophrenia or diagnoses within the schizophrenia group.

Personality disorder and outcome

Personality status was recorded using the short version of the Personality Assessment Schedule (PAS-Q) before randomization. Those with personality disorder and psycho-

sis (dual diagnosis) were compared with those for psychoses alone (a) at baseline, (b) after 2 years.

The results of the baseline data are shown in *Table 9.6*. The results are generally similar to those of other studies, suggesting that the PAS-Q was indeed accessing premorbid personality status rather than consequences of illness. Symptoms, as recorded by the Comprehensive Psychopathological Rating Scale (CPRS), disability (recorded using the DAS), both met and unmet needs (recorded using the Camberwell Assessment of Need (CAN)) (Phelan *et al.*, 1995) and quality of life (using the Lancashire Quality of Life Scale) (Oliver *et al.*, 1997) were significantly greater in the patients with personality disorder at baseline. In evaluating the outcome after 2 years it was therefore important to adjust for these baseline differences.

The influence of personality status on outcome after 2 years was still substantial despite these baseline differences. The most marked difference was in the poorer quality of life of those with increasingly severe personality disorder, but symptomatic outcome was also worse, and patient dissatisfaction was greater in those with greater personality disturbance (*Table 9.7*). The results also show a generally linear change across the range of personality disorder which, despite the lessened sensitivity of the PAS-Q compared with the full PAS, suggests that the gradation of severity is a valid one.

The results of the study confirm yet again that the measurement of personality status in psychotic patients before treatment is a major predictor of outcome although many of the differences are present at baseline and must be adjusted for in studying the effects of personality disorder on outcome.

Affective psychoses

The nomenclature of personality in patients with affective psychoses is confused. In retrospect, it seems highly likely that many of the personality labels such as *melancholic* and *cyclothymic* described the disorder more accurately than the personality although there are some authorities (e.g. Glatzel, 1974; von Zerssen, 1982; von Zerssen and Akiskal, 1998) who disagree. It has also been noted on many

Table 9.6 Baseline data separated by personality status (UK700 project)

Variable		PAS-Q category				P-value[1,2]
		no disorder	difficulty	simple disorder	diffuse (complex) disorder	
No. of patients		259	225	118	68	
Age	Mean (sd)	38 (12)	39 (12)	37 (11)	38 (11)	0.35
	Range	17, 64	19, 65	19, 65	19, 65	
Female	%	44	43	40	47	0.80
OPCS ethnicity						0.68
Black Caribbean	%	29	25	26	31	
Age first psychiatric symptoms	Mean (sd)	26 (9)	26 (9)	24 (6)	25 (8)	0.11
	Range	14, 58	11, 59	15, 42	16, 53	
Months psychiatric inpatient since onset	Median (quartiles)	8	8	10	13.5	0.002
	Range	(4, 17)	(4, 16)	(4.75, 22)	(7, 29)	
		1,323	1,350	1,247	2,144	
Course type at baseline						0.03
episodic – no episode >6m	%	58	47	53	47	
continuous – no remission >6m	%	32	39	34	49	
neither	%	10	15	13	4	
CPRS at baseline	Mean (sd)	15.0 (11.3)	18.4 (12.0)	21.2 (12.0)	30.9 (15.0)	<0.001
	Range	0, 67	0, 71	1, 51	3, 79	
Quality of life at baseline	Mean (sd)	4.4 (0.7)	4.3 (0.8)	4.2 (0.7)	3.9 (0.6)	<0.001
	Range	2.2, 6.3	1.2, 6.5	1.8, 5.9	2.7, 5.7	
Unmet needs (CAN) at baseline	Mean (sd)	2.2 (2.1)	2.7 (2.4)	3.0 (2.5)	3.8 (2.3)	<0.001
	Range	0, 12	0, 11	0, 10	0, 11	
DAS total at baseline	Mean (sd)	0.91 (0.82)	1.12 (0.78)	1.38 (0.84)	1.82 (0.87)	<0.001
	Range	0, 4.71	0, 3.60	0.13, 4.75	0.29, 4.00	
Patient (dis)satisfaction at baseline	Mean (sd)	17.8 (4.9)	18.7 (4.6)	19.7 (4.7)	20.3 (4.2)	<0.001
	Range	9, 33	9, 36	9, 36	13, 33	

[1] Where percentages reported the Chi-Squared test was used, where means reported analysis of variance was used and where medians presented Kruskal Wallis test was used.
[2] Test of linear association with baseline CPRS, $P < 0.001$; baseline quality of life, $P < 0.001$; baseline unmet needs (CAN), $P < 0.001$; baseline DAS total, $P < 0.001$; baseline service (dis)satisfaction, $P < 0.001$.

Table 9.7 Comparison of 2-year clinical assessments between personality groups – analyses adjusted for baseline scores on outcome

Outcome	PAS-Q classification									P-value
	No personality disorder	n	Personality difficulty	n	Personality disorder	n	Diffuse disorder	n		
CPRS, mean (95% CI)	16.5 (14.7, 18.3)	202	19.4 (17.6, 21.2)	189	20.0 (17.5, 22.5)	96	16.3 (12.9, 19.7)	60		0.03
Quality of life, mean (95% CI)	4.72 (4.62, 4.81)	185	4.51 (4.42, 4.61)	172	4.45 (4.31, 4.59)	82	4.45 (4.26, 4.63)	50		0.002
Unmet needs (CAN), mean (95% CI)	1.73 (1.40, 2.06)	202	2.07 (1.74, 2.40)	195	2.17 (1.69, 2.65)	94	1.96 (1.36, 2.56)	60		0.38
DAS total, mean (95% CI)	1.00 (0.90, 1.10)	203	1.12 (1.02, 1.22)	191	1.22 (1.08, 1.36)	94	1.15 (0.95, 1.34)	55		0.08
Patient (dis)satisfaction (95% CI)	16.3 (15.6, 17.1)	146	17.1 (16.3, 17.9)	134	18.0 (16.9, 19.1)	65	18.0 (16.7, 19.2)	50		0.05

occasions in earlier chapters that personality characteristics appear to change during the course of an affective disorder and that questionnaires (which have been used mainly in outcome studies) are suspect for this reason. Thus studies that demonstrate a worse outcome in depressive illness in patients with high neuroticism scores on the Maudsley Personality Inventory (MPI) (e.g. Weissman and Klerman, 1977) could be criticized on methodological grounds.

Nevertheless, the findings are supported by one study that used the SIDP interview schedule (Pfohl *et al.*, 1982). Patients with severe depressive illness who required electroconvulsive therapy (ECT) as treatment for their depressive disturbance were assessed with the SIDP before treatment. Patients were assessed on their immediate response to the treatment and followed up 6 months later. It was found that there was no difference in initial response to ECT in patients with and without personality disorder, but at followup those patients who had been diagnosed as having personality disorder had experienced significantly greater numbers of depressive episodes in the 6 months than those without personality disorder (Zimmerman *et al.*, 1986). Although the numbers were small, the type of personality disorder did not have a major influence on this finding. Another unpublished study of depressed patients (Pfohl, personal communication) yielded similar findings with regard to antidepressant drug therapy; patients with personality disorder received more drug treatment over followup. It is, therefore, reasonable to conclude that personality disorder handicaps the outcome of affective disorder in a similar way to schizophrenia. The relationship is complicated because severe psychotic illness, both affective and schizophrenic, can create personality change which can then be interpreted as disorder.

Recognition of personality change as a diagnostic category is formalized in ICD-10 (F62.1). Akiskal and his colleagues (Akiskal *et al.*, 1980, 1983; Akiskal, 1983) have argued strongly for the view that some of the features of borderline personality disorder are postdepressive complications, in which case they should not really be classified as personality disorders. The position of dysthymic disorder is also problematical. If, indeed, there is a form of depressive disturbance that begins in early adult life and persists more or less to old age (Akiskal, 1983) then it would seem more reasonable to regard this as a personality disorder, probably equivalent to dysthymic personality disorder in the PAS classification. However, further outcome studies are needed to resolve this issue.

It should also be recognized that response to treatment in other forms of depression are also adversely affected by the presence of personality disorder, including typical major depressive episodes (Shea *et al.*, 1992), depression presenting as crisis (Andreoli *et al.*, 1993) and in day hospital psychotherapy (Piper *et al.*, 1994). These findings emphasize the need to 'develop treatment packages that are tailored to a patient's personality as well as the Axis I diagnosis' (Vize and Tyrer, 1994). One, probably inappropriate, outcome is prolonged attendance over many years at an outpatient clinic; many such patients may have other named psychiatric disorders but they appear to have predominant personality problems (Pomeroy and Ricketts, 1985).

Alcohol and drug dependence

There is considerable argument over the existence of an 'alcoholic personality' and the general view, established before adequate personality assessment procedures, is that such a personality does not exist (Barnes, 1979). Whether one accepts or disputes that personality disturbance is more common among patients with alcohol dependence, there is general agreement that there is not one type of personality that is specific to alcohol dependence and abuse. Outcome studies have suggested that certain personality types are more prone to become dependent on alcohol, although these have not been formalized in terms of personality disorder. In general, those who have personality characteristics that are aggressive, impulsive and anti-authoritarian are at greater risk of developing alcohol dependence and having a poor response to treatment than other types of personality (Cahalan and Room, 1974; Williams, 1976; DeJong *et al.*, 1993).

There have been few satisfactory studies of outcome in which initial assessment of personality could be regarded as independent of

current drinking state. There are also important differences between alcoholic populations depending on the type of service available. Personality classification based on the Minnesota Multiphasic Personality Inventory (MMPI) shows that, in addition to the impulsive and antisocial personality group, there is an anxious or fearful personality type (Goldstein and Linden, 1969; Whitelock *et al.*, 1971; Løberg, 1981). These personality types are fundamentally different and the presence of the fearful group gives credence to the notion that many with mild affective disturbance turn to alcohol for relief of symptoms in the first instance but then become dependent.

There have been several studies of the outcome of alcohol dependence using the newer structured interview schedules for assessing personality disorder since an early study using the PAS (Griggs and Tyrer, 1981). This was a small study involving 33 consecutively admitted patients with alcohol dependence who had their personality and social adjustment assessed immediately after admission. Outcome was assessed after a further 2 months, which is unsatisfactorily short. All the patients had been discharged from hospital by the time of follow-up. The findings were unusual in that there was evidence that one type of personality disorder, schizoid personality disorder, was associated with a significantly better outcome than other personality types, including normal personality. Patients with personality disorders in the sociopathic group did badly. There was only one patient in each of the passive–dependent and anankastic personality groups and both of these did well. The authors concluded that non-sociopathic abnormal personalities had drinking problems that had 'some of the features of symptomatic drinking, and is therefore more likely to respond to measures that generally improve social adjustment and life situation'. The relatively large proportion of schizoid personalities in the population was somewhat unexpected but a similar group has been identified using the MMPI (Goldstein and Linden, 1969).

Interestingly, there are several studies in the substance use literature that show no difference between the outcome of patients with substance misuse only and those with the dual diagnosis of substance misuse and personality disorder. Several studies have shown no difference in outcome between substance abusers with or without personality disorder (Clopton *et al.*, 1993; Darke *et al.*, 1994; Hoffman *et al.*, 1994) and these studies are noteworthy in demonstrating a trend against the general notion that personality disorder hinders response to treatment in all psychiatric disorders.

As with the other conditions described in this section, the distinction between alcohol dependence as a mental state disorder and abnormal personality is often difficult to maintain. Alcohol dependence has less status as an 'illness' than schizophrenia and the affective psychoses, and can be regarded as a behavioural problem that is a consequence of a personality disorder. Nevertheless, there is sufficient reason to believe that personality status is important both in the management and outcome of alcohol dependence and that some of the argument over the existence of the alcoholic personality is unproductive. There appear to be several types of personality abnormality that can be associated with alcohol dependence; these need to be delineated more carefully and studied with regard to outcome.

Summary

In the first edition of this book we commented 'the almost universal finding in studies of outcome of mental illness is that personality disorder of any type exerts a malign and negative influence' and that 'the individual nature of the personality disorder appears to be much less important than its severity in affecting outcome' (Tyrer and Seivewright, 1988). This broad brush statement may still be true in the general sense, but we are getting an increasing number of exceptions to the rule and some potentially important interactions between treatment and personality disorder that have a major influence on outcome. The finding that psychological treatments only tend to lead to a successful outcome in neurotic disorder when there is no personality disturbance, and that this factor is much less important in drug treatment, would be of great clinical value if the finding was replicated in other studies.

We have moved a long way since personality disorder was diagnosed in so many people *after* they had failed to respond to intervention and became synonymous with untreatability. However, until we assess all people coming for assessment for treatment with approaches that allow us to assess their personality status with some degree of confidence we cannot avoid this error and will continue to need reassurance that personality disorder is not being equated simply with a chronic course. Despite this caveat, the consistency of the findings suggests that personality disorder is indeed a major prognostic factor in all forms of mental illness. Study of disorders in which no established treatment exists is an excellent way of determining outcome and until we can identify which conditions improve or persist there is no yardstick by which we can measure the effectiveness of our interventions. Only after we have a clear knowledge of the natural history of a disorder can we judge where and when new treatments should be focused. Good outcome in personality disorder may be attainable, and whether it is achieved through time, treatment or the two together is immaterial, provided we know which is which.

10

Challenges for the future

Peter Tyrer

In the first edition of this book we concluded that five clear statements could be made about personality disorder but their full implications needed to be explored further:

1. Personality disorder is a necessary concept in clinical psychiatry because it describes a class of abnormality not included elsewhere in classification.
2. Personality disorder is a common accompaniment of mental state disorders and generally becomes more frequent with increasing severity of psychiatric illness.
3. The classification of personality disorder is unsatisfactory, but improving, and currently has too many categories.
4. Personality disorder is relatively enduring but there are different natural histories with different disorders.
5. Personality disorder generally has a negative effect on the outcome of other mental state disorders.

I think these are worth repeating because they do not seem out of date. In the last few years there has been a great deal of progress made in understanding personality disorders and it is now a much more prominent subject in both professional and lay minds than it was at the time of our first edition. Nonetheless, although advances have been made, the fundamental statements above are still worth repeating and the areas of dissatisfaction with the subject also remain the same. These are now asked in the form of questions that are

put by so many when they encounter this curious field of endeavour.

Can personality disorder be assessed reliably?

Although the answer to this question is a qualified 'yes' we have only made limited progress in the past 10 years. On the positive side we have seldom come across the old criticism that personality disorder is a pejorative term with no meaning apart from an indication of negative personal interaction. We also have much more reliable measures of recording the presence and absence of personality disorder than we had in the past but it is still much more difficult to get good agreement than for many other disorders in psychiatry. However, it has also become clear that the dividing line between 'normal' and 'disordered' personality is not a clear-cut one and there are many advantages in conceptualizing personality disorder as a dimensional condition, ranging from normal personality through to more severe personality disorders (Tyrer and Johnson, 1996).

The argument against the categorical and for a dimensional system have been put cogently by many who have been acknowledged in this volume, but of whom Lee Anna Clark and John Livesley are perhaps the most prominent and certainly among the most industrious. During the course of this they, and others such as Thomas Widiger and Ted Millon, contend that the DSM and ICD classifications of personality disorder are seriously flawed. They believe they are flawed because:

1. They are unreliable. The decision as to whether someone has a personality disorder or not in the broader sense is much more reliably assessed than the presence or absence of an individual disorder and sometimes the agreement between assessments for individual disorders are laughably poor (e.g. Perry, 1992; Bronisch and Mombour, 1994).
2. The diagnostic criteria are not specific, often address more than one trait, are difficult to define clearly, and only succeed when they describe traits rather than what are called 'prototypic behaviours' (Blashfield *et al.*, 1985).
3. There is so much overlap between the personality disorder categories where possession of several personality disorders is the norm and that of a single entity noteworthy through its rarity, that the validity of these categories is seriously in doubt.
4. The ability to separate personality status from mental state is still difficult, particularly in the presence of chronic illness, so the ability to discriminate between those aspects of disorder which are a consequence of personality and those which are secondary to mental state cannot be achieved by operational criteria alone.
5. The distinction between 'normal' and 'abnormal' personality is to a great extent artificial, as the same structure of personality is shown in populations with or without personality disorder (Tyrer and Alexander, 1979; Schroeder and Livesley, 1991).

Predicting the way forward is far from easy. What is clear is that the system of classification based on operational criteria for personality disorder is, if not already dead, in terminal decline, although, like all classifications that reach acceptance through painful compromise and debate, it will take a long time before it officially leaves the scene. It looks most likely to be replaced by one of two options. The first is to eliminate Axis II from the DSM classification (it is still classified with mental state disorders in ICD-10) and replace the personality axis by a set of higher and lower order dimensional characteristics along the lines suggested by the work of Livesley *et al.* (1998). There is no doubt that this would lead to a more reliable system of classification that would allow every individual to be classified for major personality traits, but it would be somewhat cumbersome to use in practice and, perhaps unfairly, would be resisted by practitioners. The second is to abandon most of the individual categories of personality disorder and reform them into the three or four major groups and to score each of them in a dimensional format, probably covering four to five categories. The three clusters of the DSM classification personality disorders; A (odd or eccentric), B (flamboyant or dramatic) and C (anxious or fearful) would be obvious candidates but, as a number of factor analytical and cluster analysis studies have shown, a fourth group of obsessional or anankastic personalities also merits separate status (Tyrer and Alexander, 1979; Schroeder and Livesley, 1991; Mulder and Joyce, 1995). This latter system would effectively combine dimensional and categorical classifications but would be confined to a much more limited number of personality disorders. It may also have the advantage of destigmatizing the diagnostic label 'personality disorder' by emphasizing that all these conditions are on a continuum.

In the course of this debate it would help greatly if there was an internationally accepted assessment for personality disorder. Unfortunately, the presence of so many different instruments for recording personality disorder indicates that none can be really satisfactory and the lack of agreement between them (Reich, 1987; Perry, 1992) is so poor that it is extremely difficult to achieve international comparisons.

At the Third European Congress for the Study of Personality Disorders in July 1998 the following targets were set by the Executive Committee during the course of the meeting (Tyrer, 1998b):

1. The routine assessment of personality status in all patients presenting to psychiatric services using an internationally accepted procedure.
2. Separate recognition of those with severe personality disorder requiring specialized interventions, also using an internationally accepted procedure.
3. At least one centre of excellence devoted to

the study and treatment of personality disorder.

4. At least one centre of excellence devoted to research into personality disorder.

5. At least one national centre devoted to the training of all staff involved in the treatment of severe personality disorder with the establishment of a formal qualification to achieve common standards and competence.

6. The establishment of audit and monitoring systems for all specialized services involved in the treatment of personality disorders so that competence and standards of care and treatment are maintained.

The first two of these are heavily dependent on achieving rationalization in assessment of personality disorder. Because of the increasing use of the term 'severe personality disorder' it becomes even more important to get the classification system right. One of the reasons why severe personality disorder has become so important is that it has now been adopted by planners and politicians in trying to identify this small group of individuals who cause major problems to society as a consequence of personality disturbance. It is a relatively safe prediction that in the next 10 years we will have better identification of what constitutes severe personality disorder and more robust ways of assessing it.

Is personality disorder persistent?

According to the ICD-10 and DSM-IV classifications personality disorder is 'stable and of long duration, having its onset in late childhood or adolescence' and 'pervasive' (World Health Organization, 1993; American Psychiatric Association, 1994). The data from a large number of sources now suggest that personality disorder (and almost certainly personality in normal individuals) changes significantly over the course of time but this should be measured in years rather than months or weeks. It would therefore be quite wrong to assume that, for example, some treatment measure given to a group of people with personality disorders would necessarily be responsible for improvement in that personality disorder if assessment was made, say, 2 years later. To establish efficacy of the intervention a control group not exposed to that intervention would be necessary. Unfortunately such controlled studies have not been carried out and suggestions that such improvement is a consequence of treatment, such as has been the case of many studies of psychoanalytical psychotherapy, should be regarded as premature. The conclusions that might be drawn from the data available to date are summarized in *Table 10.1*.

It is reasonable to conclude that the time course of the three clusters shows differences

Table 10.1 Developmental history of personality disorders

Cluster of personality disorder	Individual personality categories	Change over time
A (Odd and eccentric)	Schizoid Schizotypal (DSM only) Paranoid	Relatively persistent with possible tendency to increase with advancing age; however, if the features of disorder are very marked initially there is more likely to be improvement over time
B (Flamboyant or dramatic)	Antisocial (dissocial) Borderline Impulsive Histrionic Narcissistic	Significant improvement by age of 40 or 50, sometimes with full resolution of disorder
C (Anxious or fearful sometimes including obsessive–compulsive also)	Anxious (Avoidant) Dependent (Hypochondriacal) (Dysthymic) (Depressive)	Usually shows improvements if traits in personality disorder marked in early life but in others tends to persist at mild or moderate levels of severity

and that in general the findings support the view that it is useful to conceptualize personality disorders in this way. There is even some support for the existence of the fourth cluster of obsessionality or compulsivity in that this group of symptoms is more likely to be persistent than the other conditions in cluster C. The notion of universal persistence of personality disorders cannot be sustained, however, and it is worth while spreading the word that these disorders are not necessarily brands for life and can change.

It is also possible to think of these three groups in developmental terms. The cluster B personality features, occurring early in life and often maturing in middle age, can be viewed as either 'immature personality disorders' as suggested in the first edition of this book (Tyrer and Seivewright, 1988) or as disorders of arrested development that retain many of the primitive egotistical features of personality until they have completed the full cycle of maturation.

What is severe personality disorder?

Sometimes descriptions that are considered unscientific and invalid become so much part of common parlance that in the end it is impossible to ignore them. Although the lay tail should not wag the scientific dog a practical and effective classification has to take notice. It is probably true of severe personality disorder. Although no psychiatric classification exists for this concept it is being used widely by dozens of agencies and by those who are not immediately concerned with diagnostic practice but find it necessary to separate one group from the main body of those with personality disturbance. In one way the persistence of this term demonstrates the failure of the current classification system. A good classification is one that is clinically useful and when a term turns out to be clinically useful but not in the classification the rules may have to be changed.

In Chapter 4 it was argued that a classification based on severity in which the different clusters of personality disorder become significant through their number rather than their type, is the best way of recording severity. Severe personality disorder is characterized by gross societal disturbance and it is surely right that this should be at least a putative group within the classification of personality disorder. Of course, it may not achieve satisfactory reliability and validity at its first attempt but there seems little doubt that this term is likely to stay no matter how many at present may be antagonized by it.

The Personality Assessment Schedule (PAS), based on a quantitative assessment of traits and their impact on social functioning, relies on a computer algorithm to create the diagnosis of severe personality disorder. The diagnosis is made in a setting of a full personality assessment and is an advance for diagnostic guidelines or operational criteria for just making the separation between severe personality disorders and all other groups, including all the 'non-severe' personality disorders. In *Table 10.2*, the suggested characteristics that should separate the two groups are listed; they just represent a checklist at this point and may merit further examination.

Table 10.2 Differences between severe and other personality disorders

Severe personality disorder	All other personality disorders
Affects many people (usually more than 50)	Affects fewer than 20 people except under special circumstances
Is usually associated with antisocial behaviour	Usually associated with problems in relationships independently of antisocial behaviour
Represents a threat to society	Is not a threat to society
Serious law-breaking behaviour is common and, if detected, leads to criminal conviction	If law-breaking shown, less often involved with criminal conviction
Significant danger of violence towards others and self as a consequence of personality disorder	Little danger of violence to others, but self-harm often a significant problem
Severe disruption in all relationships and behaviour as a consequence of personality disorder	Despite problems in relationships and behaviour there are usually islands of normal function

Deciding what constitutes severe personality disorder is an important clinical question and will have to remain categorical in most countries if services are to operate effectively. It is likely that units for those with severe personality disorder are going to increase rather than decrease in number and, if the diagnosis is to have any meaning, it should be robust enough to determine admission to such units. At present the diagnosis is made in an idiosyncratic way and often decided upon after an episode of disturbed behaviour rather than before. Further work also needs to be done on the vexed issue of risk assessment. From the point of view of the public this assessment primarily concerns the risk of violence and until we have a clear idea of the circumstances which reduce or increase the risk in any particular circumstance, we will not know whether any intervention is successful.

Can personality disorder be separated cleanly from mental state disorders?

This will be one of the major battlefields in personality disorder research in the next 10 years. The two armies are equally matched and it is difficult to foresee the outcome. At the outset, however, it is now generally accepted that the present system of classification and attempted separation has failed and cannot long be sustained. However, like all juggernauts of great weight, it will take some time before it is arrested and subsequently dismantled. In its place we will either have a hierarchical or dimensional system of classification.

The hierarchical system is one that combines simplified categorical systems linked to severity of disorder. As other sections of this book suggest, this is a model that we would prefer to see for several reasons:

1. It allows a full range of personality disturbance to be classified in a clinically useful way.
2. It allows the severity of personality to be classified as well as the type.
3. It simplifies the current classification and reduces inappropriate overlap (comorbidity).

4. It continues to emphasize that personality disorder is a different dimension of classification from mental state disorders so that disorders of personality are always considered in classification.

Provided that assessment gives an accurate description of personality status the hierarchical system offers the opportunity to classify intermediate levels of personality abnormality in such a way that the diagnosis of 'personality disorder' is destigmatized to some extent. By confining diagnoses to the four major clusters of personality disorder (possibly refined since they do not fit the empirical evidence derived from dimensions entirely) (Schroeder and Livesley, 1991), the amount of overlap between diagnoses is kept to a minimum and any comorbidity is also recognized in the severity of classification. The system also allows a gradual change in the straitjacket imposed by the current classifications of DSM-IV and ICD-10 without abandoning the old system entirely.

The dimensional system has been promulgated strongly by Thomas Widiger, John Livesley and Lee Anna Clark. They point to the much greater reliability achieved in personality assessment when personality traits are assessed and judged that the best form of classification is one that assesses all these traits on a separate axis but does not include diagnostic categories as these have demonstrably failed to be of value in the current system. The value of the dimensional approach is that:

1. It is demonstrably more reliable than the categorical system.
2. It avoids the problem of comorbidity between Axis I and Axis II disorders as the first will now be recorded by categorical diagnoses and the second by a separate dimensional one.
3. It completely destigmatizes personality assessment as everyone, no matter whether non-disordered or having a severe personality disorder, would have a score on the scale.

Although this model is one that provides the 'best fit' for existing data it may not recommend itself to the average clinicians. I sometimes repeat the unfair answer to the question, 'what is the difference between the psychologist and the psychiatrist?', to which the answer is 'a psychiatrist thinks in categories and a psychologist in dimensions'. Although this is an exaggeration there is no doubt that psychiatrists, and indeed all doctors, find categories much easier to understand and, when executive decisions are necessary, much more appropriate. There is also uncertainty in the dimensional system whether Axis II (in DSM-VI and beyond) will be retained for personality disorder. Certainly there is no other part of the classification of medicine in which dimensions are used in a diagnostic system, and it is certainly unlikely that the *International Classification of Disease* would allow one to exist.

Whatever system is chosen it will still be important to identify personality as a separate component of possible pathology independently from mental state assessment. In this process, illustrated in the flow chart (*Figure 10.1*), several forms of assessment, ranging from the medium of the semi-structured interview through to information derived from past records, will be necessary.

Can personality disorder be successfully treated, both as a primary and secondary condition?

It is a common truism that diagnoses that are considered untreatable possess the most degree of stigma and those that respond well have the least. This was demonstrated dramatically in the early 1960s after the introduction of successful antidepressants. The diagnosis of depression, formerly in the doldrums, became extremely popular and all sorts of conditions became re-labelled as depression in order to allow them to be treated with antidepressants. The ultimate example of this

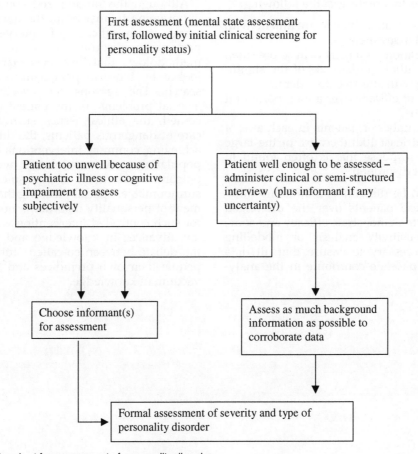

Figure 10.1 Flowchart for assessment of personality disorder

was the Italian condition 'depressione sine depressione' (depression without depression) which seemed to allow practitioners to make the diagnosis of depression for almost everyone who consulted them.

If any treatment for personality could be proved to be demonstrably effective, or indeed reliably improve the prognosis of a mental state disorder comorbid with personality disorder, it would represent a seismic advance in the subject. At present, despite many encouraging preliminary studies, no treatment has been found to be effective. The best examples of 'near-efficacy' are the studies of new antidepressants (selective serotonin re-uptake inhibitors – SSRIs) in the treatment of borderline personality disorder (Markowitz *et al.*, 1991; Fava *et al.*, 1994; Salzman *et al.*, 1995; Verkes *et al.*, 1998a) and studies using therapeutic community methods (Menzies *et al.*, 1993; Dolan *et al.*, 1996, 1997). However, such studies will have to be rigorous ones that require *all* the following:

1. Randomized allocation to treatment with independent assessment.
2. Demonstration of efficacy in more than borderline pathology (because of the significant overlap with affective disorders).
3. Evidence of efficacy over a long period (at least 3 months).
4. A large number of patients in each arm of the study (at least 100) (because of the large variance in response that is often found in this group of disorders).

It might also be difficult to maintain follow-up with these patients over the prolonged time period to demonstrate efficacy and some forms of sensitivity analysis or modelling might be necessary to ensure that all data after initial baseline contribute in the analysis.

Although it is sometimes stated by those involved in personality disorder research that these requirements are impossible to achieve in this difficult population I think it would be a great mistake to abandon tried and tested methods, whatever their difficulties in execution, for something which will almost certainly be second rate by comparison.

The generally poor outcome of comorbid personality disorders and mental state conditions also needs attention using the mechanism of the randomized controlled trial. This may be an easier obstacle to overcome, and if methods of treatment can be introduced which will offset the negative impact of personality disorder on outcome they will be of extreme value. Obvious ones include aids to compliance in this group, including the recently introduced compliance therapy (Kemp *et al.*, 1996, 1998) and the behavioural techniques for dialectical behaviour therapy introduced by Linehan (1995).

Although the randomized controlled trial is not going to answer all the questions concerned with efficacy of interventions for personality disorder it is an important methodology that has been largely overlooked by those in personality disorder research. The reasons for rejecting it, the 'special problems' of the patient group concerned, the ethical issues surrounding the care of dangerous patients, the difficulties in achieving common interventions in a fickle population, and uncertainties over primary outcomes and choice of assessments, are all surmountable. Special pleading that the treatment of personality disorder is not yet ready for such controlled intervention will only delay advances in knowledge and perpetuate the debate between so-called 'authorities' to peddle their own prejudices and beliefs in a vacuum of knowledge.

Appendix 1

Personality Assessment Schedule (PAS) – original version

Peter Tyrer, John Alexander and Brian Ferguson

This schedule is designed to formalize the assessment of personality disorder and may be used with any subject irrespective of psychiatric status. The way in which the schedule is used will depend on the current mental state of the patient and an assessment of this is a necessary precursor to the personality ratings. It is recommended that the screening schedule of the Present State Examination or SCID (Structured Clinical Interview for DSM-III) be used for the mental state examination, but, if this is not possible, sufficient information should be obtained from the history and examination to make a diagnostic formulation of any psychiatric problems, which should be recorded on the assessment form. If this is not carried out there is a danger that the personality ratings will be contaminated by the mental state.

There are 24 personality variables to be assessed in the schedule. Each of these can be rated by interview with the subject and interview with an informant.

An interview with an informant is desirable in all cases. The interview with the subject is not necessary if he or she is unable to give coherent answers to questions because of gross abnormalities in mental state; the interview with the informant indicates that there has been a marked *qualitative* change in the subject's personality so that replies to questions about past personality are unlikely to be correct; the subject displays severe memory disturbance, whether of organic or psychological origin, and is unable to recall aspects of his premorbid state. If an interview with an informant is not possible, additional independent information about personality may be obtained from other sources (e.g. general practitioner, social worker, probation officer), if this information is considered valid. If several informants are available the final score can be a composite of those in which the most reliable informant carried the greatest weight.

Use of the schedule

(1) The initial questions for each personality variable are obligatory. The questions preceded by an asterisk are amplifying questions which may be asked in response to the subject's initial reply. The questions in brackets are direct closed questions which may be asked if replies to other questions have been evasive, contradictory or vague. Although the questions are confined to a specific personality variable there is sometimes overlap with other variables. It may therefore be necessary to re-rate the variable later in the interview.

(2) *Ratings of severity:* The ratings are made on a nine-point scale for all variables. The number is recorded in the appropriate box at the side of each item or an accompanying sheet. The scale is specifically designed to record abnormal personality traits and most normal variation will occur between scores 0 and 3. The greater the severity of the trait the greater will be the rating. In addition to the specific points mentioned for each scale, the following general principles should be used to determine the score for a particular trait. (The word trait is synonymous with personality variable in this account, although it is less often used for severe personality disturbance.)

0 Trait absent. Presence of the trait is undetected both in respect of feelings and behaviour.

1 Subject recognizes the presence of the trait but it is shown chiefly in terms of feelings rather than behaviour. When the trait does affect behaviour, it is not an habitual response so much as a tendency to indulge more in that type of behaviour when several choices are open. Knowledge of how the subject spends spare time may help with this rating, as it is in spare time activities that the element of choice is most obviously shown. (An informant is unlikely to make a distinction between 0 and 1 ratings.)

2 Personality trait is definitely present and affects behaviour, but only to a limited extent. It is not associated with problems in occupational, social and interpersonal life. The changes in behaviour produced by the trait are such that those close to the subject will notice them but most friends and acquaintances would not.

3 The personality trait markedly affects feelings and behaviour. The presence of the trait may be noticed by others who are not closely related to the subject and may occasionally give rise to the problems in occupational, social and interpersonal life. However, these problems will seldom be persistent and those around the subject can normally accommodate to them without much difficulty.

4 The personality trait is marked and is apparent to the subject and to most people who have frequent contact with the subject. The trait produces some difficulties in occupational, social and interpersonal adjustment and this tends to be of a mild but persistent nature.

5 The personality trait is marked to both the subject and most people who come into contact with the subject. It has a marked influence on behaviour and leads to problems in occupational, social and interpersonal relationships. This rating differs from 4 in that the problems lead to more serious difficulties in adjustment in society and marked underachievement (e.g. inability to settle in one job, refusal to meet people, episodic aggression).

6 Personality trait has a major influence on behaviour and tends to affect all aspects of life. The problems in occupational, social and interpersonal relationship are such that major breakdown occurs (e.g. divorce, social isolation, prolonged unemployment), as a direct result of the personality abnormality.

7 The personality trait is so marked that it is noticed by almost all who come in contact with the subject, even those who only see the subject once. Independent life in the community is impossible because of the severity in occupational, social and interpersonal relationships so some form of supervision or continuous support is necessary.

8 The personality trait dominates behaviour completely (therefore it cannot be given to more than one rating in the schedule). The disturbance produced by the trait is so marked that prolonged periods of institutional care (e.g. hospital, prison, nursing home) take up a large part of the life history in the absence of any formal illness.

Note: most normal variation is accounted for between the ratings of 0 and 3. Only a small number of individuals rate higher scores than 3. The key issues in deciding whether a score of more than 3 is justified are:

(*a*) The production of problems in daily living because of the severity of the trait.
(*b*) The suffering and underachievement that the trait produces.
(*c*) The inability of those around the subject to deal with these problems without asking for additional (often professional) help.

An informant's information is primarily of value for ratings of 3 and upwards. A reliable subject is best fitted to rate lower ratings as these have little or no persistent effect on behaviour.

(3) In all instances of abnormal personality traits try and get the subject or informant to provide examples of the problems produced by the trait.
(4) Assess the reliability of the subjects' and informants' replies at the end of interview and score on the nine-point scale. Wherever the informants' and subjects' ratings for an item differ by three or more points ask further questions, and where possible, obtain independent information about the trait in question.

Additional notes on PAS

Procedure for scoring

It will be noticed on the final scoring sheet there is a space for 'the final score'. If the reliability of the informant's ratings is considered to be greater than the subject's ratings or equal to them, the final score will normally consist of the informant's ratings alone. If, however, the difference between informant's and subject's ratings for a personality attribute is greater than two points, it is advisable to ask further questions to establish the reasons for the discrepancy, possibly with both informant and subject present together. On an individual item it may also be considered that the subject's ratings are more reliable than those of the informant even though the rest of the ratings may be more accurately determined by the informant. In such instances the scoring may more closely approximate to the subject's ratings for that item.

If the subject's ratings are to be considered more reliable than those of the informant (which is particularly likely if the informant is not a close relative and has only known the subject for a limited period), the subject's ratings will take greater precedence in the final scoring. However, any informant rating that is greater than 3 must be carefully followed up by further questioning if it significantly disagrees with that of the subject. This is because any abnormal behaviour as a consequence of the personality attribute is likely to be more accurately detected by the informant than by the subject.

If an informant is not available, the subject's ratings alone can be used although this is much less satisfactory than having the informant's ratings also. If the subject's ratings are to be used, as much independent information as possible about premorbid personality is needed to corroborate the subject's ratings. This may be possible from past medical or social records but useful facts (p. 143) recording major life events may also be useful. This is administered before the PAS, preferably with other independent information as well, and any relevant positive findings introduced at the appropriate point in the PAS when this is administered subsequently. The subject will then have to explain the reasons for the apparently abnormal behaviour and, if the abnormality is judged to be related to a personality attribute, it will be scored appropriately. The additional schedule therefore serves in some way as a lie schedule.

When scoring each rating use the notes below each personality trait for guidance only. The scoring should follow the principles outlined in pages 133 and 134 for all traits.

Comparison of scores in different subgroups of patients

The individual scores for personality attributes can be compared separately by the usual statistical methods. The investigator may, however, wish to know to which category of personality each patient belongs. A program based on cluster analysis is available, which places each patient into one of five personality groups: normal, sociopathic, passive–dependent, anankastic or schizoid (Tyrer and Alexander, 1979). If investigators would like to know how their patients are classified according to their system they may either obtain a copy of the program (Tyrer and Tyrer, 1997) from Peter Tyrer at the Paterson Centre, London W2 1PD, or, alternatively, use the scoring system on pages 156 to 159 to categorize the disorders. Additional classification with modified questions suitable for DSM-III diagnostic categories is also available from the above address if required. Details of hand scoring of schedules are also available for those who do not have access to a computer; these are given on pp. 164–167.

Useful facts

Sometimes both subjects and informants have a distorted impression of previous personality and make it sound more favourable than it really was. The rater therefore needs as much information as possible about the patient's past experience so that these can be introduced into the questioning at relevant points in the interview. Below is a list of some of the important events that are affected frequently by personality characteristics. The rater should have information about these events, preferably obtained independently, before the interview. If this is not possible questions should be put to both subject and informant during the interview. It would be wrong to assume that any of these events are necessarily associated with personality abnormality but they are useful anchor points around which questions about personality can be asked. If there are serious discrepancies between independent evidence of these events and the subject's or informant's responses the rater should resolve these before making a final score for that personality item. As in other parts of the schedule independently derived information is given greater weight when making this decision.

(1) *Marital relationship* – if unmarried has the subject ever cohabited? If married or divorced how many times have the couple separated for any reason during marriage?

(2) *Child care.* Have there been any problems with the children of the patient? Have any children been involved with the police or official agencies and have they ever been in care?

(3) *Has the subject ever been in debt?* What were the circumstances?

(4) *Employment.* How many jobs has the subject had since leaving school? What were the circumstances of leaving these jobs? Was the subject ever sacked from a job or did they leave because of problems with colleagues?

(5) *Legal.* Has the subject ever been convicted of an offence? If so, what was the offence and outcome?

(6) *Does the subject drink alcohol, take illegal drugs or gamble?* If so, have any problems arisen as a consequence of these activities?

(7) *Housing.* How many addresses has the subject had in the last 10 years? What were the reasons for moving? Has the subject ever been homeless?

(8) *Adolescent problems.* Did the subject have any problems when attending school after the age of 11? If so, what was the outcome?

Interview procedure

It is helpful to have a check list of ratings of severity for each personality trait and the 'useful facts' above when interviewing the patient or informant. These are appended and may be detached for ease of reference when interviewing. The list of facts may be completed after the interview if necessary.

Subject
I am going to ask you some questions about the type of person you are normally.

*I am trying to find out what you were like before your present problems began.

In answering these questions I would therefore like you to think about your personality as it has been throughout your life. I am going to ask you some more questions about this but first of all how would you describe your personality in a few words? (Note main features and record on sheet at end of schedule.)

Informant
I am going to ask you some questions about the type of person S is normally.

*I am trying to find out what S was like before his/her present problems began.

In answering these questions I would therefore like you to think about S's personality as it has been throughout his/her life. I am going to ask you some more questions about this but first of all how would you describe S's personality in a few words? (Note main features and record on sheet at end of schedule.)

1. PESSIMISM

Subject
Do you get depressed easily or are you reasonably cheerful?
Are you pessimistic or optimistic about the future or do you just take it as it comes?

(1)

*Have you always felt depressed and low spirited, or has this only happened recently?
*Do other people notice it? (Give examples)

(Has this affected you at work, at home and with friends? In what way?)
(Have you ever thought seriously about suicide?)

Further questions may be needed to separate episodes of depressive illness from persistent depressive attitudes and behaviour.

Informant
Does S get depressed easily or is he/she reasonably cheerful?
Is he/she pessimistic or optimistic about the future or does he/she just take it as it comes?

☐
(2)

*Has S always felt depressed and low spirited or has this only happened recently?
*Does S appear gloomy to other people?

(Has this affected him/her at work, at home and with friends? In what way?)
(Do people avoid S because he/she is so miserable?)

Subject/Informant

Note	Ratings 1–3	A pessimistic outlook on life with no effect on behaviour.
	Ratings 4–6	Depressive behaviour including social withdrawal and morbid depression to the extent that others notice and are affected by the behaviour.
	Ratings 7–8	Persistent pessimism and depressive behaviour with almost complete withdrawal and isolation.

Ratings of 5 and above are only justified when depressive feelings and behaviour, associated with hopelessness about the future, are present or have been present in the absence of formal psychiatric illness. Do not include recurrent depressive illness in this category unless the personality between episodes is also abnormal or there is evidence that S has been clinically depressed all his/her life. Short periods of pessimism or depressed feelings of less than two weeks should be regarded as evidence of lability of mood rather than evidence of abnormal pessimism. If in doubt delay rating until lability trait scored.

2. WORTHLESSNESS

Subject
How do you think of yourself in relation to other people? Do you feel better, worse, or about the same?

☐
(3)

*Do you feel inferior to others? In what way? For how long?
*How does it affect you?

(Have you always felt like this or only just recently?)

*Do you think your life would have been different if you did not feel inferior to others? In what way?

(Do you feel useless or worthless most of the time?)
(Have you ever thought you deserved more out of life?)
(How would you feel if you were promoted at work?)

Informant
How does S think of himself/herself in relation to other people?
Does he/she feel better, worse, or about the same?

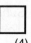
(4)

*Does he/she feel inferior to others?
*Do others notice this?

(Has he/she always felt like this or only just recently?)

*Does he/she think his/her life would have been different if he/she did not feel inferior to others? In what way?

(Does S feel useless or worthless most of the time?)

Subject/Informant

Note	Ratings 1–3	Mild feelings of inferiority, fully compensated and not obviously apparent to others.
	Ratings 4–6	Strong feelings of inferiority, affecting behaviour. Subject will not do things he/she is capable of because of abnormally low self-esteem. At least some impairment at work and social adjustment.
	Ratings 7–8	Strong feelings of inferiority amounting to worthlessness. Because of these feelings subject requires continuous reassurance and support. Not able to work regularly or make any useful relationship.

Do not confuse worthlessness with depression although the two often coexist.

3. OPTIMISM

Subject
I asked earlier whether you were normally a cheerful person. (Refer to answer)

(5)

*Are you more or less cheerful than most other people?
Have you always felt very cheerful no matter what has been happening in your life?

*Sometimes cheerfulness and over-confidence can lead to difficulties in life, such as overspending or making plans to do something which cannot succeed. Is this true of you?
*Would you describe yourself as too optimistic? (Examples of problems associated with optimism.)

*Have you any special abilities that make you feel optimistic and successful?

(Have you ever been in debt or got into trouble in any way because of over-confidence?)

Exclude problems associated with irresponsibility or childishness.

Informant
I asked earlier whether S was normally a cheerful person. Do you think of S as cheerful? Would others describe him/her as cheerful? Has S always felt very cheerful no matter what has been happening in his/her life?

(6)

*Sometimes even cheerfulness can lead to difficulties in life, such as overspending or making plans to do something which cannot succeed.
*Would you describe S as too optimistic? (Examples of problems associated with optimism.)

*Does S think of himself/herself as a special person who is bound to succeed?
(Has S ever been in debt or got into trouble in any way because of over-confidence?)

Subject/Informant

Note	Ratings 1–3	Subject is more cheerful than most others and is capable of communicating his/her cheerfulness to them.

Ratings 4–6   Over-cheerfulness leads to unrealistic ambitions and aspirations, including overspending, over-confidence and impaired judgement, so subject may be sacked from work or be in serious debt. Subject remains optimistic and self-important in spite of these problems.

Ratings 7–8   Breakdown in relationships, inability to maintain stability in any aspect of social, occupational or interpersonal life because of abnormal cheerfulness, over-optimism and self-importance.

To merit a high rating the optimism has to be more or less continuous and not part of the manic phase of manic depressive illness. Short periods of abnormal optimism of less than 2 weeks should be regarded as evidence of lability of mood rather than evidence of abnormal optimism. If in doubt delay rating till lability trait scored.

4. LABILITY

Subject

Do your spirits ⎫ change from day to day or week to week, or do they/does it remain more
Does your mood ⎭ or less the same

☐

(7)

*Are these changes connected with what is going on in your life or are they separate?

*How long do they last?
*Do they lead to problems?
(Can you predict your changes in mood?)
(How often do you laugh and cry?)

Informant
Does S's mood change from day to day or week to week, or does it remain more or less the same?

☐

(8)

*Are these changes connected with what is going on in his/her life or are they independent?
*How long do they last?
*Do other people notice these changes? Do they lead to problems?

(Is S unpredictable because of these sudden changes in mood?)
(How often does he/she laugh and cry?)
(Do you ever feel that he/she can turn these feelings on when he/she wants?)

Subject/Informant
Note   Ratings 1–3   A tendency towards mild exaggeration of mood swings in response to life changes.

             Ratings 4–6   Marked lability, noticeable to others and leading to problems because of strength of mood swings. Most mood changes responsive to life events but may be independent. Unpredictability of subject's behaviour because of mood change also a source of difficulties.

             Ratings 7–8   Breakdown in social, occupational and personal relationship because of abnormal swings in mood. In these instances it would be more likely that the changes are independent of life events so that they cannot be manipulated in any way. What is known as 'cyclothymia' will be included here if the swings in mood occur at least as frequently as once every 2 weeks. If they occur less frequently than this, but still produce important personality problems, then the relevant rating should be included under the pessimism and optimism scales.

5. ANXIOUSNESS

Subject

Are you normally an anxious or a calm person?
When things go wrong in your life (e.g. illness in family, accident) do you get more nervous, the same or less nervous than most people?

(9)

*Do you ever worry about things that most people would not be concerned about?
(Give examples)
*Do you show your nervousness to other people or do you cover it up?
*Have you always been an anxious person?

(Do you worry about something or someone most of the time?)
(Has your anxiety ever led to problems?) (Specify)

Informant

Is S normally an anxious or a calm person?
When things go wrong in his/her life (e.g. illness in family, accident) does he/she get more nervous, the same or less nervous than most people?

(10)

*Does S every worry about things that most people would not be concerned about?
(Give examples)
*Do other people notice that S is an anxious person or does he/she keep it to himself/herself?
*How has this worrying affected S?

(Does S worry about something or someone most of the time?)

Subject/Informant

Note	Ratings 1–3	Mild anxiety-proneness which is normally suppressed so that others are not aware of it.
	Ratings 4–6	Anxiety noticeable to others, leading to changes in behaviour.
	Ratings 7–8	Frequent or continuous free-floating anxiety of such severity that breakdown in social adjustment occurs.

Life-long phobic anxiety may contribute to this rating but the severity of the rating would depend on the same categories mentioned in the outline to scoring (i.e. it is the extent to which it interferes with personal and social adjustment that determines the rating).

6. SUSPICIOUSNESS

Subject

How well in general do you get on with other people?
Do you normally trust them or are you suspicious of them, at least at first?
How long does it take for you to get to know people before you will trust them?

(11)

*Do you tend to worry what is going on behind your back?
*Do you ever think that other people might be against you or criticize you unfairly?

(Have you many friends?)
(Are you worried in case someone might find out what you have been saying to me?)

Informant

How well in general does S get on with other people?
Does S normally trust them or is he/she suspicious of them, at least at first?
How long does it take for him/her to get to know people before he/she will trust them?

(12)

*Would you say that S is a suspicious person?
*Does he/she have many friends? (If yes) Is this because he/she will not trust anybody?
*Is S a jealous person?

Subject/Informant

Note	Ratings 1–3	Mild feelings of suspiciousness, not noticed by others. Subject tends to have relatively few friends but is capable of close relationships and will trust those he/she knows well.
	Ratings 4–6	Problems in social adjustment because of abnormal suspiciousness. Takes a very long time to get to know people and only trusts a very small number of people. Feels that others criticize him/her without adequate cause.
	Ratings 7–8	Breakdown in relationships and social adjustment because of abnormal suspiciousness. At extreme ratings the patient is completely isolated because he/she feels all are against him/her.

7. INTROSPECTION

Subject

Do you think a great deal about how you feel and what you do or do you think about them very little?
Do you prefer being on your own to being with other people?

(13)

*Are you a person who spends a lot of time thinking? (If yes) What about?
*Are you an introvert?
*Are you like this all the time or only when there is a problem on your mind?

Informant

Does S think a great deal about how he/she feels and what he/she does or does he/she think about them very little?
Does S prefer being alone to being with other people?

(14)

*Is S an introvert?
*Is S ever completely bound up in himself/herself? How often?
*Does S appear to live in a world of his/her own?
*How does this affect his/her relationships with other people?
*Do other people notice that S is like this?

Subject/Informant

Note	Ratings 1–3	Mild introspection and introversion, not noticeable to others.
	Ratings 4–6	Problems in adjustment because of excessive rumination and introspection, often with a tendency to indulge in fantasy. These feelings may lead to problems by indecision, impaired judgement and poor relationships.
	Ratings 7–8	Completely bound up in self to the exclusion of other matters, indulges in much fantasy. Self-neglect frequent.

8. SHYNESS

Subject
Are you normally a shy person or are you confident with other people?
Do you get to know people quickly or do you take a long time before feeling at ease with them?
Do you lack self-confidence?

(15)

*Do you ever go out of your way to avoid people because of shyness?
*Do you have difficulty in making friends because you are shy?
*Would you like to feel more at ease with people? Has shyness caused problems for you?

(Do you feel uncomfortable even in the presence of friends?)
(Are you feeling shy or uncomfortable now?)

Informant
Does S get to know people quickly or does he/she take a long time before feeling at ease with them?
Is S normally a shy person or does he/she have no difficulty getting on with people?
Is S a self-confident person?

(16)

*Does he/she ever go out of his/her way to avoid people because of shyness?
*Does S have difficulty in making friends because S is shy?
*Do other people notice that S is shy?
*Has shyness caused problems for S?

(Does S feel uncomfortable even in the presence of friends?)

Subject/Informant

Note	Ratings 1–3	Mild shyness, but this is compensated and others do not notice it.
	Ratings 4–6	Excessive shyness and lack of self-confidence leading to avoidance of people and personal discomfort when with people.
	Ratings 7–8	Very marked shyness leading to breakdown in social adjustment. Subject unable to work adequately or make relationships because of symptoms. In severe cases may be completely isolated.

It is important to exclude natural aloofness and detachment from shyness – the former group are not distressed in the company of other people, shyness is always associated with some feelings of anxiety.

9. ALOOFNESS

Subject
Are you a person who likes to stay apart from other people or do you like to have close relationships?
Have you any really close relationships? (If no, does this bother you?)
Do you need people in any way or can you do without them?

(17)

(Would you mind living entirely on your own without any contact with other people?)
(Do others ever say you are stand-offish or aloof?)

Informant
Is S an {isolated/aloof} person who likes to stay apart from other people or does he/she like to have close relationships?
Has he/she any really close relationships?

(18)

*Does S ever appear stand-offish or detached to other people?
*Is S happier when he/she is on his/her own?

(Do other people tend to stay apart from S?)
(Has this tendency to be aloof led to any problems in S's life?)

Subject/Informant

Note	Ratings 1–3	Mild detachment leading to a reluctance to involve subject in close relationships. Not noticeable to others and adequate relationships made with close friends and relatives.
	Ratings 4–6	Abnormal aloofness noticeable to others and leading to problems in social adjustment, mainly in interpersonal relationships.
	Ratings 7–8	Excessive detachment and lack of interest in other people. No close relationships. Indifference to other people's feelings and opinions.

Lack of interest in other people is unrelated to shyness or psychiatric symptomatology such as social fears. Subject does not feel distressed with other people and merely has no interest in them.

10. SENSITIVITY

Subject
Are you a {touchy/sensitive} person or does it take a lot to upset you?
How do you react to criticism? (Give examples)

(19)

*Do people ever say you are too touchy?
*How long does it take for you to get over criticism?

(Have any of my questions upset or disturbed you in any way?)
(Do you tend to take things personally?)

Informant
Is S a {touchy/sensitive} person or does it take a lot to upset him/her?
How does S react to criticism? (Give examples)

(20)

*Have people to be careful what they say to S in order not to upset him/her?
*Do people ever say S is too touchy?
*Does he/she take a long time to get over criticism?

(Has this sensitivity led to problems in S's relationships with others?)

Subject/Informant

Note	Ratings 1–3	Mild sensitivity. May be upset easily but does not show it except to close friends and relatives.
	Ratings 4–6	Excessive personal sensitivity with a tendency to self-reference (e.g. feels people are being critical when they are not). This leads to problems in social adjustment (e.g. frequent changes of job, broken relationships).
	Ratings 7–8	Excessive sensitivity leads to breakdown in social performance. Extreme tendency to self-reference.

Sensitivity to the feelings of others is not an abnormal phenomenon and should not be included in this rating. This rating is concerned with personal sensitivity and touchiness. If in doubt about this rating, delay till ratings of vulnerability and irritability are made. Also differentiate between sensitivity and suspiciousness. Although the two may overlap, sensitivity leads to emotional distress whereas suspiciousness is usually independent and may frequently be prominent in insensitive people.

11. VULNERABILITY

Subject
Do you find that when things go wrong in your life it disturbs you a great deal or do you remain on an even keel?
Does it take you a short time or a long time to get back to normal after some mishap (e.g. illness in family, accident, loss of job)?

(21)

(How do you think you would cope with a crisis such as death in the family, car accident or loss of your job?)

Informant
Does S find that when things go wrong in his/her life it disturbs him/her a great deal or does he/she remain on an even keel?
Does it take S a short time or a long time to get back to normal after some mishap (e.g. illness in family, accident, loss of job)?

(22)

*Does S need to be protected from unpleasant things because others know he/she will take them very badly? (If yes) Could you give an example?
*Are other people aware that S is vulnerable? How do they show it?

(Do you protect S from unpleasant events?)

Subject/Informant

Note	Ratings 1–3	Reacts more than most to adversity but does not show these feelings to others.
	Ratings 4–6	Abnormally vulnerable, reacts excessively to adversity, so leading to social maladjustment for a prolonged period. Eventually, however, more normal functioning is resumed until the next adverse episode.
	Ratings 7–8	Subject vulnerable to even the minor stresses of life to which he/she reacts as though they were major problems. Breakdown in social adjustment because of this.

It is important to separate vulnerabiity from sensitivity and resourcelessness. Although all three may be present in one individual, the characteristics are separate. The sensitive person is touchy and reacts easily to implied criticism, the vulnerable person reacts to major life events by feelings of distress which may take a long time to resolve and are not commonly associated with compensatory action, and the resourceless person reacts to adversity by not coping and just giving up. When assessing vulnerability do not include sensitivity and resourcelessness.

12. IRRITABILITY

Subject
Are you an irritable or a placid person?
Are you impatient at times? Under what kind of circumstances?
How do you show it?

(23)

*Do you keep it to yourself or do other people notice that you are impatient and irritable?
*Does this lead to problems in your relationships with other people?

(When was the last time you were really irritable?)
(How did you show this?)

Informant
Is S an irritable or a placid person?
Is he/she impatient at times? Under what kind of circumstances? How does he/she show it?

(24)

*Does he/she keep it to himself/herself or do other people notice that S is impatient and irritable?
*Does this lead to problems in S's relationships with other people? (Specify)

Subject/Informant

Note	Ratings 1–3	Mild irritability, kept under control.
	Ratings 4–6	Abnormally irritable, leading to social adjustment problems (e.g. poor relationships with others).
	Ratings 7–8	Severe irritability, making it very difficult for subject to make adequate relationships with others. Inability of the subject to cope in any environment which involves sudden changes because of severe irritability.

In making this rating, impulsiveness and aggression should be excluded. An impulsive act is followed by regret. Irritability is largely shown in verbal responses and does not include physical violence, which should be scored under aggression. 'Passive–aggressive' features may be included here if the irritability leads to procrastination, obstruction and delay in completing tasks.

13. IMPULSIVENESS

Subject
Do you always think carefully before you do something or do you act on impulse?

(25)

*Have you ever done things on impulse and regretted them afterwards? (Give examples)
*Have you ever been in trouble because you are impulsive? (Give examples)
*When you have been impulsive has it ever harmed other people?

If 'Useful facts' section (p. 143) suggests impulsivity is a problem (e.g. criminal offences) mention them here if subject answers negatively.

Informant
Does S think carefully before he/she does something or does he/she act on impulse?

(26)

*Does he/she ever do things on impulse and regret that afterwards?
*Has S ever been in trouble because he/she is impulsive? (Give examples)
*Has his/her impulsiveness ever harmed other people?

(Has S had problems with drugs or drink because he/she is impulsive?)

Subject/Informant

Note	Ratings 1–3	Mild impulsiveness, not noticeable to others, or causing no problems in social adjustment.
	Ratings 4–6	Impulsiveness associated with regret which has led to problems of social adjustment (e.g. loss of job).
	Ratings 7–8	Frequent impulsiveness leading to criminal behaviour and/or breakdown in social functioning throughout adult life.

As impulsiveness may sometimes be associated with aggression, this rating may be delayed until aggression is assessed.

14. AGGRESSION

Subject
Do you lose you temper easily or does it take a lot to make you angry?
When you get angry how do you show it?

(27)

*Have you ever lost control completely?
*Are you normally like this or only on certain occasions (e.g. after heavy drinking)?

(Do you ever react by physical violence?)
(Have you ever been in trouble with the law?)

Informant
Does S get angry easily or is he/she generally placid?
When S does get angry how does he/she show it?

(28)

*Has he/she ever lost control completely?
*Is he/she normally like this or only on certain occasions (e.g. after heavy drinking)?
*How do other people react to S's violence? What problems does it cause?

(Does he/she ever react by physical violence or does he/she keep it to himself/herself?)
(Has S ever been in trouble with police/law?)

Subject/Informant

Note	Ratings 1–3	Anger and aggression felt frequently but kept to himself/herself. Passive aggression to be included here.
	Ratings 4–6	Aggression abnormal and leads to social difficulties (e.g. trouble with police), and violence at home. Do not rate criminal offences here unless they are a direct consequence of aggressiveness.
	Ratings 7–8	Breakdown of social adjustment with long history of antisocial behaviour, usually with criminal record.

15. CALLOUSNESS

Subject
Are you easily affected by other people's feelings or can you ignore them?

(29)

*Do you care much about other people? (Do you care at all?)

(Do you find it difficult to sympathize with and understand other people's feelings?)
(Have you ever enjoyed hurting other people?)

Informant
Is S easily affected by other people's feelings or can S ignore them?

(30)

*Does S care much about other people?

Does S find it difficult to sympathize with and understand other people's feelings?

*Does he/she ever appear to get pleasure from hurting people in any way?
*How does this affect his/her relationships with other people?

(Has he/she ever hurt people (physically or mentally) deliberately?)
(Give examples)
(Is S callous or sadistic?)

Subject/Informant

Note	Ratings 1–3	Mild insensitivity and indifference to others' feelings.
	Ratings 4–6	Cold and indifferent to the extent that S is only capable of a few relationships, and these are rarely close.
	Ratings 7–8	Marked callousness with or without sadistic behaviour, leading to breakdown in social functioning, and frequent criminal involvement.

16. IRRESPONSIBILITY

Subject

Do you ever do things without caring about the consequences or are you always careful in what you do?
Would you describe yourself as a responsible or an irresponsible person?

(31)

Do you ever get into serious difficulties because of irresponsibility (e.g. into debt, criminal acts, sexual difficulties)? How has irresponsibility affected your life? (Give examples). Bring up any information derived from the section 'Useful facts' if negative answers given but past history suggests irresponsibility.

Informant

Does S ever do things without caring about the consequences or is S always careful in what he/she does?
Would you describe S as a responsible or an irresponsible person?

(32)

*Does he/she ever get into serious difficulties because of irresponsibility (e.g. into debt, criminal acts, sexual difficulties)?
*How does this affect his/her relationships with others? How has irresponsibility affected his/her life? Has it caused serious problems?

Subject/Informant

Note	Ratings 1–3	Mildly irresponsible, feelings kept under control, not noticed by others or, if manifest, not causing real problems.
	Ratings 4–6	Highly irresponsible, takes risks repeatedly, problems in social adjustment (e.g. in debt, frequent accidents, unwanted pregnancies). Do not rate criminal offences automatically unless they stem from irresponsibility.
	Ratings 7–8	Irresponsibility so great that S needs to be constantly supervised and cannot live independently because of this.

17. CHILDISHNESS

Subject

Do you ever act in a childish way or would you regard yourself as fairly mature?
Do you ever manipulate people to get your own way?

(33)

*Do you like being the centre of attention?
*Have you ever acted selfishly, only thinking of yourself?
(Has this led to problems?)

Informant
Does S ever act in childish ways or would you regard him/her as fairly mature?
Does he/she ever manipulate people to get his/her own way?
Has this ever led to problems?

☐

(34)

*Is S a selfish person who only cares about himself/herself?
*Does he/she appear to be younger than his/her years?
*Does he/she like being the centre of attention?

(How does this affect his/her relationships with others?)
(Has he/she any mature relationships?)
(Do other people tend to treat S as a child?)

Subject/Informant
Note   Ratings 1–3   Self-centred attitudes with occasional childish behaviour but this is seldom noticeable to others.

Ratings 4–6   Immature behaviour and marked selfishness leading to social adjustment problems.

Ratings 7–8   Severe childishness, cannot live independently because of this. All relationships involve others supervising or caring for S.

18. RESOURCELESSNESS

Subject
When you are faced with a challenge do you usually respond to it well or do you give in to it?
When there are problems in your life do you usually tackle them alone?
Are you somebody who can normally solve your own problems?

☐

(35)

*How have you coped with major problems in the past? (Get examples)

(When was the last time you coped with a serious problem on you own?)

Informant
When S is faced with a challenge does he/she usually respond to it well or does S give in to it?
When there are problems in S's life does he/she usually tackle them alone or does S need help from others?

☐

(36)

*Does S constantly need support to cope with life's problems?
*How does this affect his/her relationships with others?
*How has S coped with major problems in the past?

Subject/Informant
Note   Ratings 1–3   Copes with problems with some difficulty but does not involve others to an unnecessary extent.

Ratings 4–6   Others involved in coping with S's problems, impairing social functioning. Frequent problems in work.

Ratings 7–8   Unable to cope with life's practical difficulties without continuous support. Not able to live independently because of this.

19. DEPENDENCE

Subject
Do you rely on other people a great deal or are you an independent person?

*Do you find it difficult to make up your mind without involving others?
*How would you like to live and/or work alone?

(Who do you depend on most?) (In what way?)
(Would you like to be less dependent?)
(Has your dependence led to problems in your relationships?)

Informant
Does S rely on other people a great deal or is he/she usually independent?

(38)

*Does he/she find it difficult to make up his/her mind without involving others?
*Do you think S could cope with living and/or working alone? What would happen?

(Do you think S is too dependent? On whom?)
(Does this lead to problems?) (Give examples)
(Has he/she always been like this?)

Subject/Informant

Note	Ratings 1–3	Some dependence in excessive need for advice and reassurance from close relatives or friends but behaviour seldom abnormal.
	Ratings 4–6	Excessive reliance on others, leading to social adjustment problems.
	Ratings 7–8	Completely dependent on individual group or institution. Unable to work or function independently at any level.

20. SUBMISSIVENESS

Subject
Do you give in easily to others or do you stand up for yourself?

(39)

*Do you go along with decisions made by others even if you feel it is the wrong decision?
*Do you prefer to avoid arguments?
*Do people ever take advantage of you? (Give examples)

(Are you easily dominated?)
(Do you wish you could stand up for yourself better?)

Informant
Does S give in easily to others or does S stand up for himself/herself?

(40)

*Does S go along with decisions made by others even if he/she feels they are the wrong decisions?
*How does this affect relationships with others?
*Do people ever take advantage of S because they know he/she will not retaliate?

(Is S easily dominated?)
(Is he/she afraid to say what he/she really thinks?)

Subject/Informant

Note	Ratings 1–3	Mild submissiveness and compliance, but stands firm on major issues.
	Ratings 4–6	Very submissive, unwilling to express own views, is dominated in most relationships.
	Ratings 7–8	Gives in to everybody, no independent function, exploited by others. Breakdown in social functioning.

21. CONSCIENTIOUSNESS

Subject

Are you normally a fussy or a carefree person?
Do you plan everything down to the last detail or do you seldom plan anything in life?

(41)

*Do people ever say you are too fussy or conscientious, or even a perfectionist?
*Do you wish you were less conscientious?
*Are you a person with high standards?
*Does conscientiousness ever lead to problems in your life? (Specify)

(Did you worry that you might be late today?)
(If I had been late would it have upset your routine?)
(Do you think you work harder than the average person?)

Informant

Is S normally a fussy or a carefree person?
Does he/she plan everything down to the last detail or does he/she seldom plan anything in life?

(42)

*Do people ever say S is too fussy or conscientious, or even a perfectionist?
*How does this affect his/her relationships with others?
*Is he/she a person with high standards?

Subject/Informant

Note	Ratings 1–3	Over-fussy and conscientious, preoccupied with routine and excessively meticulous, but no social adjustment problems.
	Ratings 4–6	Conscientiousness abnormal, plans excessively far ahead, adjustment problems because of need for meticulous planning.
	Ratings 7–8	Excessive conscientiousness accompanied by doubt. Unable to achieve anything as the smallest of tasks becomes a major enterprise. Unable to work or use leisure, leads to interpersonal breakdown. In severe cases subject will usually have many obsessional symptoms.

In making a rating do not include obsessional symptoms (i.e. symptoms which the subject recognizes to be silly and consciously tries to overcome), unless these are part of the underlying personality of the subject. Also recognize that conscientiousness is thought to be a favourable personality trait and may be exaggerated by S or informant.

22. RIGIDITY

Subject

Do you find difficulty in adjusting to new situations or are you an adaptable person?
Do you get upset if your plans are changed for any reason or are you flexible?

(43)

*Can you adjust to others who act or feel differently from you (e.g. at work, with family)?

(Do you always have to have your own way?)

Informant

Does S find difficulty in adjusting to new situations or is S an adaptable person?
Does he/she get upset if his/her plans are changed for any reason or is S flexible?

(44)

*Can he/she adjust to others who act or feel differently from him/her (e.g. at work, with family)?
*Is he/she a person of fixed ideas?
*Do other people get upset with S because he/she is inflexible?
(Give examples of problems caused by inflexibility)

Subject/Informant

Note	Ratings 1–3	Rigidity present but attempted compensation by subject leads to no social adjustment problems.
	Ratings 4–6	Rigidity extreme, refuses to change, often dominating others. Marked problems in social adjustment because of rigidity, although if subject is driving and energetic he/she may appear successful initially.
	Ratings 7–8	Inflexibility so severe that life is completely ritualistic and impairment of adjustment so marked that independent life is impossible.

23. ECCENTRICITY

Subject

Do you think you are very different from other people? In what way?

(45)

*Have you any unusual habits or interests? What are they?
*Have you any unusual beliefs in things like telepathy and mind control?
(Have these beliefs caused problems in your life?)

(Direct questions may be asked about any eccentric features noted at interview.)

Informant

Do others ever regard S as eccentric in any way? In what way?

(46)

*Has he/she any unusual habits or interests? What are they?
*Does he/she tend to conform with other people or is he/she unaware of them?
*Does he/she deliberately set out to shock people by being unconventional?
*Has he/she any unusual beliefs about telepathy and mind control?
(Do you find his/her thoughts and speech difficult to follow?)
(Can you give examples and problems they have caused?)

Subject/Informant

Note	Ratings 1–3	Mild eccentricity, often deliberately stressed because it does not conform, but no social adjustment problems.
	Ratings 4–6	Marked eccentricity. S unable or unwilling to conform, recognized as odd by others, marked social impairment. Has odd thinking, speech and beliefs that cause problems in adjustment.
	Ratings 7–8	Behaviour and attitudes so bizarre that life in society impossible without supervision.

A low rating should be given if the subject acts in an eccentric way to attract attention. The true eccentric is oblivious to others' reactions. Any unusual beliefs or perceptions may only be rated if they are independent of mental illness such as schizophrenia.

24. HYPOCHONDRIASIS

Subject
Do you worry a great deal about your health or do you seldom give it a thought?

*When you have been ill have you worried that it might be more severe than it turned out to be?
*Are you more concerned about your health than most other people?

(How often do you visit the doctor? What for?)
(Have you ever been really well?)

Informant
Does S worry a great deal about his/her health or does S seldom give it a thought?

(48)

*When he/she has been ill has he/she worried that it might be more severe than it turned out to be?
*Is S more concerned about his/her health than most other people?
*Do you or other people think of S as a hypochrondriac?

Subject/Informant
Note | Ratings 1–3 | Mild hypochondriasis. Over-concerned about minor illness and health (e.g. takes vitamins or health foods regularly).
| Ratings 4–6 | Hypochondriasis marked. S frequently considered himself/herself to be ill even when physically healthy. Social adjustment problems; hypochondriasis affects behaviour and relationships.
| Ratings 7–8 | Hypochondriasis dominates S's life. Considers himself/herself to be ill despite contrary evidence. Unable to live independently because fears about health dominate behaviour.

Many people with a history of mental illness are naturally concerned about its likely recurrence and its effects on other people. Do not rate such concern as abnormal unless it is excessive.

Reliability of subject

On the basis of your interview, do you consider the subject to have been a reliable witness?
Note | Rating 0 | Highly reliable witness. Evidence from behaviour and demeanour at interview and any previous knowledge of witness all consistent.

(49)

| Ratings 1–3 | Probably a reliable witness but independent information lacking.
| Ratings 4–6 | Possibly an unreliable witness from demeanour at interview but no independent evidence of this.
| Ratings 7–8 | Unreliable witness. Report inconsistent with previous knowledge of witness and evidence of incorrect report from demeanour at interview.

Reliability of informant

On the basis of your interview, do you consider the informant to have been a reliable witness?
Note | Rating 0 | Highly reliable witness. Evidence from behaviour and demeanour at interview and any previous knowledge of witness all consistent.

(50)

| Ratings 1–3 | Probably a reliable witness but independent information lacking.
| Ratings 4–6 | Possibly an unreliable witness from demeanour at interview but no independent evidence of this.
| Ratings 7–8 | Unreliable witness. Report inconsistent with previous knowledge of witness and evidence of incorrect report from demeanour at interview.

Please check that you have rated all the items. Note here any additional personality characteristics that have not been rated elsewhere.

_____

_____

_____

_____

_____

_____

_____

_____

_____

_____

_____

_____

_____

_____

_____

_____

_____

_____

_____

_____

_____

_____

_____

_____

_____

_____

_____

_____

_____

_____

_____

_____

_____

Combining subject and informant information

The following procedure is used when both subject and informant versions are available and the assessor wishes to combine them:

(i) If both informant and subject receive the same ratings the combined score is the same;

(ii) If the informant scores differ from the subject on one or more ratings decide the 'most accurate' score based on (a) item being tested (e.g. aggression towards others more likely to be rated better by informant, wish to be solitary more likely to be rated better by subject), (b) level of severity (high scores (4 or above)) more likely to be rated accurately by the informant, low scores of 2 or less more likely to be rated accurately by subject (since expression of trait not always shown in general behaviour);

(iii) If more than one informant has completed scores combine informant ratings in a similar way but ensure that more credence is given to assessments that (a) include knowledge of subject in premorbid (i.e. before mental state diagnosis) state, (b) are dispassionate and independent of personal animosity towards the subject, (c) are based on contact with the subject in a range of situations, not just one (e.g. workplace).

Personality Assessment Schedule

Name of interviewer .... Date ....

Name of subject .... Place of interview................................

Age of subject..................................... Previous acquaintance of subject and

Interviewer: YES/NO ....

Name of informant................................ Age of informant.................................

Relationship to subject .... Duration of acquaintance of subject and informant:

....

Details of psychiatric treatment of subject (if any)

Year	Inpatient Outpatient Day patient	Duration of treatment
....	....	....
....	....	....
....	....	....

Current diagnostic formulation...................

.... ICD code..

.... DSM code.......................................

Current treatment (if any) ....

....

Main personality features described spontaneously at beginning of interview

Subject ....

Informant...

Scoring

Variable	No.	Box no.	Write rating 0–8 in appropriate box Sub.	Box no.	Inf.	Final score
Pessimism	1	1		2		
Worthlessness	2	3		4		
Optimism	3	5		6		
Lability	4	7		8		
Anxiousness	5	9		10		
Suspiciousness	6	11		12		
Introspection	7	13		14		
Shyness	8	15		16		
Aloofness	9	17		18		
Sensitivity	10	19		20		
Vulnerability	11	21		22		
Irritability	12	23		24		
Impulsiveness	13	25		26		
Aggression	14	27		28		
Callousness	15	29		30		
Irresponsibility	16	31		32		
Childishness	17	33		34		
Resourcelessness	18	35		36		
Dependence	19	37		38		
Submissiveness	20	39		40		
Conscientiousness	21	41		42		
Rigidity	22	43		44		
Eccentricity	23	45		46		
Hypochondriasis	24	47		48		
Reliability of information		49		50		

COMMENTS (Problems in scoring to be noted here) ....

....

....

Revised classification of personality disorder using PAS

The schedule is scored in the usual way and a final score decided for each personality variable before embarking on classification.

Stage 1
Examine all 24 scores. If none is greater than 2 code as 'normal personality' and do not proceed further.

Stage 2
Compute scores for individual personality groupings as follows:
(1)   *Sociopathic – add* scores for variables 12, 13, 14, 15 and 16, divide total by 5 and subtract from this the sum of scores for variables 2, 21 and 23 divided by 30.
(2)   *Passive–dependent – add* scores for variables 5, 11, 17, 18 and 19, divide total by 5 and then subtract from this the sum of scores for variables 15, 22 and 23 divided by 30.
(3)   *Anankastic – add* scores for variables 7, 10, 21, 22 and 24, divide total by 5 and then subtract from this the sum of scores for variables 13, 15 and 16 divided by 30.
(4)   *Schizoid – add* scores for variables 6, 7, 8, 9 and 23, divide total by 5 and subtract from this the sum of scores for variables 4, 12 and 14 divided by 30.
(5)   *Explosive – add* together the scores for variables 12, 13, 14 and 16, divide total by 4 and subtract from this the total of scores for variables 2, 8, 20 and 21, divided by 40.
(6)   *Sensitive–aggressive – add* together the scores for variables 6, 10, 12 and 14, divide by 4 and subtract from this the total of scores for variables 3, 23 and 24 divided by 30.
(7)   *Histrionic – add* together the scores for variables 4, 11, 17 and 19, divide total by 4 and subtract from this the scores for variables 9, 15, 22 and 23 divided by 40.
(8)   *Asthenic – add* together the scores for variables 5, 10, 18 and 20, divide total by 4 and subtract from this the totals for variables 3, 14 and 15 divided by 30.
(9)   *Anxious – add* together the scores for variables 5, 8, 20 and 21, divide total by 4 and subtract from this the totals for variables 3, 14 and 15 divided by 30.
(10)   *Paranoid – add* together the scores for variables 5, 6, 10 and 11, divide total by 4 and subtract from this the total for variables 2, 15 and 23 divided by 30.
(11)   *Hypochondriacal – add* together the scores for variables 5, 19, 21 and 24, divide total by 4 and subtract from this the total for variables 3, 16, 20 and 23 divided by 40.
(12)   *Dysthymic – add* together the scores for variables 2, 8, 9 and 21, divide total by 4 and subtract from this the total score for variables 3 and 14 divided by 20.
(13)   *Avoidant – add* together the scores for variables 5, 7, 8 and 11, divide total by 4 and subtract from this the total scores for variables 10, 12, 14 and 23 divided by 40.

Rating of severity of personality disturbance

The 'adjusted' score for each of the 13 personality types is used. For the first four types (sociopathic, passive–dependent, anankastic and schizoid), a score of 2.5 or more indicates simple personality disorder, and a score of 2–2.49 indicates personality difficulty. For the remaining nine personality types (explosive, sensitive–aggressive, histrionic, asthenic, anxious, paranoid, hypochondriacal, dysthymic and avoidant), a score of 2.75 or more indicates personality disorder, and 2.25–2.74 indicates personality difficulties. When a score in one cluster (the four groups above) only is 3.75 or greater the personality disturbance is also classed as personality disorder. When a score of 2.75 or greater is found in more than one cluster the personality disturbance is classified as complex personality disorder unless there is a mean difference of 1.0 or greater between the highest score in one cluster and the highest score in either of the remaining ones. (This reflects the overlap between traits, when very high scores can affect several clusters.)

Severe personality disorder

This is decided by a two-stage process. A score of 4.0 or more for one of the flamboyant cluster personalities (sociopathic, impulsive, sensitive–aggressive) together with a score of 3.0 in one of the other personality disorders (except histrionic) suggests severe personality disorder. In the second stage the assessor has to decide the following:

(i) Does the personality disorder create significant distress and dysfunction not only to immediate friends, family or household members but also to wider society (defined as all other people apart from friends, household and family members)?

(ii) Is the extent of such distress to be great enough to affect at least 50 other individuals apart from family members and close friends as a direct consequence of the personality disorder (e.g. people alter the times of arriving and leaving their houses in order to avoid encountering the individual)?

(iii) Is there clear evidence that threat is created by the pattern of personality characteristics in that fear of mental or physical harm is an intrinsic part of the distress or discomfiture created by the personality abnormality (e.g. fear of unprovoked violence)?

If the answers to all these questions are positive the individual can be described as having severe personality disorder.

In obtaining this information it is important to use more than one source, as individuals with these disorders are unlikely to admit all these negative characteristics readily or spontaneously. It is also important for the assessor to make their own judgement as to whether the fears and concerns of the individuals concerned are justified and not based on stigma or prejudice.

Combining diagnoses

In some studies it may be necessary to combine the diagnoses to obtain numbers large enough for analysis. This can be done by reducing the numbers of personality types to four: antisocial, dependent, inhibited and withdrawn.

These are combined according to the scheme below.

Sociopathic
Explosive
Sensitive–aggressive } Antisocial group
Passive–dependent

Histrionic
Asthenic } Dependent group
Anankastic

Anxious
Hypochondriacal } Inhibited group
Dysthymic

Schizoid
Paranoid } Withdrawn group
Avoidant

Key traits

For some studies research workers prefer to use a dimensional assessment of personality rather than a categorical one. This has the advantage that all subjects being tested with the schedule will have a key trait score for each of the main personality groups and this may be useful in studies that are looking at personality traits and characteristics rather than specific personality disorder. Key traits score for each of the four major personality types is calculated as follows:

(1) *Sociopathic* – add scores for variables 12, 13, 14, 15 and 16, and divide total by 5.
(2) *Passive–dependent* – add scores for variables 5, 11, 17, 18 and 19, and divide total by 5.
(3) *Anankastic* – add scores for variables 7, 10, 21, 22 and 24, and divide total by 5.
(4) *Schizoid* – add scores for variables 6, 7, 8, 9 and 23, and divide total by 5.

The nine sub-categories of personality disorder can also have their key traits scores calculated in a similar way. However, it should be noted that many of these overlap as they are sub-categories of the main ones and therefore their key traits scores will be similar. Explosive (impulsive) and sensitive–aggressive personalities are subtypes of the sociopathic group, histrionic and asthenic personalities are subtypes of the passive–dependent group, anxious, hypochondriacal and dysthymic personalities are subtypes of the anankastic group, and paranoid and avoidant personalities are subtypes of the schizoid group.

(5) *Explosive (impulsive)* – *add* together the scores for variables 12, 13, 14 and 16, and divide total by 4.

(6) *Sensitive–aggressive* – *add* together the scores for variables 6, 10, 12 and 14, and divide total by 4.

(7) *Histrionic* – *add* together the scores for variables 4, 11, 17 and 19, and divide total by 4.

(8) *Asthenic* – *add* together the score for variables 5, 10, 18 and 20, and divide total by 4.

(9) *Anxious* – *add* together the scores for variables 5, 8, 20 and 21, and divide total by 4.

(10) *Paranoid* – *add* together the scores for variables 5, 6, 10 and 11, and divide total by 4.

(11) *Hypochondriacal* – *add* together the scores for variables 5, 19, 21 and 24, and divide total by 4.

(12) *Dysthymic* – *add* together the scores for variables 2, 8, 9 and 21, and divide total by 4.

(13) *Avoidant* – *add* together the scores for variables 5, 7, 8 and 11, and divide total by 4.

Personality Assessment Schedule: DSM-IV version

Although the PAS was developed before DSM-III was introduced and includes some items that are not present in DSM personality disorders (e.g. hypochondriasis) there is still a considerable degree of overlap between the personalities derived from the PAS and those in DSM-IV. The scoring system below is suitable for reaching a DSM-IV diagnosis with the PAS. This is a simple procedure that can be done by hand as well as using a short computer program.

Add the ratings for each of the four variables and divide by four to get the mean score. A mean score of 2.75 or greater indicates a DSM personality disorder. Simultaneous presence of several personality disorders is permitted in DSM-IV, but the personality type with the highest score could be regarded as the most serious.

DSM-IV Personality type coding

301.00   Paranoid – suspiciousness + sensitivity + vulnerability + irritability (6 + 10 + 11 + 12)

301.2   Schizoid – introspection + aloofness + eccentricity + pessimism (7 + 9 + 23 + 1)

301.22   Schizotypal – shyness + eccentricity + suspiciousness + aloofness (8 + 23 + 6 + 9)

301.5   Histrionic – lability + dependence + childishness + irresponsibility (4 + 19 + 17 + 16)

301.7   Antisocial   –   callousness + aggression + impulsiveness + irresponsibility   (15 + 14 + 13 + 16)

301.8   Borderline – lability + impulsiveness + aggression + worthlessness (4 + 13 + 14 + 2)

301.82   Avoidant – vulnerability + shyness + anxiousness + submissiveness (11 + 8 + 5 + 20)

301.6   Dependent   –   dependence + submissiveness + resourcelessness + sensitivity   (19 + 20 + 18 + 10)

301.4   Obsessive–compulsive – conscientiousness + rigidity + introspection + anxiousness (21 + 22 + 7 + 5)

[301.81   Narcissistic – childishness + vulnerability + optimism + irritability (17 + 11 + 3 + 12)]

[301.84   Passive–aggressive – irritability + resourcelessness + rigidity + childishness (12 + 18 + 22 + 17)]

ICD-10

ICD-10 personality disorders show a close relationship with the PAS subclassification. The following diagnoses can be regarded as equivalent:

Sociopathic	(PAS)	and	Dissocial	(ICD-10)
Passive–dependent	(PAS)	and	Dependent	(ICD-10)
Explosive	(PAS)	and	Impulsive	(ICD-10)
Sensitive–aggressive	(PAS)	and	Dissocial	(ICD-10)
Histrionic	(PAS)	and	Histrionic	(ICD-10)
Asthenic	(PAS)	and	Dependent	(ICD-10)

Avoidant	(PAS)	and	Anxious	(ICD-10)
Schizoid	(PAS)	and	Schizoid	(ICD-10)
Paranoid	(PAS)	and	Paranoid	(ICD-10)
Anankastic	(PAS)	and	Anankastic	(ICD-10)

Other diagnoses in the PAS can be categorized under 'Personality Disorder – other' in ICD-10.

Appendix 2

Personality Assessment Schedule PAS-I (ICD-10 version)

Subject version

(The informant version is similar except that the questions are put in the third person)

Preliminary information

The aim of the PAS is to identify personality features that are enduring and independent of any current mental illness. The more information that is available about a patient the less likely is the assessment to be distorted by any current mental health problems. If little or no information exists it is suggested that the following probing questions be asked before passing on to the main questions involved in the PAS. The following procedure is suggested but this could be modified and changed under the circumstances of the interview and with the individuals concerned.

I should like to find out what sort of person you were like before your present problems began. Could you tell me in a few words how you would describe yourself in this respect?
(record response and have available as an aide memoire during interview)

I wonder if you could tell me a bit more information about yourself. Are you married or have you ever been married? Have you any children? Where are they living now?
(elucidate to what extent relationships have been unstable and whether there have been any difficulties in close relationships. This will also determine whether the person has any interest in close relationships)

Are you working at present, if not, when was the last time you were in work? What are the jobs you have been mainly involved in since leaving school? What were the circumstances in which you left or lost your last job(s)?
(determine if personality characteristics rather than just adverse circumstances might have been involved in loss of job)

Have you ever been in trouble with the law? What was the problem? Were you arrested?
(ask sensitively to avoid false negatives – determine nature of offence and circumstances)

Have you ever had any problems with alcohol or drugs? Have you ever felt that these take over your life and you can't control them? Do you gamble? Has this been a problem?
(general questions concerning addictions and substance misuse, as if these are not known the questions on personality status may be misinterpreted)

How many times have you moved house in the last 10 years? What were the reasons for moving? Have you ever been homeless?
(determine if relationship and personal difficulties involved here)

NAME ....   PATIENT NUMBER ....

RATER ....   DATE..

Screening questions

The full PAS includes screening questions which then lead on to other questions which eventually lead to a scoring of the characteristics in question. In deciding whether the question is being answered honestly please take into account the information derived from the interview carried out above. It is appreciated that on many occasions the screening question may lead to a positive response which then turns out to be negative when further questions are asked. In rating whether or not social impairment is present in the specific ICD-10 questions note that the same criteria for severity of social impairment are used as in the main schedule (i.e. the equivalent of a score of 4 or more for any question in the main schedule would lead to a score of 2 if replicated in the answer to a specific ICD-10 criterion).

For all sections:
Only ask the questions in bold type.
Only ask the questions in italics if the answers to the first questions suggest a positive response.

SECTION A

SUSPICIOUSNESS
How well in general do you get on with other people?
Do you normally trust them or are you suspicious of them, at least at first?
How long does it normally take for you to get to know people before you trust them?

Do you tend to worry about what is going on behind your back?
Do you ever think that other people might be against you or criticize you unfairly?

(Have you many friends?)
(Are you worried in case someone might find out what you have been saying to me?)

Ratings 1–3:	Mild feelings of suspiciousness, not noticed by others. Subject tends to have relatively few friends but is capable of close relationships and will trust those that he/she knows well.
Ratings 4–6:	Problems in social adjustment because of abnormal suspiciousness. Takes a very long time to get to know people and only trusts a very small number of people. Feels that others criticize him/her without adequate cause.
Ratings 7–8:	Breakdown in relationships and social adjustment because of abnormal suspiciousness. At extreme ratings patient is completely isolated because he/she feels all are against him/her.

Take into account relevant answers to questions about close relationships in the previous section, 'preliminary information'.

Tick if characteristic suspected:

□

SENSITIVITY
Are you a touchy or sensitive person or does it take a lot to upset you?
Does it bother you when people criticize you? How do you normally react?

Do people ever say you are too touchy?
How long does it take for you to get over criticism?

(Have any of my questions upset or disturbed you in any way?)
(Do you tend to take things personally?)

Ratings 1–3:	Mild sensitivity. May be upset easily but does not show it except to close friends and relatives.
Ratings 4–6:	Excessive personal sensitivity with a tendency to self-reference (e.g. feels people are being critical when they are not). This leads to problems in social adjustment (e.g. frequent changes of job, broken relationships).
Ratings 7–8:	Excessive sensitivity leads to breakdown in social performance. Extreme tendency to self-reference.

Sensitivity to the feelings of others is not an abnormal phenomenon and should not be included in this rating. This rating is concerned with personal sensitivity and touchiness. If in doubt about this rating delay till ratings of vulnerability and irritability are made. Also differentiate between sensitivity and suspiciousness. Although the two may overlap, sensitivity leads to emotional distress whereas suspiciousness is usually independent and may frequently be prominent in insensitive people.

Take into account relevant answers to questions about close relationships in the previous section, 'preliminary information'.

Tick if characteristic suspected:

(1) **No evidence of suspiciousness or sensitivity**   **GO TO SECTION C**

(2) **Possible suspiciousness or sensitivity**   **GO TO SECTION B**

SECTION B

1. Are you sensitive to setbacks in life?
(0) Not sensitive to setbacks
(1) Sensitive to setbacks but no impairment of social function
(2) Sensitive to setbacks with impairment of social function

☐

2. Do you tend to bear grudges against people?
(0) No tendency to bear grudges
(1) Tendency to bear grudges but no social impairment
(2) Tendency to bear grudges with impairment of social function

☐

3. Do you feel other people criticize you or want to harm you for no good reason?
(0) No suspiciousness of others
(1) Hostility/criticism present but no impairment of social function
(2) Hostility/criticism present with impairment of social function

☐

4. Do you always have to stand up for your rights?
(0) No, not at all
(1) Defends rights but no impairment of social function
(2) Defends rights persistently with impairment of social function

☐

5. Are you abnormally jealous?
(0) Not jealous at all
(1) Jealous to some extent but no impairment of social function
(2) Abnormally jealous leading to problems in relationships

☐

6. Do you feel people tend to talk about you or refer to you in other ways?
(0) No tendency to self-reference
(1) Some self-reference, no social impairment
(2) Self-reference common with impairment in social functioning

☐

7. Do you think groups of people are out to get you?
(0) No evidence of conspiracy
(1) Tends to detect conspiracy but no social impairment
(2) Detects conspiracy and this leads to social impairment

☐

☐

TOTAL SCORE

SECTION C

ALOOFNESS
Are you a person who likes to stay apart from other people or do you prefer to have close relationships?
Do you have any really close relationships? Does it trouble you that you don't have more?
(Note: if subject has few close relationships but definitely desires more this item should not be scored)

Do you need people in any way or can you do without them?

(Would you mind living entirely on your own without any contact with other people?)
(Do others ever say you are stand-offish or aloof?)

Ratings 1–3:   Mild detachment leading to a reluctance to become involved in close relationships. Not noticeable to others and adequate relationships made with close friends and relatives.
Ratings 4–6:   Abnormal aloofness noticeable to others and leading to problems in social adjustment, mainly in interpersonal relationships.
Ratings 7–8:   Excessive detachment and lack of interest in other people. No close relationships. Indifference to other people's feelings and opinions.

Lack of interest in people is unrelated to shyness or psychiatric symptomatology such as social fears. Subject does not feel distressed with other people and merely has no interest in them.

Take into account relevant answers to questions about close relationships in the previous section, 'preliminary information'.

Tick if characteristic suspected:

ECCENTRICITY
Do you have any unusual habits or interests which make you different from other people?
(Note: some people who show this characteristic are not aware of its effect on others, so the interviewer's observations of eccentric characteristics will be relevant when scoring the item)

Do you think you are very different from other people? In what way?
Have you any unusual habits or interests? What are they?
Have you any unusual beliefs in things like telepathy and mind control?

(Have these beliefs caused problems in your life?)
(Direct questions may be asked about any eccentric features noted at interview)
Note that eccentricity in this respect is quite separate from histrionic flamboyance)

Ratings 1–3:   Mild eccentricity, often deliberately stressed because it does not conform, but no social adjustment problems.
Ratings 4–6:   Marked eccentricity. Subject unable or unwilling to conform, recognized as odd by others, marked social impairment. Has odd thinking speech and beliefs that cause problems in adjustment.
Ratings 7–8:   Behaviour and attitudes so bizarre that life in society impossible without supervision.

A low rating should be given if the subject acts in an eccentric way to attract attention. The true eccentric is oblivious to others' reactions. Any unusual beliefs or perceptions may only be rated if they are independent of mental illness such as schizophrenia.

Take into account relevant answers to questions about close relationships in the previous section, 'preliminary information'.

Tick if characteristic suspected:

(3) No evidence of aloofness or eccentricity

(4) Possible aloofness or eccentricity

GO TO SECTION E

GO TO SECTION D

SECTION D

1. Have you ever enjoyed anything?
(0) Pleasure experienced
(1) Little or no experience of pleasure but no social impairment
(2) No pleasure experienced with impairment of social function

☐

2. Do you have any feelings for other people?
(0) Yes, feelings for others experienced
(1) Little or no feelings for others but no social impairment
(2) No feelings for others with social impairment

☐

3. How do you react when people praise or criticize you?
(0) Normal pleasure or anger experienced
(1) Little response but no social impairment
(2) Little response with definite social impairment

☐

4. Have you ever had any sexual interests?
(0) Yes, normal interest (with either sex) at some time
(1) Little interest but no social impairment
(2) Little interest with definite social impairment

☐

5. Do you prefer to be alone?
(0) No, prefers some company
(1) Prefers being alone, but no social impairment
(2) Strong wishes to be alone with social impairment

☐

Do you think a great deal about how you feel and what you do or do you think about them very little?
* Are you a person who spends a lot of time thinking? If yes what about?
* Are you an introvert?
* Are you like this all the time or only when there is a problem on your mind?

6. Have you any close personal relationships?
(0) Yes, definite close relationships
(1) None, or only one close relationship but no social impairment
(2) No close relationships with social impairment

☐

7. Do you take notice of other people and the way they react to you?
(0) Normal acceptance of social convention
(1) Little notice of social convention, but no social impairment
(2) Little or no notice taken of social convention with social impairment

☐

TOTAL SCORE

☐

SECTION E

AGGRESSION
Do you lose your temper easily or does it take a lot to make you angry?
How do you react when you get angry?

Have you ever lost control completely?
Are you normally like this or only on certain occasions (e.g. after heavy drinking)?

(Do you ever react by physical violence?)
(Have you ever been in trouble with the law?)

Ratings 1–3:	Anger and aggression felt frequently but kept to himself/herself. Passive aggression to be included here.
Ratings 4–6:	Aggression abnormal and leads to social difficulties (e.g. trouble with police), and violence at home. Do not rate criminal offences here unless they are a direct consequence of aggressiveness.
Ratings 7–8:	Breakdown of social adjustment with long history of antisocial behaviour, usually with criminal record.

Take into account relevant answers to questions about problems with the law in the previous section, 'preliminary information'. Note that many criminal offences are independent of personality disorder

Tick if characteristic suspected:

CALLOUSNESS
Are you easily affected by other people's feelings or can you ignore them?
Do you care about other people?

(Do you find it difficult to sympathize with and understand other people's feelings?)
(Have you enjoyed hurting other people?)

Ratings 1–3:	Mild insensitivity and indifference to others' feelings.
Ratings 4–6:	Cold and indifferent to the extent that subject is only capable of a few relationships, and these are rarely close.
Ratings 7–8:	Marked callousness with or without sadistic behaviour, leading to breakdown in social functioning, and frequent criminal involvement.

Take into account relevant answers to questions about problems with the law in the previous section, 'preliminary information'. Note that many criminal offences are independent of personality disorder

Tick if characteristic suspected:

(5) No evidence of aggression or callousness   GO TO SECTION G

(6) Possible aggression or callousness   GO TO SECTION F

SECTION F

1. Do you care about the needs of other people?
(0) Normal concern for others
(1) Little concern but no social impairment
(2) Little concern with social impairment

☐

2. Do you take notice of rules in society or are you antisocial?
(0) Not antisocial
(1) Some antisocial acts but no social impairment
(2) Antisocial behaviour with social impairment

☐

3. Do you find it difficult to keep close relationships?
(0) No difficulty
(1) Some difficulty in keeping relationships but no social impairment
(2) Difficulty in keeping relationships and consequent social impairment

☐

4. Do you lose your temper easily?
(0) No tendency to aggression
(1) Some aggression but no social impairment
(2) Aggressive behaviour with social impairment

☐

5. Do you regret your behaviour?
(0) Normal guilt or few negative experiences
(1) No guilt about past behaviour but no social impairment
(2) No guilt and no benefit from experience, with social impairment

☐

6. Are other people to blame for your troubles in society?
(0) Does not blame others
(1) Blames others but no social impairment
(2) Blames others with social impairment

☐

7. Are you irritable most of the time?
(0) No, not at all
(1) Is irritable but no social impairment
(2) Irritable with social impairment

☐

TOTAL SCORE

☐

SECTION G

IMPULSIVENESS
Do you always think carefully before you do something or do you act on impulse?
Have you ever done things on impulse and regretted them afterwards?

Have you ever been in trouble because you are impulsive? (Give examples)
When you have been impulsive has it ever harmed other people?

Ratings 1–3:	Mild impulsiveness, not noticeable to others, or causing no problems in social adjustment.
Ratings 4–6:	Impulsiveness associated with regret which has led to problems of social adjustment (e.g. loss of job).
Ratings 7–8:	Frequent impulsiveness leading to criminal behaviour and/or breakdown in social functioning throughout adult life.

Take into account relevant answers to questions about changes in job and housing in the previous section, 'preliminary information'. If preliminary information suggests impulsivity is a problem (e.g. criminal offences, problems with drugs or drink) mention them here if subject answers negatively.

Tick if characteristic suspected:

IRRESPONSIBILITY
Do you ever do things without caring about the consequences or are you always careful in what you do?
Would you describe yourself as a responsible or irresponsible person?

Do you ever get into serious difficulties because of irresponsibility (e.g. get into debt, criminal acts, sexual difficulties)?
How has irresponsibility affected your life? (Give examples)

Ratings 1–3:	Mildly irresponsible, feelings kept under control, not noticed by others, or if manifest, not causing real problems.
Ratings 4–6:	Highly irresponsible, takes risks repeatedly, problems in social adjustment (e.g. in debt, frequent accidents, unwanted pregnancies). Do not rate criminal offences automatically unless they stem from irresponsibility.
Ratings 7–8:	Irresponsibility so great that subject needs to be constantly supervised and cannot live independently because of this.

Take into account relevant answers to questions about changes in job and housing in the previous section, 'preliminary information'. If preliminary information suggests irresponsibility is a problem (e.g. criminal offences, sexual difficulties, getting into debt) mention them here if subject answers negatively.

Tick if characteristic suspected:

These questions cover both borderline and impulsive personality disorder (emotionally unstable personality disorder). In both these impulsivity is a prominent feature but in borderline personality disorder there is uncertainty over identity with unstable relationships and rapid mood swings with threats or actual self harm.

(7) No evidence of impulsiveness or irresponsibility   **GO TO SECTION K**

(8) Possible impulsiveness or irresponsibility   **GO TO SECTION H**

SECTION H

1. Do you act unexpectedly without thinking about the consequences?
(0) No impulsiveness
(1) Impulsiveness with no social impairment
(2) Impulsiveness followed by quarrelsome behaviour and social impairment

2. When you decide to do something do you plan ahead and consider the consequences?
(0) Able to plan ahead
(1) Difficulty in planning ahead but no social impairment
(2) Unable to predict consequences of actions, leading to social impairment

3. Can you keep doing a task even when there is no reward immediately?
(0) No difficulty in maintaining task
(1) Some problems in maintaining tasks but no social impairment
(2) Major difficulty in maintaining tasks with social impairment

4. Do your spirits (moods) change suddenly for no reason?
(0) No problems with mood variation
(1) Mood variability but no social impairment
(2) Mood variability with social impairment

Are these changes connected with what is going on in your life or are they separate?
How long do they last?
Do they lead to problems?
(Can you predict your changes in mood?)
(How often do you laugh and cry?)

5. Do you often feel uncertain about yourself as a person?
(0) No uncertainty about self-image and preferences
(1) Uncertain about self but no social impairment
(2) Uncertain about self with social impairment

6. Do you often get involved in strong relationships which keep breaking down?
(0) No fragile relationships
(1) Some relationships unstable but no social impairment
(2) Relationships intense and unstable but no social impairment

7. Do you often harm, or threaten to harm yourself?
(0) No suicidal threats
(1) Some suicidal threats but no social impairment
(2) Frequent suicidal threats but no social impairment

TOTAL SCORE

SECTION K

CHILDISHNESS
Do you ever act in a childish way or would you regard yourself as fairly mature?

Do you ever manipulate people to get your own way?
Do you like being the centre of attention?
Have you ever acted selfishly, only thinking of yourself? (Has this led to problems?)

Ratings 1–3:   Self-centred attitudes with occasional childish behaviour but this is seldom noticeable to others.

Ratings 4–6:   Immature behaviour and marked selfishness leading to social adjustment problems.

Ratings 7–8:   Severe childishness, cannot live independently because of this. All relationships involve others supervising or caring for subject.

Take into account relevant answers to questions about habit and relationships in the previous section, 'preliminary information'.

Tick if characteristic suspected:

LABILITY
Do your spirits change from day to day or week to week, or do they stay more or less the same?

Are these changes connected with what is going on in your life or are they separate?
How long do they last?
Do they lead to problems?
(Can you predict your changes in mood?)
(How often do you laugh and cry?)

Ratings 1–3:   A tendency towards mild exaggeration of mood swings in response to life changes.

Ratings 4–6:   Marked lability, noticeable to others and leading to problems because of strength of mood swings. Most changes responsive to life events but may be independent. Unpredictability of subject's behaviour because of mood swings also a source of difficulties.

Ratings 7–8:   Breakdown of social, occupational and personal relationships because of abnormal swings in mood. In these instances it would be more likely that the changes are independent of life events so that they cannot be manipulated in any way. What is known as 'cyclothymia' will be included here if the swings in mood occur at least as frequently as once every two weeks. If they occur less frequently than this, but still produce important personality problems, then the relevant rating should be included under the pessimism and optimism scales.

Take into account relevant answers to questions about habit and relationships in the previous section, 'preliminary information'.

Tick if characteristic suspected:

(9) **No evidence of childishness or lability**   GO TO SECTION N

(10) **Possible childishness or lability**   GO TO SECTION M

SECTION M

1. Are you more emotional than most other people?
(0) No exaggeration of emotions
(1) Self-dramatization and exaggerated emotions but no social impairment
(2) Self-dramatization and exaggeration of emotions with social impairment

☐

2. Are you easily influenced by other people?
(0) No, not suggestible
(1) Yes, usually influenced and suggestible but no social impairment
(2) Yes, usually influenced and suggestible with social impairment

☐

3. Are you a very changeable person?
(0) No, mood stable
(1) Yes, shallow and labile affectivity with no social impairment
(2) Yes, shallow and labile affectivity with social impairment

☐

4. Are your needs the only important ones in life?
(0) No, not egocentric or self-indulgent
(1) Defends rights but no impairment of social function
(2) Defends rights persistently with impairment of social function

☐

5. Is it important for you to be liked by others?
(0) No, not important
(1) Yes, longs for appreciation but no social impairment
(2) Yes, continual yearning to be liked, with social impairment

6. Do you always need to be the centre of attention?
(0) No, not at all
(1) Yes, often needs to be the centre of attention but no social impairment
(2) Yes, continual need to be the centre of attention leads to social impairment

☐

7. Do you manipulate others to get what you want in life?
(0) No, not manipulative
(1) Yes, manipulative behaviour but no social impairment
(2) Yes, manipulative behaviour leads to social impairment

☐

☐

TOTAL SCORE

☐

SECTION N

CONSCIENTIOUSNESS
Are you normally a fussy or a carefree person?
Do you plan everything in detail or do you seldom plan anything in life?

Do people ever say you are too fussy or conscientious, or even a perfectionist?
Do you wish you were less conscientious?
Are you a person with high standards?
Does conscientiousness ever lead to problems in your life? (Specify)

(Did you worry that you might be late today?)
(If I had been late would it have upset your routine?)
(Do you think you work harder than the average person?)

Ratings 1–3:	Over fussy and conscientious, preoccupied with routine and excessively meticulous, but no social adjustment problems.
Ratings 4–6:	Conscientiousness abnormal, plans excessively far ahead, adjustment problems because of need for meticulous planning.
Ratings 7–8:	Excessive conscientiousness accompanied by doubt. Unable to achieve anything as the smallest of tasks becomes a major enterprise. Unable to work or use leisure, leads to interpersonal breakdown. In severe cases subject will have many obsessional symptoms.

Take into account relevant answers to questions about working history in the previous section, 'preliminary information'.

In making a rating do not include obsessional symptoms (i.e. symptoms which the subject recognizes to be silly and consciously tries to overcome), unless these are part of the underlying personality of the subject. Also recognize that conscientiousness is thought to be a favourable personality trait and may be exaggerated by the subject or informant.

Tick if characteristic suspected:

$$\square$$

RIGIDITY
Do you find it difficult to adjust to new situations or are you an adaptable person?
Do you get upset if your plans are changed for any reason?

Can you adjust to others who act or feel differently from you (e.g. at work, with family)?
Do you always have to have your own way?

Ratings 1–3:	Rigidity present but attempted compensation by subject leads to no social adjustment problems.
Ratings 4–6:	Rigidity extreme, refuses to change, often dominating others. Marked problems in social adjustment because of rigidity, although if subject is driving and energetic he/she may appear successful initially.
Ratings 7–8:	Inflexibility so severe that life is completely ritualistic and impairment of adjustment so marked that independent life is impossible.

Take into account relevant answers to questions about working history in the previous section, 'preliminary information'.

Tick if characteristic suspected:

$$\square$$

(11) No evidence of conscientiousness or rigidity	**GO TO SECTION Q**
(12) Possible conscientiousness or rigidity	**GO TO SECTION P**

SECTION P

1. Do you have problems making up your mind about what to do?
(0) No indecisiveness
(1) Yes, indecisive and caution but no social impairment
(2) Yes, indecisiveness, doubt and caution lead to social impairment

☐

2. Do you always have to get the details of things you do exactly right?
(0) No, no perfectionism
(1) Yes, some perfectionism with excessive preoccupation with detail but no social impairment
(2) Yes, perfectionist and excessively preoccupied with detail, with social impairment

☐

3. Are you excessively conscientious?
(0) No, not particularly conscientious
(1) Yes, conscientious not leading to social impairment
(2) Yes, excessive conscientiousness with concern over doing things absolutely right
leading to social impairment

☐

4. Are you excessively conventional in your relationships with other people?
(0) No, not abnormally conventional
(1) Yes, conventional and inhibited relationships but no social impairment
(2) Yes, abnormally conventional with problems expressing feelings leading
to social impairment

☐

5. Do you insist that others fit in with your way of doing things?
(0) No, no abnormal rigidity
(1) Yes, some rigidity and stubbornness but no social impairment
(2) Yes, abnormally rigid and stubborn leading to social impairment

☐

6. Do you usually have thoughts and impulses that you cannot get out of your mind?
(0) No, no abnormal thoughts or impulses
(1) Yes, unwelcome thoughts and impulses but no social impairment
(2) Yes, unwelcome thoughts and impulses that lead to social impairment

☐

7. Do you have to plan everything far ahead and in great detail?
(0) No, no excessive planning
(1) Yes, plans things excessively but no social impairment
(2) Yes, plans things excessively and in great detail leading to social impairment

☐

TOTAL SCORE

☐

SECTION Q

ANXIOUSNESS
Are you normally an anxious or a calm person?
Are you less nervous, about the same, or more nervous than most other people?

Do you ever worry about things that most people would not be concerned about? (Give examples)
Do you show your nervousness to other people or do you cover it up?
Have you always been an anxious person?

(Do you ever worry about something or someone most of the time?)
(Has your anxiety ever led to problems?) (Specify)

Ratings 1–3:   Mild anxiety-proneness which is normally suppressed so that others are not aware of it.
Ratings 4–6:   Anxiety noticeable to others, leading to changes in behaviour.
Ratings 7–8:   Frequent or continuous free-floating anxiety of such severity that breakdown in social adjustment occurs.

Life-long phobic anxiety may contribute to this rating but the severity of the rating would depend on the same categories mentioned in the outline to scoring (i.e. it is the extent to which it interferes with personal and social adjustment that determines the rating).

Take into account relevant answers to questions about personal relationships in the previous section, 'preliminary information'. Anxious personalities restrict their lifestyles to avoid anxiety.

Tick if characteristic suspected:

SHYNESS
Are you normally a shy person or are you confident with other people?
Do you lack self-confidence?
Do you get to know people quickly or does it take a long time before feeling at ease with them?
Do you ever go out of your way to avoid people because of shyness?
Do you have difficulty in making friends because you are shy?
Would you like to feel more at ease with people? Has shyness caused problems for you?
(Do you feel uncomfortable even in the presence of friends?)
(Are you feeling shy or uncomfortable now?)

Ratings 1–3:   Mild shyness, but this is compensated and others do not notice it.
Ratings 4–6:   Excessive shyness and lack of self-confidence leading to avoidance of people and personal discomfort when with people.
Ratings 7–8:   Very marked shyness leading to breakdown in social adjustment. Subject unable to work adequately or make relationships because of symptoms. In severe cases may be completely isolated.

It is important to exclude natural aloofness and detachment from shyness – the former group are not distressed in the company of other people, shyness is always associated with some feelings of anxiety.
Take into account relevant answers to questions about personal relationships in the previous section, 'preliminary information'. Anxious personalities restrict their lifestyles to avoid anxiety.

Tick if characteristic suspected:

(13) No evidence of anxiousness or shyness   **GO TO SECTION S**

(14) Possible anxiousness or shyness   **GO TO SECTION R**

SECTION R

1. Do you feel anxious and tense all the time?
(0) No, not anxious continuously
(1) Yes, persistent anxiety and tense but no social impairment
(2) Persistently anxious and tense with social impairment

2. Do you feel self-conscious and inferior to other people?
(0) No, not abnormally self-conscious
(1) Yes, feels self-conscious and inferior but no social impairment
(2) Yes, persistent need to be liked and accepted, leading to social impairment

3. Do you always want to be liked and accepted by people?
(0) No, not at all
(1) Yes, needs to be liked and accepted but no social impairment
(2) Yes, persistent need to be liked and accepted but no social impairment

4. Are you very sensitive to people criticizing or rejecting you?
(0) No, not especially sensitive to criticism or rejection
(1) Yes, sensitive to criticism and rejection but no social impairment
(2) Sensitive to criticism and rejection with social impairment

5. Do you avoid getting involved with other people in case you might not be accepted?
(0) No, does not avoid relationships
(1) Yes, unwilling to enter relationships because of fear of acceptance but no social mpairment
(2) Unwilling to enter relationships because of fear of acceptance leading to impaired social function

6. Have you always tended to avoid certain activities and situations (e.g. like going on a bus) because you think they might be dangerous?
(0) No, no avoidance
(1) Yes, tends to avoid situations because of exaggerated risks, but no social impairment
(2) Persistent avoidance of certain situations, leading to social impairment

7. Do you restrict what you do in life because you need to have everything organized and secure?
(0) No, no restriction of lifestyle
(1) Yes, restricted lifestyle but no social impairment
(2) Yes, restricted lifestyle because of need for security with social impairment

TOTAL SCORE

SECTION S

RESOURCELESSNESS
When you are faced with a challenge do you usually respond to it well or do you give in to it?
Are you someone who can normally tackle problems in life alone or do you need other people's help?

How have you coped with major problems in the past? (Give examples)
(When was the last time you coped with a serious problem on your own?)

Ratings 1–3:	Copes with problems with some difficulty but does not involve others to an unnecessary extent.
Ratings 4–6:	Others involved in coping with subject's problems, impairing social functioning. Frequent problems in work.
Ratings 7–8:	Unable to cope with life's practical difficulties without continuous support. Not able to live independently because of this.

Take into account relevant answers to questions about drug and alcohol use and nature of close relationships in the previous section, 'preliminary information'.

Tick if characteristic suspected:

VULNERABILITY
Do you find that when things go wrong in your life (e.g. loss of job, death in family) you are disturbed a great deal, or do you cope with them well?
Does it usually take a short or long time to get back to normal after upsets in your life?

(How do you think you would cope with a crisis such as death in the family, car accident or loss of your job?)

Ratings 1–3:	Reacts more than most to adversity but does not show these feelings to others.
Ratings 4–6:	Abnormally vulnerable, reacts excessively to adversity, so leading to social maladjustment for a prolonged period. Eventually, however, more normal functioning is resumed until the next adverse episode.
Ratings 7–8:	Subject vulnerable to even the minor stresses of life to which he/she reacts as though they were major problems. Breakdown in social adjustment because of this.

It is important to separate vulnerability from sensitivity and resourcelessness. Although all three may be present in one individual, the characteristics are separate. The sensitive person is touchy and reacts easily to implied criticism, the vulnerable person reacts to major life events by feelings of distress which may take a long time to resolve and are not commonly associated with compensatory action, and the resourceless person reacts to adversity by not coping and just giving up. When assessing vulnerability do not include sensitivity and resourcelessness.

Take into account relevant answers to questions about drug and alcohol use and nature of close relationships in the previous section, 'preliminary information'.

Tick if characteristic suspected:

(15) No evidence of resourcelessness or vulnerability   **GO TO SECTION X**

(16) Possible resourcelessness or vulnerability   **GO TO SECTION U**

SECTION U

1. Do you let others decide most of your responsibilities for you?
(0) No, no significant transfer of responsibilities
(1) Yes, others assume responsibility but no social impairment
(2) Yes, significant transfer of responsibilities with social impairment

2. Do you allow others to decide what is best for you?
(0) No, no undue submissiveness
(1) Yes, is submissive to others but no social impairment
(2) Yes, undue submissiveness and compliance with social impairment

3. Do you find it dificult to make demands on the people you depend on?
(0) No difficulty in making demands
(1) Yes, difficulty in making demands but no social impairment
(2) Yes, difficulty in making demands with social impairment

4. Do you think you are less able to do things and have less stamina than other people?
(0) No, no difficulties in coping
(1) Yes, is less competent and lacks stamina but no social impairment
(2) Yes, is helpless and lacks stamina and this leads to social impairment

5. Are you afraid of being abandoned or left alone?
(0) No, no fear
(1) Yes, afraid of being abandoned and of being left alone but no social impairment
(2) Yes, afraid of being abandoned and left alone with social impairment

6. Do you feel completely helpless whenever a relationship ends?
(0) No, able to cope with ending of relationship
(1) Feels devastated and helpless after relationship ends but no social impairment
(2) Yes, feels devastated and helpless after relationship ends with social impairment

7. When things go wrong in your life do others normally have to help you get over them?
(0) No, not at all
(1) Yes, needs help from others but no social impairment
(2) Yes, needs help from others which leads to social impairment

TOTAL SCORE

SECTION X
SCORESHEET
TRANSCRIBE SCORES FROM SECTIONS B, D, F, H, M, P, R AND U

Paranoid personality score (section B) ☐

Schizoid personality score (section D) ☐

Dissocial personality score (section F) ☐

Emotionally unstable (impulsive) score (section H) ☐

Emotionally unstable (borderline) score (section H) ☐

Histrionic personality score (section M) ☐

Anankastic personality score (section P) ☐

Anxious personality score (section R) ☐

Dependent personality score (section U) ☐

Total score for any personality category 0–3 (no personality disorder); 4–6 (personality difficulty), 7 or greater (personality disorder). For ratings of severity score 0 if no categories score greater than 3, score 1 (personality difficulty) if 1 to 3 categories score between 4 and 6, score 2 (simple personality disorder) if 4 or more categories score between 4 and 6, or if any one category scores 7 or more, and score 3 (complex personality disorder) if two or more categories from different clusters (cluster A = paranoid and schizoid); cluster B = dissocial, emotionally unstable and histrionic; cluster C = anankastic, anxious or dependent) score 7 or more. Score 4 (severe personality disorder) if there is a score of 8 or more for dissocial personality disorder or for one of the emotionally unstable personality disorders together with a score of 7 or more for one of the cluster A or C personality disorders.

Code severity score (0–4) ☐

List major personality abnormality ....

....

....

....

....

Appendix 3

Quick Personality Assessment Schedule (PAS-Q)

The PAS-Q is a quick form of the Personality Assessment Schedule that is best carried out by assessors who have already been trained in the full PAS. It is assumed from the following that this training has already been carried out.

Preliminary information

The aim of the PAS and PAS-Q is to identify personality features that are enduring and independent of any current mental illness. The more information that is available about a patient the less likely is the assessment to be distorted by any current mental health problems. If little or no information exists it is suggested that the following probing questions be asked before passing on to the main questions involved in the PAS-Q. The following procedure is suggested but this could be modified and changed under the circumstances of the interview and with the individuals concerned.

I should like to find out what sort of person you were like before your present problems began. Could you tell me in a few words how you would describe yourself in this respect?
(Record response and ask further questions if neutral response only (e.g. 'I'm easy going, get on well with everybody)

I wonder if you could tell me a bit more information about yourself.
Are you married or have you ever been married? Have you any children?
Where are they living now?
(Elucidate to what extent relationships have been unstable and whether there have been any difficulties in close relationships. This will also determine whether the person has any interest in close relationships)

Are you working at present, if not, when was the last time you were in work?
What are the jobs you have been mainly involved in since leaving school?
What were the circumstances in which you left your last job(s)?
(Determine if behaviour or relationships were related to change or loss of job)

Have you ever been in trouble with the law?
What was the problem?
Were you arrested?
(Enquire about circumstances bearing in mind that they are likely to be underplayed)

How much do you drink?
Have you ever had any problems with alcohol or drugs?
Have you ever felt that these take over your life and you can't control them?
Do you gamble? Has this been a problem?
How many times have you moved house in the last 10 years?
What were the reasons for moving?
Have you ever been homeless?

Screening questions for PAS

The full PAS includes screening questions which then lead on to other questions which eventually lead to a scoring of the characteristics in question. In the PAS-Q only the screening questions are asked. In deciding whether the question is being answered honestly please take into account the information derived from the interview carried out above. It is appreciated that on many occasions the screening question may lead to a positive response which then turns out to be negative when further questions are asked.

For all sections:
Only ask the questions in bold type.
Only ask the questions in italics if the answers to the first questions suggest a positive response.

SECTION A

SUSPICIOUSNESS
How well in general do you get on with other people?
Do you normally trust them or are you suspicious of them, at least at first?
How long does it normally take for you to get to know people before you trust them?

Do you tend to worry what is going on behind your back?
Do you ever think that other people might be against you or criticize you unfairly?

(Have you many friends?)
(Are you worried in case someone might find out what you have been saying to me?)

SENSITIVITY
Are you a touchy or sensitive person or does it take a lot to upset you?
Does it bother you when people criticize you? How do you normally react?

Do people ever say you are too touchy?
How long does it take for you to get over criticism?

(Have any of my questions upset or disturbed you in any way?)
(Do you tend to take things personally?)

Take into account relevant answers to questions about close relationships in the previous section, 'preliminary information'.

Please record if no significant paranoid personality features (0), paranoid personality difficulty (1) if these traits are present but not causing serious social dysfunction; paranoid personality disorder (2) if they are causing serious social dysfunction (using PAS guidelines).

Group	Characteristic	Main Features	Personality Type	Rating of Severity
		(N.B. these should be persistent and independent of mental state disorder to be scored)	(ICD-10 equivalent)	(0–2)
Withdrawn	Suspiciousness Sensitivity	Touchiness, refusal to trust people, frequent fears of conspiracy, persistent blaming of others	Paranoid	

SECTION B

ALOOFNESS
Are you a person who likes to stay apart from other people or do you prefer to have close relationships?
Do you have any really close relationships? Does it trouble you that you don't have more?
(Note: if subject has few close relationships but defiantly desires more this item should not be scored)

Do you need people in any way or can you do without them?

(Would you mind living entirely on your own without any contact with other people?)
(Do others ever say you are stand-offish or aloof?)

ECCENTRICITY
Do you have any unusual habits or interests which make you different form other people?
(Note: some people who show this characteristic are not aware of its effect on others, so the interviewer's observations of eccentric characteristics will be relevant when scoring the item)

Do you think you are very different from other people? In what way?
Have you any unusual habits or interests? What are they?
Have you any unusual beliefs in things like telepathy and mind control?

(Have these beliefs caused problems in your life?)
(Direct questions may be asked about any eccentric features noted at interview)
(Note that eccentricity in this respect is quite separate from histrionic flamboyance)

Take into account relevant answers to questions about close relationships in the previous section, 'preliminary information'.

Please record if no significant paranoid personality features (0), schizoid personality difficulty (1) if these traits are present but not causing serious social dysfunction; record schizoid personality disorder (2) if they are causing serious social dysfunction (using PAS guidelines).

Group	Characteristic	Main Features	Personality Type	Rating of Severity
		(N.B. these should be persistent and independent of mental state disorder to be scored)	(ICD-10 equivalent)	(0–2)
Withdrawn	Aloofness Eccentricity	Social withdrawal and voluntary isolation, few or no close relationships, ignorance of social conventions	Schizoid	

SECTION C

AGGRESSION
Do you lose your temper easily or does it take a lot to make you angry?
How do you react when you get angry?

Have you ever lost control completely?
Are you normally like this or only on certain occasions (e.g. after heavy drinking)?

(Do you ever react by physical violence?)
(Have you ever been in trouble with the law?)

CALLOUSNESS
Are you easily affected by other people's feelings or can you ignore them?
Do you care about other people?

(Do you find it difficult to sympathize with and understand other people's feelings?)
(Have you enjoyed hurting other people?)

Take into account relevant answers to questions about problems with the law in the previous section, 'preliminary information'. Note that many criminal offences are independent of personality disorder.

Please record if no significant dissocial personality features (0), dissocial personality difficulty (1) if these traits are present but not causing serious social dysfunction; and dissocial personality disorder (2) if they are causing serious social dysfunction (using PAS guidelines).

Group	Characteristic	Main Features	Personality Type	Rating of Severity
		(N.B. these should be persistent and independent of mental state disorder to be scored)	(ICD-10 equivalent)	(0–2)
Flamboyant	Aggression Callousness	Short-tempered, tendency to react by physical violence, insensitivity to feelings of others, absence of guilt, excessive irritability	Dissocial and antisocial	

SECTION D

IMPULSIVENESS
Do you always think carefully before you do something or do you act on impulse?
Have you ever done things on impulse and regretted them afterwards?

Have you ever been in trouble because you are impulsive? (Give examples)
When you have been impulsive has it ever harmed other people?

IRRESPONSIBILITY
Do you ever do things without caring about the consequences or are you always careful in what you do?
Would you describe yourself as a responsible or irresponsible person?

Do you ever get into serious difficulties because of irresponsibility (e.g. get into debt, criminal acts, sexual difficulties)?
How has irresponsibility affected your life? (Give examples)

Take into account relevant answers to questions about changes in job and housing in the previous section, 'preliminary information'.

These questions cover both borderline and impulsive personality disorder (emotionally unstable personality disorder). In both these impulsivity is a prominent feature but in borderline personality disorder there is uncertainty over identity with unstable relationships and rapid mood swings with threats or actual self harm.

Please record if no significant paranoid personality features (0), borderline personality difficulty (1) if these traits are present but not causing serious social dysfunction; and borderline personality disorder (2) if they are causing serious social dysfunction (using PAS guidelines).

Group	Characteristic	Main Features	Personality Type	Rating of Severity
		(N.B. these should be persistent and independent of mental state disorder to be scored)	(ICD-10 equivalent)	(0–2)
Flamboyant	Impulsiveness Irresponsibility	Tendency to act on impulse followed by regrets because of negative consequences, failure to plan ahead or to anticipate consequences of behaviour	Impulsive	
		Inability to maintain close relationships which are often intense, uncertain self image	Borderline	

SECTION E

CHILDISHNESS
Do you ever act in a childish way or would you regard yourself as fairly mature?

Do you ever manipulate people to get your own way?
Do you like being the centre of attention?
Have you ever acted selfishly, only thinking of yourself? (Has this led to problems?)

LABILITY
Do your spirits change from day to day or week to week, or do they stay more or less the same?

Take into account relevant answers to questions about habit and relationships in the previous section, 'preliminary information'.

Please record if no significant histrionic personality features (0), histrionic personality difficulty (1) if these traits are present but not causing serious social dysfunction; and histrionic personality disorder (2) if they are causing serious social dysfunction (using PAS guidelines).

Group	Characteristic	Main Features	Personality Type	Rating of Severity
		(N.B. these should be persistent and independent of mental state disorder to be scored)	(ICD-10 equivalent)	(0–2)
Flamboyant	Childishness Lability	Self-centred, tendency to dramatization and manipulative behaviour, shallow and labile in feelings, easily influenced by others	Histrionic	

SECTION F

CONSCIENTIOUSNESS
Are you normally a fussy or a carefree person?
Do you plan everything in detail or do you seldom plan anything in life?

Do people ever say you are too fussy or conscientious, or even a perfectionist?
Do you wish you were less conscientious?
Are you a person with high standards?
Does conscientiousness ever lead to problems in your life? (Specify)

(Did you worry that you might be late today?)
(If I had been late would it have upset your routine?)
(Do you think you work harder than the average person?)

RIGIDITY
Do you find it difficult to adjust to new situations or are you an adaptable person?
Do you get upset if your plans are changed for any reason?

Can you adjust to others who act or feel differently from you (e.g. at work, with family)?
Do you always have to have your own way?

Take into account relevant answers to questions about working history in the previous section, 'preliminary information'.

Please record no obsessional personality features (0) if score 0, obsessional personality difficulty (1) if these traits are present but not causing serious social dysfunction; and obsessional personality disorder (2) if they are causing serious social dysfunction (using PAS guidelines).

Group	Characteristic	Main Features	Personality Type	Rating of Severity
Fearful	Conscientiousness Rigidity	Excessive conscientiousness in everyday activities, tendency to plan everything in great detail, unable to alter plans to suit changing needs, excessively stubborn	Anankastic	(0–2)

SECTION G

ANXIOUSNESS
Are you normally an anxious or a calm person?
Are you less nervous, about the same, or more nervous than most other people?

Do you ever worry about things that most people would not be concerned about? (Give examples)
Do you show your nervousness to other people or do you cover it up?
Have you always been an anxious person?

(Do you ever worry about something or someone most of the time?)
(Has your anxiety ever led to problems?) (Specify)

SHYNESS
Are you normally a shy person or are you confident with other people?
Do you lack self-confidence?

Do you get to know people quickly or does it take a long time before feeling at ease with them?
Do you ever go out of your way to avoid people because of shyness?
Do you have difficulty in making friends because you are shy?
Would you like to feel more at ease with people? Has shyness caused problems for you?

(Do you feel uncomfortable even in the presence of friends?)
(Are you feeling shy or uncomfortable now?)

Take into account relevant answers to questions about personal relationships in the previous section, 'preliminary information'. Anxious personalities restrict their lifestyles to avoid anxiety.

Please record no anxious personality abnormality (0) if scores both 0, anxious personality difficulty (1) if these traits are present but not causing serious social dysfunction; and anxious personality disorder (2) if they are causing serious social dysfunction (using PAS guidelines).

Group	Characteristic	Main Features	Personality Type	Rating of Severity
		(N.B. these should be persistent and independent of mental state disorder to be scored)	(ICD equivalent)	(0–2)
Fearful	Anxiousness Shyness	Persistent tension and anxiety, excessive self-consciousness, tendency to avoid social contacts	Anxious	

SECTION H

RESOURCELESSNESS
When you are faced with a challenge do you usually respond to it well or do you give in to it?
Are you someone who can normally tackle problems in life alone or do you need other people's help?

How have you coped with major problems in the past? (Give examples)

(When was the last time you coped with a serious problem on your own?)

VULNERABILITY
Do you find that when things go wrong in your life (e.g. loss of job, death in family) you are disturbed a great deal, or do you cope with them well?
Does it usually take a short or long time to get back to normal after upsets in your life?

(How do you think you would cope with a crisis such as death in the family, car accident or loss of your job?)

Take into account relevant answers to questions about drug and alcohol use and nature of close relationships in the previous section, 'preliminary information'.

Please record no dependent personality abnormality (0) if score 0, dependent personality difficulty (1) if these traits are present but not causing serious social dysfunction; and dependent personality disorder (2) if they are causing serious social dysfunction (using PAS guidelines).

Group	Characteristic	Main Features	Personality Type	Rating of Severity
		(N.B. these should be persistent and independent of mental state disorder to be scored)	(ICD equivalent)	(0–2)
Fearful	Resourcelessness Vulnerability	Inability to function without help from others, difficulty adjusting to negative events, excessive dependence on and submissiveness to others	Dependent	

References

Adler G. (1979) The myth of the alliance with borderline patients. *American Journal of Psychiatry*, **136**, 642–645.

Adlington, R. (1925) (Ed. and Trans.) *A Book of Characters*. London: George Rutledge and Sons Ltd; New York: E. P. Dutton and Co.

Akiskal, H. S. (1983) Dysthymic disorder: psychopathology of proposed chronic depressive subtypes. *American Journal of Psychiatry*, **140**, 11–20.

Akiskal, H. S., Hirschfeld, R. M. A. and Yerevanian, B. L. (1983) The relationship of personality to affective disorders: a critical review. *Archives of General Psychiatry*, **40**, 801–810.

Akiskal, H. S., Rosenthal, T. L., Haykal, R. F. *et al.* (1980) Characterological depressions: Clinical and sleep EEG findings separating 'subaffective dysthymias' from character spectrum disorders. *Archives of General Psychiatry*, **37**, 777–783.

Alexander, F. (1930) The neurotic character. *International Journal of Psychoanalysis*, **11**, 291–311.

Allport, G. W. (1937) *Personality: a Psychological Interpretation*, p. 558. New York: Holt, Rinehart and Winston.

Allport, G. W. and Odbert, H. S. (1936) Trait names: a psycholexical study. *Psychological Monographs*, **47**, No. 211.

Alnaes, R. and Torgersen, S. (1988) The relationship between DSM-III symptom disorders (Axis I) and personality disorders (Axis II) in an outpatient population. *Acta Psychiatrica Scandinavica*, **78**, 348–355.

Alpert, J. E., Uebelacker, L. A., Mclean, N. E. *et al.* (1997) Social phobia, avoidant personality disorder and atypical depression: co-occurrence and clinical implications. *Psychological Medicine*, **27**, 627–633.

American Psychiatric Association (1952) *Diagnostic and Statistical Manual of Mental Disorders*, 1st edn. Washington DC: American Psychiatric Association.

American Psychiatric Association (1968) *Diagnostic and Statistical Manual of Mental Disorders*, 2nd edn. Washington DC: American Psychiatric Association.

American Psychiatric Association (1980) *Diagnostic and Statistical Manual of Mental Disorders*, 3rd edn. Washington DC: American Psychiatric Association.

American Psychiatric Association (1987) *Diagnostic and Statistical Manual of Mental Disorders*, 3rd edn revised. Washington DC: American Psychiatric Association.

American Psychiatric Association (1994) *Diagnostic and Statistical Manual of Mental Disorders*, 4th Edition. Washington DC: American Psychiatric Association.

Andreoli, A., Frances, A., Gex-Fabry, M. *et al.* (1993) Crisis intervention in depressed patients with and without DSM-III-R personality disorders. *Journal of Nervous and Mental Disease*, **181**, 721–737.

Andrews, G. (1991) The essential psychotherapies. *British Journal of Psychiatry*, **162**, 447–451.

Andrews, G., Stewart, G., Morris-Yates, A. (1990) Evidence for a general neurotic syndrome. *British Journal of Psychiatry*, **157**, 6–12.

Ansseau, M., Troisfontaines, B., Papart, P., *et al.* (1991) Compulsive personality as predictor of response to serotonergic antidepressants. *British Medical Journal*, **303**, 760–761.

Åsberg, M., Montgomery, S., Perris, C. *et al.* (1978) A comprehensive psychopathological rating scale *Acta Psychiatrica Scandinavia*, **suppl 271**, 5–29.

Aubuchon, P. G. and Malatesta, V. J. (1994) Obsessive compulsive patients with comorbid personality disorder: associated problems and response to a comprehensive behavior therapy. *Journal of Clinical Psychiatry*, **55**, 448–453.

Baer, L. (1994) Factor analysis of symptom subtypes of obsessive compulsive disorder and their relation to personality and tic disorders. *Journal of Clinical Psychiatry*, **55 Suppl**, 18–23.

Ballinger, B. R. and Reid, A. H. (1987) A standardized assessment of personality disorder in mental handicap. *British Journal of Psychiatry*, **150**, 108–109.

Barbato, N. and Hafner, R. J. (1998) Comorbidity of bipolar and personality disorder. *Australia and New Zealand Journal of Psychiatry*, **32**, 276–280.

Barnes, G. F. (1979) The alcoholic personality: a re-analysis of the literature. *Journal of Studies on Alcohol*, **40**, 571–634.

Baron, M. (1981) *Schedule for Interviewing Borderlines*. New York: New York State Psychiatric Institute.

Baron, M., Asnis, L. and Gruen, R. (1981) The Schedule for Schizotypal Personalities (SSP): A diagnostic interview for schizotypal features. *Journal of Psychiatric Research*, **4**, 213–228.

Barrash, J., Kroll, J. and Casey, K. (1983) Discriminating borderline from other personality disorders. *Archives of General Psychiatry*, **40**, 1297–1302.

Barsky, A. J., Barnett, M. C. and Cleary, P. D. (1994) Hypochondriasis and panic disorder. Boundary and overlap. *Archives of General Psychiatry*, **51**, 918–925.

Barsky, A. J., Wyshak, G. and Klerman, G. L. (1992) Psychiatric comorbidity in DSM-III-R hypochondriasis. *Arch. Gen. Psychiatry*, **49**, 101–108.

Barton, R. (1959) *Institutional neurosis*. Bristol: John Wright.

Beck, A. T., Freeman, A. and associates (1990) *Cognitive therapy of personality disorders*. New York: The Guilford Press.

Beck, J. S. (1996) Cognitive therapy for personality disorders. In Salkovskis P. M. (ed.) *Frontiers of cognitive therapy*. The Guilford Press, New York, London.

Bejerot, S., Ekselius, L. and von Knorring, L. (1998) Comorbidity between obsessive-compulsive disorder (OCD) and personality disorders. *Acta Psychiatrica Scandinavia*, **97**, 398–402.

Bell, M. (1981) *Bell Object Relations Self-Report Scale*. West Haven, Connecticut: Veterans Administration Medical Center.

Benjamin, L. S. (1993) *Interpersonal Diagnosis and Treatment of Personality Disorders*. New York: The Guilford Press.

Benjamin, L. S. (1997) Special feature: personality disorders: models for treatment and strategies for treatment development. *Journal of Personality Disorders*, **11**, 307–324.

Bennie, E. H. and Kinnell, H. G. (1975) Dangerous offenders. *Lancet*, **ii**, 1303.

Berne, E. (1970) *Games People Play*. London: Penguin.

Bianchi, G. (1971) Origins of disease phobia. *Australia and New Zealand Journal of Psychiatry*, **5**, 241–257.

Bianchi, G. N. and Fergusson, D. M. (1977) The effect of mental state on EPI scores. *British Journal of Psychiatry*, **131**, 306–309.

Black, D. W., Warrack, G. and Winokur, G. (1985) The Iowa record-linkage study: 1. Suicides and accidental deaths among psychiatric patients. *Archives of General Psychiatry*, **42**, 71–75.

Black, D. W. and Moyer, T. (1998) Clinical features and psychiatric comorbidity of subjects with pathological gambling behavior. *Psychiatric Services*, **49**, 1434–1439.

Black, D. W., Noyes, R. J., Pfohl, B., Goldstein, R. B. and Blum, N. (1993) Personality disorder in obsessive-compulsive volunteers, well comparison subjects, and their first-degree relatives. *American Journal of Psychiatry*, **150**, 1226–1232.

Bland, R. C., Newman, S. C., Dyck, R. J. *et al.* (1990) Prevalence of psychiatric disorders in a prison population. *Canadian Journal of Psychiatry*. **35**, 407–413.

Blashfield, R., Noyes, R., Reich, J. *et al.* (1994) Personality disorder traits in generalized anxiety and panic disorder patients. *Comprehensive Psychiatry*, **35**, 329–334.

Blashfield, R., Sprock, J., Pinkston, K. and Hodgin, J. (1985) Exemplar prototypes of personality disorder diagnoses. *Comprehensive Psychiatry*, **26**, 11–21.

Blazer, D., George, L. K., Landerman, *et al.* (1985) Psychiatric disorders. A rural/urban comparison. *Archives of General Psychiatry*, **42**, 651–656.

Bleuler, M. (1941) *Course of illness, personality and family history in schizophrenics*. Liepzig: Thième.

Bluglass, R. S. (1977) A Psychiatric Study of Scottish Prisoners. *MD Thesis*, St Andrew's University.

Bowden, P. (1978) Men remanded into custody for medical reports: the selection for treatment. *British Journal of Psychiatry*, **133**, 320–331.

Bowlby, J. (1973) *Attachment and Loss, Volume 2 – Separation: Anxiety and Anger*. London: Hogarth Press.

Bowman, M. J. and Sturgeon, D. A. (1977) A clinic within a general hospital for the assessment of urgent psychiatric problems. *Lancet*, **ii**, 1067–1068.

Bridges, K. W. and Goldberg, D. P. (1985) Somatic presentation of DSM-III psychiatric disorders in primary care. *Journal of Psychosomatic Research*, **29**, 563–569.

Brinkley, J. R., Beitman, B. D. and Friedel, R. O. (1979) Low dose neuroleptic regimes in the treatment of borderline patients. *Archives of General Psychiatry*, **36**, 319–326.

Briquet, P. (1859) *Traité clinique et thérapeutique de l'hystérie*. Paris: Baillière.

Bronisch, T. and Mombour, W. (1994) Comparison of a diagnostic checklist with a structured interview for the assessment of DSM-III-R and ICD-10 personality disorders. *Psychopathology*, **27**, 312–320.

Brooner, R. K., Herbst, J. H., Schmidt, C. W. *et al.* (1993) Antisocial personality disorder among drug abusers. Relations to other personality diagnoses and the five-factor model of personality. *Journal of Nervous and Mental Disease*, **181**, 313–319.

Brooner, R. K., King, V. L., Kidorf, M. *et al.* (1997) Psychiatric and substance use comorbidity among treatment-seeking opioid abusers. *Archives of General Psychiatry*, **54**, 71–80.

Brothwell, J., Casey, P. R. and Tyrer, P. (1992) Who gives the most reliable account of a psychiatric patient's personality? *Irish Journal of Psychological Medicine*, **9**, 90–93.

Burke, K. C., Burke, J. D. J., Regier, D. A. and Rae, D. S. (1990) Age at onset of selected mental disorders in five community populations. *Archives of General Psychiatry*, **47**, 511–518.

Buss, A. H. and Plomin, R. (1975) *A Temperament Theory of Personality*. New York: Wiley.

Cahalan, D. and Room, R. (1974) *Problem Drinking among American Men*. New Brunswick, NJ: Rutgers Center of Alcohol Studies.

Campling, P. (1999) Boundaries: discussion of a difficult transition. In: *Therapeutic Communities: Past, Present and Future*, eds Campling, P. and Haigh, R., pp. 90–98. London: Jessica Kingsley.

Caplan, P. J. (1987) The Psychiatric Association's failure to meet its own standards: the dangers of self-defeating personality as a category. *Journal of Personality Disorders*, **1**, 178–182.

Casey, P. R. (1985) Psychiatric morbidity in general practice: A diagnostic approach. *MD Thesis*, University College, Cork, Ireland.

Casey, P. R. (1989) Personality disorder and suicide intent. *Acta Psychiatrica Scandinavica*. **79**, 290–295.

Casey, P. and Tyrer, P. (1986) Personality, functioning and symptomatology. *Journal of Psychiatric Research*, **20**, 363–374.

Casey, P. and Butler, E. (1995) The effects of personality on response to ECT in major depression. *Journal of Personality Disorder*, **9**, 134–142.

Casey, P., Dillon, S. and Tyrer, P. (1984) The diagnostic status of patients with conspicuous psychiatric morbidity in primary care. *Psychological Medicine*, **14**, 673–681.

Caspi, A. (1996) Personality development across the life course. *Handbook of Child Psychology*, 5th Edn Vol 3 Chap. 6, eds W. Dawson and N. Eisenberg, New York: Wiley.

Castaneda, R. and Franco, H. (1985) Sex and ethnic distribution of borderline personality disorder in an inpatient sample. *American Journal of Psychiatry*, **142**, 1202–1203.

Cattell, R. B. (1965) *The Scientific Analysis of Personality*. Harmondsworth: Penguin Books Ltd.

Chodoff, P. and Lyons, H. (1958) Hysteria, the hysterical personality and 'hysterical' conversion. *American Journal of Psychiatry*, **114**, 734–740.

Christiansen, K. O. (1970) Crime in the Danish twin population. *Acta Geneticae Medicae et Gemellogiae*, **19**, 323–326.

Cicchetti, D. V. (1976) Assessing inter-rater reliability for rating scales: Resolving some basic issues. *British Journal of Psychiatry*, **129**, 452–456.

Cicchetti, D. V. and Sparrow, S. S. (1981) Developing criteria for establishing the interrater reliability of specific items in a given inventory. *American Journal of Mental Deficiency*, **86**, 127–137.

Cicchetti, D. V., Aivano, S. L. and Vitale, J. (1977) Computer programs for assessing rater agreement and rater bias for qualitative data. *Educational and Psychological Measurement*, **37**, 195–201.

Cicchetti, D. V., Lee, C., Fontana, A. F. and Dowds, B. N. (1978) A computer program for assessing specific category rater agreement for qualitative data. *Educational and Psychological Measurement*, **38**, 805–813.

Cicchetti, D. V., Heavens, R., Didriksen, J. and Showalter, D. (1984) A computer program for assessing the reliability of nominal scales using varying sets of multiple raters. *Educational and Psychological Measurement*, **44**, 671–675.

Cicchetti, D. V., Showalter, D. and Tyrer, P. (1985) The effects of number of rating scale categories on levels of inter-rater reliability: a Monte Carlo investigation. *Applied Psychological Measurement*, **9**, 31–36.

Ciompi, L. (1969) Follow-up studies on the evolution of former neurotic and depressive states in old age: clinical and psychodynamic aspects. *Journal of Geriatric Psychiatry*, **3**, 90–106.

Clark, D. H. (1965) The therapeutic community concept: practice and future. *British Journal of Psychiatry*, **106**, 947–954.

Clark, L. A. (1990) *Schedule for Normal and Abnormal Personality (SCAN)*. Department of Psychiatry, University of Iowa.

Clark, L. A. (1992) Resolving taxonomic issues in personality disorders. *Journal of Personality Disorders*, **6**, 360–376.

Clark, L. A., Watson, D. and Reynolds, S. (1995) Diagnosis and classification of psychopathology: challenges to the current system and future directions. *Annual Review of Psychology*, **46**, 121–153.

Clark, L. A., Livesley, W. J., Schroeder, M. L. and Irish, S. L. (1996) Convergence of two systems for assessing personality disorders. *Psychological Assessment*, **8**, 294–303.

Cleckley, H. (1941) *The Mask of Sanity*. London: Henry Kimpton.

Cloninger, C. R. (1987) A systematic method for clinical description and classification of personality variants. *Archives of General Psychiatry*, **44**, 573–588.

Cloninger, C. R. and Guze, S. B. (1970) Psychiatric illness in female criminality: the role of sociopathy and hysteria in the antisocial woman. *American Journal of Psychiatry*, **127**, 303–311.

Cloninger, C. R., Reich, T. and Guze, S. B. (1975) A multifactorial model of disease transmission. III: familial relationships between sociopathy and hysteria (Briquet's syndrome) *British Journal of Psychiatry*, **127**, 23–32.

Cloninger, C. R., Svrakic, D. M. and Pryzbeck, T. R. (1993) A psychobiological model of temperament and character. *Archives of General Psychiatry*, **50**, 975–990.

Clopton, J. R., Weddige, R. L., Contreras, S. A., et al. (1993) Treatment outcome for substance misuse patients with personality disorder. *International Journal of Addiction*, **28**, 1147–1153.

Cohen, J. (1968) Weighted kappa: Nominal scale agreement with provision for scaled disagreement or partial credit. *Psychological Bulletin*, **70**, 213–320.

Coid, J. (1993) Current concepts and classification of psychopathic disorder. In '*Personality Disorders Reviewed*' (eds P. Tyrer and G. S. Stein) pp. 113–164. London: Gaskell.

Coid, J., Robertson, G. and Gunn, J. (1991) A psychiatric study of inmates in Parkhurst Special Unit in *Managing Difficult Prisoners*. Ed. R. Walmsley, Home Office Research Study 122, London: HMSO.

Conte, H., Plutchik, R., Karasu, T. B. and Jerret, I. (1980) A self-report borderline scale, discriminative validity and preliminary norms. *Journal of Nervous and Mental Disease*, **168**, 428–435.

Cooney, J. M., Farren, C. K. and Clare, A. (1996) Personality disorders among first ever admissions to an Irish public and private hospital. *Irish Journal of Psychological Medicine*, **13**, 6–8.

Cooper, B. (1965) A study of one hundred chronic psychiatric patients identified in general practice. *British Journal of Psychiatry*, **111**, 595–605.

Coppen, A. L. and Metcalfe, H. (1965) The effect of a depressive illness on MMPI scores. *British Journal of Psychiatry*, **111**, 236–239.

Cornelius, J. R., Soloff, P. H., Perel, J. M. *et al.* (1993) Continuation pharmacotherapy of borderline personality disorder with haloperidol and phenelzine. *American Journal of Psychiatry*, **150**, 1843–1848.

Cornell, D. G., Silk, K. R., Ludolf, P. and Lohr, N. E. (1983) The test-retest reliability of the Diagnostic Interview for Borderlines. *Archives of General Psychiatry*, **40**, 1307–1310.

Costa, P. and McCrae, R. (1992) *The NEO PI-R Professional Manual.* Psychological Assessment Resources, Odessa, Florida, USA.

Cote, G. and Hodgins, S. (1990) Co-occurring mental disorders among criminal offenders. *Bulletin of the American Academy of Psychiatry and Law*, **18**, 271–281.

Cowdry, R. W. and Garner, D. L. (1988) Pharmacotherapy of borderline personality disorder: alprazolam, carbamazepine, trifluoperazine and tranylcypromine. *Arch Gen Psychiatry*, **45**, 111–119.

Crockford, D. N. and el-Guebaly, N. (1998) Psychiatric comorbidity in pathological gambling: a critical review. *Canadian Journal of Psychiatry*, **43**, 43–50.

Cunningham-Williams, R. M., Cottler, L. B., Compton, W. M. and Spitznagel, E. L. (1998) Taking chances: problem gamblers and mental health disorders – results from the St. Louis Epidemiologic Catchment Area Study [published erratum appears in American Journal of Public Health 1998 Sep; 88(9): 1407]. *American Journal of Public Health*, **88**, 1093–1096.

Curran, D. and Mallinson, W. P. (1944) Recent progress in psychiatry: psychopathic personality. *Journal of Mental Science*, **90**, 266–287.

Curran, D. and Partridge, M. (1963) *Psychological Medicine*, 5th edn. London: E. S. Livingstone.

Cutting, J. (1985) *The Psychology of Schizophrenia.* Edinburgh: Churchill Livingstone.

Cutting, J., Cowen, P. J., Mann, A. H. and Jenkins, R. (1986) Personality and psychosis: use of the Standardized Assessment of Personality. *Acta Psychiatrica Scandinavica*, **73**, 87–92.

Dahl, A. A. (1996) The relationship between social phobia and avoidant personality disorder: workshop report 3. *International Clinical Psychopharmacology*, **11**, *Suppl 3*, 109–112.

Dale, P. G. (1980) Lithium therapy in agressive mentally subnormal patients. *British Journal of Psychiatry*, **137**, 469–474.

Dally, P. and Gomez, J. (1979) *Anorexia nervosa.* London: Heinemann.

Darke, S., Hall, W. and Swift, W. (1994) Prevalence, symptoms and correlates of antisocial personality disorder among methadone maintenance clients. *Drug and Alcohol Dependence*, **34**, 253–257.

Davidson, K. M. (2000) *Cognitive therapy for personality disorders: a treatment manual.* Oxford: Butterworth–Heinemann.

Davidson, K. M. and Tyrer, P. (1996) Cognitive therapy for antisocial and borderline personality disorders: single case series. *British Journal of Clinical Psychology*, **35**, 413–429.

Davis, D. R. (1972) *Introduction to Psychopathology*, 3rd edn. Oxford: Oxford University Press.

Davis, D. R. (1987) How useful a diagnosis is borderline personality? *British Medical Journal*, **294**, 265–266.

de Girolamo, G. and Reich, J. H. (1993) *Personality disorders.* Geneva: World Health Organisation.

DeJong, C. A., Van den Brink, W., Harteveld, F. M. and van der Wielen, E. G. (1993). Personality disorders in alcoholics and drug addicts. *Comprehensive Psychiatry*, **34**, 87–94.

Deltito, J. A. and Stam, M. (1989) Psychopharmacological treatment of avoidant personality disorder. *Comprehensive Psychiatry*, **30**, 498–504.

Department of Health and Social Security (1985) *Mental Illness Hospitals and Units in England. Results from the Mental Health Enquiry.* Statistical Bulletin, Government Statistical Service. London: HMSO.

Diaferia, G., Bianchi, I., Bianchi, M. L. *et al.* (1997) Relationship between obsessive-compulsive personality disorder and obsessive-compulsive disorder. *Comprehensive Psychiatry*, **38**, 38–42.

Dilling, H. and Weyerer, S. (1980) Incidence and prevalence of treated mental disorders. Health care planning in a small-town rural region of upper Bavaria. *Acta Psychiatrica Scandinavica*, **61**, 209–222.

Dilling, H., Weyerer, S. and Fichter, M. (1989) The Upper Bavarian Studies. *Acta Psychiatrica Scandinavica* **79** (Suppl. 348), 113–140.

Dohrenwend, B. P. and Dohrenwend, B. S. (1969) *Social status and psychological disorder: a causal inquiry.* New York: Wiley Interscience.

Dolan, B. and Coid, J. (1993) *Psychopathic and antisocial personality disorders: treatment and research issues.* Gaskell Books, Royal College of Psychiatrists, London.

Dolan, B., Evans, C., Norton, K. (1995) Multiple axis-II diagnoses of personality disorder. *British Journal of Psychiatry*, **166**, 107–112.

Dolan, B. M., Norton, K. and Warren, F. M. (1996) Cost-offset following specialist treatment of severe personality disorder. *Psychiatric Bulletin*, **20**, 413–417.

Dolan, B., Warren, F. and Norton, K. (1997) Changein borderline symptoms one year after therapeutic community treatment for severe personality disorder. *British Journal of Psychiatry*, **171**, 274–279.

Dowson, J. H. (1992a) Associations between self-induced vomiting and personality disorder in patients with a history of anorexia nervosa. *Acta Psychiatrica Scandinavica*, **86**, 399–404.

Dowson, J. H. (1992b) Assessment of DSM-III-R personality disorders by self-report questionnaires: the role of informants and a screening test for comorbid personality disorders. *British Journal of Psychiatry*, **161**, 344–352.

Dowson, J. H. and Grounds, A. T. (1995) *Personality disorders: recognition and clinical management*. Cambridge: Cambridge University Press.

Dreessen, L., Hoekstra, R. and Arntz, A. (1997) Personality disorders do not influence the results of cognitive and behavior therapy for obsessive compulsive disorder. *Journal of Anxiety Disorders*, **11**, 503–521.

Editorial (1934) Friends and enemies. *Lancet*, **ii**, 1232.

Edwards, D. J. A. (1990) Cognitive therapy and the restructuring of early memories through guided imagery. *Journal of Cognitive Psychotherapy: An International Quarterly*, **4**, 33–50.

Ekselius, L. and von Knorring, L. (1998) Personality disorder comorbidity with major depression and response to treatment with sertraline or citalopram. *International Clinical Psychopharmacology*, **13**, 205–211.

Emmanuel, J. S., Simmonds, S. and Tyrer, P. (1998) A systematic review of the outcome of anxiety and depressive disorders. *British Journal of Psychiatry*, **173**, suppl 34, 35–41.

Ennis, J., Barnes, R. A., Kennedy, S. *et al.* (1989) Depression in self-harm patients. *British Journal of Psychiatry*, **154**, 41–47.

Eronen, M., Angermeyer, M. C. and Schulze, B. (1998) The psychiatric epidemiology of violent behaviour. *Social Psychiatry and Psychiatric Epidemiology*, **33** Suppl 1, S13–23.

Essen-Möller, E. (1956) Individual traits and morbidity in a Swedish rural population. *Acta Psychiatrica Scandinavica, Supplementum*, **2**, 100.

Evans, K., Tyrer, P., Catalan, J. *et al.* (1999) Manual-assisted cognitive-behaviour therapy (MACT): a randomised controlled trial of a brief intervention with bibliotherapy in the treatment of recurrent deliberate self-harm. *Psychological Medicine*, **29**, 19–25.

Everitt, B. S. (1974) *Cluster Analysis*. London: Heinemann.

Eysenck, H. J. (1947) *Dimensions of Personality*. London: Kegan Paul.

Eysenck, H. J. (1959) *The Maudsley Personality Inventory*. University of London Press, London.

Eysenck, H. J. and Eysenck, S. B. G. (1964) *Manual of the Eysenck Personality Inventory*. London: University of London Press.

Eysenck, H. J. and Eysenck, S. B. G. (1969) *Manual of the Eysenck Personality Questionnaire (EPQ)*. London: University of London Press.

Eysenck, H. J. and Eysenck, S. B. G. (1975) *The Eysenck Personality Questionnaire*. London: University of London Press.

Fabrega, H. J., Ulrich, R., Pilkonis, P., and Mezzich, J. (1993) Personality disorders diagnosed at intake at a public psychiatric facility. *Hospital and Community Psychiatry* **44**, 159–162.

Fahy, T., Woodruff, P. and Szmukler, G. (1998) The etiology of schizophrenia. In: *Seminars in General Adult Psychiatry, Vol. 1*, eds G. Stein and G. Wilkinson Gaskell, London, pp. 321–380.

Fava, M., Bouffides, E., Pava, J. A. *et al.* (1994) Personality disorder comorbidity with major depression and response to fluoxetine treatment. *Psychotherapy and Psychosomatics*, **62**, 160–167.

Feighner, J. P., Robins, E., Guze, S. B. *et al.* (1972) Diagnostic criteria for use in psychiatric research. *Archives of General Psychiatry*, **26**, 57–63.

Feinstein, A. (1970) The pre-therapeutic classification of comorbidity in chronic disease. *Journal of Chronic Diseases*, **23**, 455–462.

Fenichel, O. (1945) *The Psychoanalytic Theory of Neurosis*. New York: Norton.

Fink, D. (1991) The comorbidity of multiple personality disorder and DSM-III-R axis II disorders. *Psychiatric Clinics of North America*, **14**, 547–566.

Fink, P. (1995) Psychiatric illness in patients with persistent somatisation. *British Journal of Psychiatry*, **166**, 93–99.

First, M. B., Spitzer, R. L., Gibbon, M. and Williams, J. B. W. (1995) The Structured Clinical Interview for DSM-III-R Personality Disorders (SCID-II): Part 1: Description. *Journal of Personality Disorders*, **9**, 83–91.

Fleiss, J. L., Nee, J. C. M. and Landis, J. R. (1979) The large sample variance of kappa in the case of different sets of raters. *Psychological Bulletin*, **86**, 974–977.

Flick, S. N., Roy-Byrne, P. P., Cowley, D. S. *et al.* (1993) DSM-III-R personality disorders in a mood and anxiety disorders clinic: prevalence, comorbidity and clinical correlates. *Journal of Affective Disorders*, **27**, 71–79.

Frances, A. (1980) The DSM-III personality disorders section: a commentary. *American Journal of Psychiatry*, **137**, 1050–1054.

Freud, S. (1908) Character and anal-eroticism. In *Collected Papers* (1933), vol. 2, p. 45. London: Hogarth Press.

Freud, S. (1914) On narcissism: an introduction. In *Collected Works* (1957), edited by J. Strachey, vol. 14, pp. 69–102. London: Hogarth Press.

Freud, S. (1916) Some character types met with in psychoanalytic work. In: *The Standard Edition of the Complete Psychological Works of Sigmund Freud*, Volume 14, pp. 309–333. London: Hogarth Press, 1974.

Freud, S. (1932) Libidinal types. In *Collected Papers* (1950), vol. 5. London: Hogarth Press.

Fromm, E. (1942) *Fear of Freedom*. London: Routledge.

Fyer, M. R., Frances, A. J. and Sullivan, T. (1988) Comorbidity of borderline personality disorder. *Archives of General Psychiatry*, **45**, 348–352.

Garside, R. F. and Roth, M. (1978) Multivariate statistical methods and problems of classification in psychiatry. *British Journal of Psychiatry*, **133**, 53–67.

Gillberg, I. C., Rastam, M., and Gillberg, C. (1995) Anorexia nervosa 6 years after onset: Part I. Personality disorders. *Comprehensive Psychiatry*, **36**, 61–69.

Glatzel, J. (1974) Kritische Anmerkurgen zum 'Typus melancholicus' Tellenbach. *Archiv für Psychiatrie und Nervenkrankheiten*, **219**, 197–206.

Goffman, E. (1956) *The presentation of self in everyday life*.

Monograph 2, Social Sciences Research Centre. Edinburgh: University of Edinburgh.

Goldberg, S. C., Shulz, S. C., Shulz, P. M. *et al.* (1986) Borderline and schizotypal personality disorders treated with low dose thiothixene versus placebo. *Archives of General Psychiatry* 43: 680–686.

Goldstein, S. G. and Linden, J. D. (1969) Multivariate classification of alcoholics by means of the MMPI. *Journal of Abnormal Psychology*, **74**, 661–669.

Graham, P. and Stevenson, J. (1987a) Temperament and psychiatric disorders – the genetic contribution of behaviour in childhood. *Australian and New Zealand Journal of Psychiatry*, **21**, 267–274.

Graham, P. J. and Stevenson, J. E. (1987b) Temperament, personality and personality disorder. *British Journal of Psychiatry*, **150**, 872–873.

Greer, H. S. & Cawley, R. H. (1966) Some observations on the natural history of neurotic illness. In *Australian Medical Association, Mervyn Archdall Medical Monograph No. 3* Glebe, Australia: Australasian Medical Publishing Company.

Griggs, S. M. L. B. and Tyrer, P. J. (1981) Personality disorder, social adjustment and treatment outcome in alcoholics. *Journal on Studies of Alcohol*, **42**, 802–805.

Guilford, J. P. and Guildord, R. B. (1939) An analysis of the factors in a typical test of introversion and extraversion. *Journal of Abnormal and Social Psychology*, **28**, 377–399.

Guilford, J. S., Zimmerman, W. S. and Guilford, J. P. (1976) *The Guilford-Zimmerman Temperament Survey Handbook*. San Diego: EDITS publishers.

Gunderson, J. G. and Singer, M. T. (1975) Defining borderline patients: An overview. *American Journal of Psychiatry*, **132**, 1–10.

Gunderson, J. G., Kolb, J. E. and Austin, V. (1981) The diagnostic interview for borderline patients, *American Journal of Psychiatry*, **138**, 896–903.

Gunderson, J. G. and Zanarini, M. C. (1987) Current overview of the borderline diagnosis. *Journal of Clinical Psychiatry*, **48**, 5–11.

Gunderson, J. G. and Phillips, K. A. (1991) A current view on the interface between borderline personality disorder and depression. *American Journal of Psychiatry*, **148**, 967–975.

Gunn, J. (1974) Disasters, asylums and plans: forensic psychiatry today. *British Medical Journal*, **3**, 611–613.

Gunn, J., Robertson, G., Dell, S. and Way, C. (1978) *Psychiatric Aspects of Imprisonment*. London: Academic Press.

Guze, S. B. (1976) *Criminality and Psychiatric Disorders*. New York: Oxford University Press.

Guze, S. B. and Goodwin, D. W. (1971) Diagnostic consistency in antisocial personality. *American Journal of Psychiatry*, **128**, 360–361.

Guze, S. B., Wolfgran, E. D., McKinney, J. K. and Cantwell, D. P. (1967) Psychiatric illness in the families of convicted criminals. A study of 519 first-degree relatives. *Diseases of the Nervous System*, **28**, 651–659.

Guze, S. B., Woodruff, R. A., J.R. and Clayton, P. J. (1971) Hysteria and antisocial behaviour: further evidence of an association. *American Journal of Psychiatry*, **127**, 957–960.

Guze, S. B., Cloninger, C. R., Martin, R. L. and Clayton, P. J. (1986) A follow-up and family study of Briquet's syndrome. *British Journal of Psychiatry*, **149**, 17–23.

Haigh, R. (1999) The quintessence of a therapeutic environment: five universal qualities. In: *Therapeutic Communities: Past, Present and Future*, eds Campling, P. and Haigh, R., pp. 246–257. London: Jessica Kingsley.

Halleck, S. L. (1967) Hysterical personality traits: psychological, social and iatrogenic determinants. *Archives of General Psychiatry*, **16**, 750–757.

Hare, R. D. (1970) *Psychopathy: Theory and Research*. New York: John Wiley.

Hare, R. D. (1980) A research scale for the assessment of psychopathy in criminal populations. *Personality and Individual Differences*, **1**, 111–117.

Hare, R. D. (1991) *The Hare Psychopathy Checklist – Revised*. Toronto: Multi-health Systems.

Harrington, R., Fudge, H., Rutter, M. *et al.* (1991) Adult outcomes of childhood and adolescent depression: II. Links with antisocial disorders. *Journal of the American Academy of Child and Adolescent Psychiatry*, **30**, 434–439.

Hassiotis, A., Tyrer, P. and Cicchetti, D. (1997) Detection of personality disorders by a community mental health team: a study of diagnostic accuracy. *Irish Journal of Psychological Medicine*, **14**, 88–91.

Heikkinen, M., Henriksson, M., Isometsa, E. *et al.* (1997) Recent life events and suicide in personality disorders. *Journal of Nervous and Mental Disease*, **185**, 373–381.

Helzer, J. E. and Pryzbeck, T. R. (1988) The co-occurrence of alcoholism with other psychiatric disorders in the general population and its impact on treatment. *Journal of Studies on Alcohol*, **49**, 219–224.

Henderson, D. K. (1939) *Psychopathic States*. New York: Norson.

Herbert, J. D., Hope, D. A. and Bellack, A. S. (1992) Validity of the distinction between generalized social phobia and avoidant personality disorder. *Journal of Abnormal Psychology*, **101**, 332–339.

Herman, J., Perry, J. and Van der Kolk, B. (1989) Childhood trauma in borderline personality disorder. *American Journal of Psychiatry*, **146**, 490–495.

Herzog, D. B., Keller, M. B., Lavori, P. W. *et al.* (1992) The prevalence of personality disorders in 210 women with eating disorders. *Journal of Clinical Psychiatry*, **53**, 147–152.

Higgitt, A. and Fonagy, P. (1992) Psychotherapy in borderline and narcissistic personality disorder. *British Journal of Psychiatry*, **161**, 23–43.

Hill, D. and Watterson, D. (1942) Electroencephalographic studies of psychopathic personalities. *Journal of Neurology and Psychiatry*, **5**, 47–52.

Hill, J., Harrington, R., Fudge, H. *et al.* (1989) Adult Personality Functioning Assessment (APFA): an investigator-based standardised interview. *British Journal of Psychiatry*, **155**, 24–35.

Hirschfeld, R. M. A. and Klerman, G. L. (1979) Personality attributes and affective disorders. *American Journal of Psychiatry*, **136**, 67–70.

Hirschfeld, R. M. A., Klerman, G. L., Clayton, P. J. *et al.* (1983) Assessing personality: effects of the depressive state on trait measurement. *American Journal of Psychiatry*, **140**, 695–699.

Hirschfeld, R. M., Holzer, C. E. (1994) Depressive personality disorder: clinical implications. *Journal of Clinical Psychiatry*, **55**, 10–17.

Hoch, P. and Polatin, P. (1949) Pseudo-neurotic forms of schizophrenia. *Psychiatric Quarterly*, **23**, 248–276.

Hoeper, E. W., Nycz, G. R., Cleary, P. D. *et al.* (1979) Estimated prevalence of RDC mental disorder in primary medical care. *International Journal of Mental Health*, **8**, 6–15.

Hoffart, A., Thornes, K. and Hedley, L. M. (1995) DSM-III-R Axis I and II disorders in agoraphobic inpatients with and without panic disorder before and after psychosocial treatment. *Psychiatry Research*, **56**, 1–9.

Hoffman, J. A., Caudill, B. D., Koman, J. J. *et al.* (1994) Comparative cocaine abuse treatment strategies: enhancing client retention and treatment exposure. *Journal of Addiction Disorders*, **13**, 115–128.

Holmboe, R. and Astrup, C. (1957) A follow-up study of 255 patients with acute schizophrenia and schizophreniform psychoses. *Acta Psychiatrica et Neurologica Scandinavica, Supplementum*, **115**.

Horney, K. (1939) *New ways in Psycho-analysis*. London: Kegan Paul.

Howard, M. O., Kivlahan, D. and Walker, R. D. (1997) Cloninger's tridimensional theory of personality and psychopathology: applications to substance use disorders. *Journal of Studies on Alcohol*, **58**, 48–66.

Hudziak, J. J., Boffeli, T. J., Kreisman, J. J. *et al.* (1996) Clinical study of the relation of borderline personality disorder to Briquet's syndrome (hysteria), somatization disorder, antisocial personality disorder, and substance abuse disorders *American Journal of Psychiatry*, **153**, 1598–1606.

Hyler, S. E. (1994) *Personality Diagnostic Questionnaire-4*. New York: New York State Psychiatric Institute.

Hyler, S. E., Reider, R. O. (1984) *Personality Diagnostic Questionnaire-revised*. New York: New York State Psychiatric Institute.

Hyler, S. E. and Lyons, M. J. (1988) Factor analysis of the DSM-III personality disorders. *Comprehensive Psychiatry*, **29**, 304–308.

Hyler, S., Reider, R., Spitzer, R. and Williams, J. B. W. (1983) *Personality Diagnostic Questionnaire (PDQ)*. New York: New York State Psychiatric Institute.

Hyler, S. E., Rieder, R. O., Williams, J. B. W., Spitzer, R. *et al.* (1988) The Personality Diagnostic Questionnaire: development and preliminary results. *Journal of Personality Disorders*, **2**, 229–237.

Innes, G. and Millar, W. M. (1970) Mortality among psychiatric patients. *Scottish Medical Journal*, **15**, 143–148.

International Committee for Standardization in Haematology (1978) Recommendations for reference method for haemoglobinometry in human blood (ICSH Standard EP 6/2: 1977) and specifications for international haemoglobincyanide reference preparation (ICSH Standard EP 6/3: 1977). *Journal of Clinical Pathology*, **31**, 139–143.

Jackson, H. J., Whiteside, H. L., Bates, G. W. *et al.* (1991) Diagnosing personality disorder in psychiatric inpatients. *Acta Psychiatrica Scandinavica*, **83**, 206–213.

Jacobson, S. and Tribe, P. (1972) Deliberate self injury (attempted suicide) in patients admitted to hospital in mid-Sussex. *British Journal of Psychiatry*, **121**, 379–386.

Jaspers, K. (1946) *Allgemeine Psychopathologie*, 4th edn. Berlin: Springer.

Johnson, E. O., van den Bree, M. B., Gupman, A. E. and Pickens, R. W. (1998) Extension of a typology of alcohol dependence based on relative genetic and environmental loading. *Alcohol Clinical and Experimental Research*, **22**, 1421–1429.

Jones, M. (1952) *Social Psychiatry: A Study of Therapeutic Communities*. London: Tavistock Press.

Jones, M. (1956) Industrial rehabilitation of mental patients still in hospital. *Lancet*, **ii**, 985–987.

Kahn, E. (1928) Psychopathic personalities. In *Buinke's Handbook of Mental Diseases*, Vol. 5, p. 227. Berlin: Springer.

Kaplan, M. (1983) A woman's view of DSM-III. *American Psychologist*, **38**, 786–792.

Kass, F., Skodol, A. E., Charles, E. *et al.* (1985) Scaled ratings of DSM-III personality disorders. *American Journal of Psychiatry*, **143**, 627–630.

Kelly, G. A. (1955) *The Psychology of Personal Constructs*. New York: Norton.

Kemp, R., Hayward, P., Applewhaite, G. *et al.* (1996) Compliance therapy in psychotic patients: randomised controlled trial. *British Medical Journal*, **312**, 345–349.

Kemp, R., Kirov, G., Applewhaite, G. *et al.* (1998) Randomised controlled trial of compliance therapy: 18 month follow-up. *British Journal of Psychiatry*, **172**, 413–419.

Kendell, R. E. (1975) *The Role of Diagnosis in Psychiatry*. Oxford: Blackwell.

Kendell, R. E. and DisCipio, W. J. (1968) Eysenck Personality Inventory scores of patients with depressive illness. *British Journal of Psychiatry*, **114**, 767–770.

Kendler, K. S., McGuire, M., Gruenberg, A. M. *et al.* (1993) The Roscommon Family Study. III. Schizophrenia-related personality disorders in relatives. *Archives of General Psychiatry*, **50**, 781–788.

Kendler, K. S., Walters, E. E., Neale, M. C., *et al.* (1995) The structure of the genetic and environmental risk factors for six major psychiatric disorders in women: phobia, generalized anxiety disorder, panic disorder, bulimia, major depression, and alcoholism. *Archives of General Psychiatry*, **52**, 374–383.

Kendler, K. S. and Prescott, C. A. (1998) Cannabis use, abuse, and dependence in a population-based sample of female twins. *American Journal of Psychiatry*, **155**, 1016–1022.

Kenyon, F. E. (1965) Hypochondriasis: a survey of some historical, clinical and social aspects. *British Journal of Medical Psychology*, **38**, 117–133.

Kernberg, O. F. (1967) Borderline personality organisation. *Journal of the American Psychoanalytical Association*, **15**, 641–685.

Kernberg, O. F. (1975) *Borderline Conditions and Pathological Narcissism*. New York: Jason Aronson.

Kernberg, O. F. (1984) *Severe Personality Disorders: Psychotherapeutic Strategies*. New Haven, Connecticut: Yale University Press.

Kernberg, O. F., Burstein, E. and Coyne, L. *et al.* (1972) Psychotherapy and psychoanalysis: final report of the Menninger Foundation's psychotherapy research project. *Bulletin of the Menninger Clinic*, **36**, 1–275.

Kerr, T. A., Roth, M. and Schapira, K. (1974) Prediction of outcome in anxiety states and depressive illnesses. *British Journal of Psychiatry*, **124**, 125–133.

Kessel, N. (1960) Psychiatric morbidity in a London general practice. *British Journal of Preventive and Social Medicine*, **14**, 16–22.

Kety, S. S., Rosenthal, D., Wender, P. H. *et al.* (1975) Mental illness in the biological and adoptive families of adopted individuals who have become schizophrenic. In *Genetic Research in Psychiatry*, ed. R. R. Fieve, D. Rosenthal and H. Brill, pp. 147–165. Baltimore: Johns Hopkins University Press.

Kingdon, D., Tyrer, P., Seivewright, N. *et al.* (1996) The Nottingham Study of Neurotic Disorder: influence of cognitive therapists on outcome. *British Journal of Psychiatry*, **169**, 93–97.

Klein, D. N., Miller, G. A. (1993) Depressive personality in non-clinical subjects. *American Journal of Psychiatry*, **150**, 1718–1724.

Klein, D. N. and Shih, J. H. (1998) Depressive personality: associations with DSM-III-R mood and personality disorders and negative and positive affectivity, 30-month stability, and prediction of course of Axis I depressive disorders. *Journal of Abnormal Psychology*, **107**, 319–327.

Klein, M. H., Benjamin, L. S., Rosenfeld, R. *et al.* (1993) The Wisconsin Personality Disorders Interview: development, reliability and validity. *Journal of Personality Disorders*, **7**, 285–303.

Klein, D. N., Riso, L. P., Donaldson, S. K. *et al.* (1995) Family study of early-onset dysthymia. Mood and personality disorders in relatives of outpatients with dysthymia and episodic major depression and normal controls. *Archives of General Psychiatry*, **52**, 487–496.

Knowles, J. B. and Kreitman, N. (1965) The Eysenck Personality Inventory: some considerations. *British Journal of Psychiatry*, **111**, 755–759.

Koch, J. L. A. (1891) *Die Psychopathischen Minderwertigkeiten*. Dorn: Ravensburg.

Kohut, H. (1971) *The Analysis of the Self*. New York: International Universities Press.

Kohut, H. (1975) *The Restoration of the Self*. New York: International Universities Press.

Kolada, J. L., Bland, R. C. and Newman, S. C. (1994) Epidemiology of psychiatric disorders in Edmonton. Obsessive-compulsive disorder. *Acta Psychiatrica Scandinavica Supplement*, **376**, 24–35.

Kolb, J. and Gunderson, J. (1980) Diagnosing borderline patients with a semi-structured interview. *Archives of General Psychiatry*, **37**, 37–41.

Kraepelin, E. (1905) *Lectures on Clinical Psychiatry*, 2nd edn, translated by T. Johnstone. London: Baillière Tindall and Co.

Kretschmer, E. (1918) *Der Sensitive Beziehungswahn*. Berlin: Springer.

Kretschmer, E. (1922) *Körperbau und Charakter*. Berlin: Springer.

Kroll, J. (1981) Borderline personality disorder: construct validity of the concept. *Archives of General Psychiatry*, **38**, 1021–1026.

Kroll, J., Pyle, R., Zarder, J., *et al.* (1981) Borderline personality disorder: Interrater reliability of the Diagnostic Interview for Borderlines. *Schizophrenia Bulletin*, **7**, 269–272.

Kroll, J., Carey, K., Lloyd, S. and Roth, M. (1982) Are there borderlines in Britain? A cross validation of US findings. *Archives of General Psychiatry*, **39**, 60–63.

Landis, J. R. and Koch, G. G. (1977a) The measurement of observer agreement for categorical data. *Biometrics*, **33**, 159–174.

Landis, J. R. and Koch, G. G. (1977b) A one-way component of variance model for categorical data. *Biometrics*, **33**, 671–679.

Langbehn, D. R., Pfohl, B. M., Reynolds, S. *et al.* (1999) The Iowa personality disorder screen: development and preliminary validation of a brief screening interview. *Journal of Personality Disorders*, **13**, 75–89.

Langevin, R. and Stoner, H. (1979) Evidence that depression rating scales primarily measure a social undesirability response set. *Acta Psychiatrica Scandinavica*, **59**, 70–79.

Langfeldt, G. (1937) *The Prognosis in Schizophrenia and the Factors Influencing the Course of the Disease*. Copenhagen: Levin and Munksgaard.

Langs, G., Quehenberger, F., Fabisch, K. *et al.* (1998) Prevalence, patterns and role of personality disorder in panic disorder patients with and without comorbid (lifetime) major depression. *Acta Psychiatrica Scandinavica*, **98**, 116–123.

Larkin, B. A., Copeland, J. R. M., Dewey, M. E. *et al.* (1992) The natural history of neurotic disorder in an elderly urban population: findings from the Liverpool study of continuing health in the community. *British Journal of Psychiatry*, **160**, 681–686.

Lazare, A., Klerman, G. L. and Armor, D. (1966) Oral, obsessive, and hysterical personality patterns. *Archives of General Psychiatry*, **14**, 624–630.

Lazarus, A. and Lazarus, C. (1991) *Multimodal Life History Inventory*, Second edition. Champaign, Illinois: Research Press.

Leighton, D. C., Harding, J. S., Macklin, D. B. *et al.* (1963) Psychiatric findings of the Stirling County Study. *American Journal of Psychiatry*, **119**, 1021–1026.

Leonhard, K. (1963) Die Prapsychotischen Temperamente bei den Monopolaren und Bipolaren Phasischen Psychosen. *Psychiatrie et Neurologie (Basel)*, **146**, 105–115.

Leonhard, K. (1968) *Akzentuierte* Personlichkeiten. Berlin: Verlag Volk und Gesundheit.

Lepine, J. P., Chignon, J. M. and Teherani, M. (1993) Suicide attempts in patients with panic disorder. *Archives of General Psychiatry*, **50**, 144–149.

Lerner, H. E. (1974) The hysterical personality: a 'woman's disease'. *Comprehensive Psychiatry*, **15**, 157–164.

Lewis, G. and Appleby, L. (1988) Personality disorder: the patients psychiatrists dislike. *British Journal of Psychiatry*, **153**, 44–49.

Lilenfeld, L. R., Kaye, W. H., Greeno, C. G. *et al.* (1998) A controlled family study of anorexia nervosa and bulimia nervosa: psychiatric disorders in first-degree relatives and effects of proband comorbidity. *Archives of General Psychiatry*, **55**, 603–610.

Lilienfeld, S. O., Van Valkenburg, C., Larntz, K. and Akiskal, H. S. (1986) The relationship of histrionic personality disorder to antisocial personality and somatisation disorders. *American Journal of Psychiatry*, **143**, 718–722.

Linehan, M. M., Armstrong, H. E., Suarez, A. *et al.* (1991) Cognitive-behavioral treatment for chronically parasuicidal borderline patients. *Archives of General Psychiatry*, **48**, 1060–1064.

Linehan, M. M. (1992) *Cognitive therapy for borderline personality disorder*. New York: Guilford Press.

Linehan, M. M., Heard, H. L. and Armstrong, H. E. (1993) Naturalistic follow-up of a behavioural treatment for chronically parasuicidal borderline patients. *Archives of General Psychiatry*, **50**, 971–974.

Linehan, M. M. (1995) Combining pharmacotherapy with psychotherapy for substance abusers with borderline personality disorder: strategies for enhancing compliance. *NIDA Research Monograph*, **150**, 129–142.

Links, P. S., Heslegrave, R. J., Mitton, J. E. *et al.* (1995) Borderline personality disorder and substance abuse: consequences of comorbidity. *Canadian Journal of Psychiatry*, **40**, 9–14.

Lion, J. R. (1981) A comparison between DSM-111 and DSM-II personality disorders. In *Personality Disorders: Diagnosis and Management*, 2nd edn, ed. J. R. Lion, pp. 1–9. Baltimore: Williams and Wilkins.

Livesley, W. J. (1986) Trait and behavioural prototypes of personality disorder. *American Journal of Psychiatry*, **143**, 728–732.

Livesley, W. J. (1987) A systematic approach to the delineation of personality disorders. *American Journal of Psychiatry*, **144**, 772–777.

Livesley, W. J. (1991) Classifying personality disorders: ideal types, prototypes, or dimensions? *Journal of Personality Disorders*, **5**, 52–59.

Livesley, W. J., Schroeder, M. L., Jackson, D. N. and Jang, K. L. (1994) Categorical distinctions in the study of personality disorder: implications for classification. *Journal of Abnormal Psychology*, **103**, 6–17.

Livesley, W. J., Jang, K. L. and Vernon, P. A. (1998) Phenotypic and genetic structure of traits delineating personality disorder. *Archives of General Psychiatry* **55**, 941–948.

Lloyd, R. and Williamson, S. (1968) *Born to Trouble*. London: Cassirer.

Løberg, T. (1981) MMPI-based personality subtypes of alcoholics: Relationships to drinking history, psychometrics and neuropsychological deficits. *Journal on Studies on Alcohol*, **42**, 766–782.

London Times (1795) The case of Miss Broderick.

Loranger, A. W., Susman, V. L., Oldham, J. M. and Russakoff, L. M. (1987a) International Personality Disorder Examination (PDE). A Structured Interview for DSM-III-R and ICD-10 personality disorders. WHO/ADAMHA version. White Plains, New York: The New York Hospital, Cornell Medical Center, Westchester Division.

Loranger, A. W., Susman, V. L., Oldham, M. M. and Russakoff, L. M. (1987b) The Personality Disorder Examination: a preliminary report. *Journal of Personality Disorders*, **1**, 1–13.

Loranger, A. W., Oldham, J. M. and Tulis, E. H. (1982) Familial transmission of DSM-III borderline personality disorders. *Archives of General Psychiatry*, **39**, 795–799.

Loranger, A. W., Oldham, J. M., Russakoff, L. M. and Susman, V. (1984) Structured interviews and borderline personality . *Archives of General Psychiatry*, **41**, 565–568.

Loranger, A. W., Susman, V. L., Oldham, J. M. and Russakoff, L. M. (1985) Personality Disorder Examination (PDE). A Structured Interview for DSM-IIIR and ICD-9 personality disorders. WHO/ADAMHA pilot version. White Plains, New York: The New York Hospital, Cornell Medical Center, Westchester Division.

Loranger, A. W. (1990) The impact of DSM-111 on diagnostic practice in a University Hospital. *Archives of General Psychiatry*, **47**, 672–675.

Loranger, A. W., Lenzegweger, M. F., Gartner, A. F. *et al.* (1991) Trait-state artifacts and the diagnosis of personality disorders. *Archives of General Psychiatry*, **48**, 720–728.

Loranger, A. W., Sartorius, N., Andreoli, A., *et al.* (1994) The International Personality Disorder Examination: the WHO/ADAMHA international pilot study of personality disorders. *Archives of General Psychiatry*, **51**, 215–224.

Lyons, M. J., Tyrer, P., Gunderson, J. and Tohen, M. (1997) Heuristic models of comorbidity of axis I and axis II disorders. *Journal of Personality Disorders*, **11**, 260–269.

MacFarlane, J. W. and Tuddenham, R. D. (1951) Problems in the validation of projective techniques. In *An Introduction to Projective Techniques*, edited by H. H. Anderson, pp. 26–54. New York: Prentice Hall.

MacLeod, A. K., Tata, P., Evans, K. *et al.* (1998) Recovery of positive future thinking within a high-risk suicide group: results from a pilot randomized controlled trial. *British Journal of Clinical Psychology*, **37**, 371–379.

Maddocks, P. D. (1970) A five-year follow-up of untreated psychopaths. *British Journal of Psychiatry*, **116**, 510–515.

Maier, W., Lichtermann, D., Klingler, T. *et al.* (1992) Prevalence of personality disorders (DSM-111-R) in the community. *Journal of Personality Disorders*, **6**, 187–196.

Manicavasagar, V., Silove, D. and Curtis, J. (1997) Separation anxiety in adulthood: a phenomenological investigation. *Comprehensive Psychiatry*, **38**, 274–282.

Mann, A. H., Jenkins, R., Cutting, J. C. and Cowen, P. J. (1981) The development and use of a standardized assessment of abnormal personality. *Psychological Medicine*, **11**, 839–847.

Mann, A. H., Raven, P., Pilgrim, J., Khanna, S. *et al.* (1999) An assessment of the Standardized Assessment of Personality as a screening instrument for the International Personality Disorder Examination: a comparison of informant and patient assessments for personality disorder. *Psychological Medicine*, **29**, 985–989.

Manning, N. (1989) The Therapeutic Community Movement: charisma and routinization. *International library of group psychotherapy and group process*. London: Routledge and Kegan Paul.

Markowitz, P., Calabrese, J., Schulz, S. and Meltzer, H. (1991) Fluoxetine in the treatment of borderline and schizotypal personality disorder. *American Journal of Psychiatry*, **148**, 1064–1067.

Marlowe, M. J., O'Neill-Byrne, K., Lowe-Ponsford, F. and Watson, J. P. (1996) The Borderline Syndrome Index: a validation study using the Personality Assessment Schedule. *British Journal of Psychiatry*, **168**, 72–75.

Martin, R. L., Cloninger, C. R., Guze, S. V. and Clayton, P. J. (1985) Mortality in a follow-up of 500 psychiatric outpatients: 1. total mortality. *Archives of General Psychiatry*, **42**, 47–54.

Masling, J. (1960) The influence of situational and interpersonal variables in projective testing. *Psychological Bulletin*, **57**, 65–85.

Masterson, J. F. (1976) *Psychotherapy of the Borderline Adult*. New York: Brunner/Maazel.

Matthews, G. and Deary, I. J. (1998) *Personality Traits*. Cambridge: Cambridge University Press.

Maudsley, H. (1868) *A Physiology and Pathology of Mind*, 2nd edn. London: MacMillan.

Mawson, D., Grounds, A. and Tantam, D. (1985) Violence and Asperger's syndrome: a case study. *British Journal of Psychiatry*, **147**, 566–569.

McCord, W. and McCord, J. (1964) *The Psychopath: an essay on the criminal mind*. Princeton, NJ: Van Nostrand.

McFarlane, A. (1988) The longitudinal course of post-traumatic morbidity: the range of outcomes and their predictors. *Journal of Nervous and Mental Disease*, **176**, 22–29.

McGlashan, T. H. (1983) The borderline syndrome: ii. Is borderline a variant of schizophrenia or affective disorder? *Archives of General Psychiatry*, **40**, 1319–1323.

McGlashan, T. H. (1984a) The Chestnut Lodge follow-up study. i. Follow-up methodology and study sample. *Archives of General Psychiatry*, **41**, 573–585.

McGlashan, T. H. (1984b) The Chestnut Lodge follow-up study. ii. Long-term outcome of schizophrenia and affective disorders. *Archives of General Psychiatry*, **41**, 586–601.

McGlashan, T. H. (1986a) The Chestnut Lodge follow-up study. iii. Long-term outcome of borderline personalities. *Archives of General Psychiatry*, **43**, 20–30.

McGlashan, T. H. (1986b) Schizotypal personality disorder. Chestnut Lodge follow-up study: vi. Long-term follow-up perspectives. *Archives of General Psychiatry*, **43**, 329–334.

McGuffin, P., Farmer, A. E. and Harvey, I. (1991) A polydiagnostic application of operational criteria in studies of psychotic illness: development and reliability of the OPCRIT system. *Archives of General Psychiatry*, **48**, 764–770.

McKeon, J., Roa, B. and Mann, A. (1984) Life events and personality traits in obsessional-compulsive neurosis. *British Journal of Psychiatry*, **144**, 185–189.

McPherson, K. (1994) The best and the enemy of the good: randomised controlled, uncertainty, and assessing the role of patient choice in medical decision making. *Journal of Epidemiology and Community Health*, **48**, 6–15.

Meehl, P. E. (1962) Schizotaxia, schizotypy, schizophrenia. *American Psychologist*, **17**, 827–838.

Mellsop, G., Varghese, F., Joshua, S. and Hicks, A. (1982) The reliability of Axis 11 of DSM-III. *American Journal of Psychiatry*, **139**, 1360–1361.

Menzies, D., Dolan, B. M. and Norton, K. (1993) Are short term savings worth long term costs? Funding treatment for personality disorders. *Psychiatric Bulletin*, **17**, 517–519.

Merry, J., Reynolds, C. M., Bailey, J. and Coppen, A. (1976) Prophylactic treatment of alcoholism by lithium carbonate. *Lancet*, **ii**, 481–482.

Merson, S., Tyrer, P., Duke, P. and Henderson, F. (1994) Inter-rater reliability of ICD-10 guidelines for the diagnosis of personality disorders. *Journal of Personality Disorders*, **8**, 89–95.

Millon, T. (1969) *Modern psychopathology: A Biosocial Approach to Maladaptive Learning and Functioning*. Philadelphia: W. B. Saunders.

Millon, T. (1981) *Disorders of personality, DSM-III. Axis II*. New York: John Wiley and Son.

Millon, T. (1987) On the nature of taxonomy in psychopathology. In *Issues in Diagnostic Research*, edited by C. G. Last and M. Hersen, pp. 3–85. New York: Plenum Press.

Millon, T., Davis, R. and Millon, C. (1997) MCMI-III manual. National Computer Systems, Minneapolis.

Mischel, W. (1968) *Personality and Assessment*. New York: John Wiley.

Mischel, W. (1973) Towards a cognitive social learning reconceptionalization of personality. *Psychological Review*, **80**, 252–283.

Mischel, W. (1979) On the interface of cognition and personality: beyond the person-situation debate. *American Psychologist*, **34**, 740–754.

Mischel, W. (1986) *Introduction to Personality: A New Look*, 4th edn, p. 497. New York: Holt, Rinehart and Winston.

Montgomery, S. and Åsberg, M. (1979) A new depression scale designed to be sensitive to change. *British Journal of Psychiatry*, **134**, 382–389.

Moos, R. H. (1973) Conceptionalisations of human environments. *American Psychologist*, **28**, 652–665.

Moran, P., Jenkins, R., Mann, A., Tylee, A., *et al.* (1999)

Personality Disorder in primary care. *Current Opinion in Psychiatry*, **12 (Suppl. 1)**, 140.

Morel, B. A. (1852) *Traité theorique et pratique des maladies mentales*. Paris: Baillière.

Morey, L., Waugh, M. and Blashfield, R. (1985) MMPI scales for DSM-III personality disorders: their derivation and correlates. *Journal of Personality Assessment*, **49**, 245–251

Morgenstern, J., Langenbucher, J., Labouvie, E. and Miller, K. J. (1997) The comorbidity of alcoholism and personality disorders in a clinical population: prevalence rates and relation to alcohol typology variables. *Journal of Abnormal Psychology*, **106**, 74–84.

Mulder, R. T., Joyce, P. R. (1995) Temperament and the structure of personality disorder symptoms. *Psychological Medicine*, **27**, 99–106.

Mulder, R. T., Joyce, P. R. and Cloninger, C. R. (1994) Temperament and early environment influence comorbidity and personality disorders in major depression. *Comprehensive Psychiatry*, **35**, 225–233.

Mullaney, J. A. and Trippett, C. J. (1979) Alcohol dependence and phobias: clinical description and relevance. *British Journal of Psychiatry*, **135**, 565–573.

Muller, J. J., Chafetz, M. E. and Blare, H. T. (1967) Acute psychiatric services in the general hospital: III, statistical survey. *American Journal of Psychiatry*, **124**, 46–56.

Murphy, S. M. and Tyrer, P. (1991) A double-blind comparison of the effects of gradual withdrawal of lorazepam, diazepam and bromazepam in benzodiazepine dependence. *British Journal of Psychiatry*, **158**, 511–516.

Myers, J. K., Weissman, M. M., Tischler, G. L. *et al.* (1984) Six month prevalence of psychiatric disorders in three communities, 1980 to 1982. *Archives of General Psychiatry*, **41**, 959–967.

National Institutes for Mental Health (1971) Biometry Branch, Survey Report Section. Statistical note no. 48. Bethesda: NIMH.

Naughton, M., Oppenheim, A. and Hill, J. (1996) Assessment of personality functioning in the transition from adolescent to adult life: preliminary findings. *British Journal of Psychiatry*, **168**, 33–37.

Norton, K. and Hinshelwood, R. D. (1996) Severe personality disorders: treatment issues and selection for inpatient psychotherapy. *British Journal of Psychiatry*, **168**, 723–731.

Noyes, R. J., Woodman, C. L., Holt, C. S. *et al.* (1995) Avoidant personality traits distinguish social phobic and panic disorder subjects. *Journal of Nervous and Mental Disease*, **183**, 145–153.

Nyman, G. E. and Marke, S. (1962) *Sjobring's Differentialla Psykologi: Analys och Skalkonstruktion*. Lund: Gleerup.

O'Rourke, D., Fahy, T. J. and Prescott, P. (1996) The Galway study of panic disorder: 4. Temporal reliability of diagnosis by Present State Examination test-retest. *British Journal of Psychiatry*, **169**, 98–104.

O'Hare, A. and Walsh, D. (1986) Activities of Irish Psychiatric Hospitals and Units, 1983. The Medico-social Research Board, Ireland.

Oldham, J. M. and Skodol, A. E. (1991) Personality disorders in the public sector. *Hospital and Community Psychiatry*, **42**, 481–487.

Oldham, J. M., Skodol, A. E., Kellman, H. D. *et al.* (1992) Diagnosis of DSM-III-R personality disorders by two semistructured interviews: patterns of comorbidity. *American Journal of Psychiatry*, **149**, 213–220.

Oliver, J. P., Huxley, P. J., Priebe, S. and Kaiser, W. (1997) Measuring the quality of life of severely mentally ill people using the Lancashire quality of life profile. *Social Psychiatry and Psychiatric Epidemiology*, **32**, 76–83.

O'Toole, B. I., Marshall, R. P., Schureck, R. J. and Dobson, M. (1998) Posttraumatic stress disorder and comorbidity in Australian Vietnam veterans: risk factors, chronicity and combat. *Australia and New Zealand Journal of Psychiatry*, **32**, 32–42.

Ovenstone, I. K. (1973) Spectrum of suicidal behaviours in Edinburgh. *British Journal of Preventive and Social Medicine*, **27**, 27–35.

Padesky, C. A. and Greenberger, D. (1995) *Clinician's guide to mind over mood*. The Guilford Press. New York, London.

Pallis, D. J. and Birtchnell, J. (1977) Seriousness of suicide attempts in relation to personality. *British Journal of Psychiatry*, **130**, 253–259.

Partridge, G. E. (1930) Personality disorder. *American Journal of Psychiatry*, **10**, 53.

Pepper, C. M., Klein, D. N., Anderson, R. L. *et al.* (1995) DSM-III-R axis II comorbidity in dysthymia and major depression. *American Journal of Psychiatry*, **152**, 239–247.

Peralta, V., Cuesta, M. J. and de Leon, J. (1991) Premorbid personality and positive and negative symptoms in schizophrenia. *Acta Psychiatrica Scandinavica*, **84**, 336–339.

Perley, M. and Guze, S. B. (1962) Hysteria: the stability and usefulness of clinical criteria. *New England Journal of Medicine*, **266**, 421–426.

Perris, C. (1966) A study of bi-polar (manic depressive) and unipolar recurrent depressive psychoses. iv: A multidimensional study of personality traits. *Acta Psychiatrica Scandinavica Supplement*, **194**, 68–82.

Perris, C., Eisemann, M., von Knorring, L. and Perris, H. (1984) Personality traits in former depressed patients and in healthy subjects without past history of depression. *Psychopathology*, **17**, 178–186.

Perry, J. (1982) *The Borderline Personality Disorder Scale (BPD-Scale)*. Cambridge, Mass: Cambridge Hospital.

Perry, J. C. (1992) Problems and considerations in the valid assessment of personality disorders. *American Journal of Psychiatry*, **149**, 1645–1653.

Persons, J. B. and Bertagnolli, A. (1994) Cognitive-behavioural treatment of multiple-problem patients: application to personality disorder. *Clinical Psychology and Psychotherapy*, **1**, 279–285.

Pfohl, B., Blum, N. and Zimmerman, M. (1995) Structured interview for DSM-IV personality: SIDP-IV. Department of Psychiatry, University of Iowa.

Pfohl, B., Coryell, W., Zimmerman, M. and Stangl, D. (1986) DSM-III personality disorders: diagnostic overlap and internal consistency of individual DSM-III criteria. *Comprehensive Psychiatry*; **27**: 21–34.

Pfohl, B., Stangl, D. and Zimmerman, M. (1982) Structured Interview for DSM-III Personality Disorders (SIDP). University of Iowa Hospitals and Clinics, Iowa City, USA.

Pfohl, B., Blum, N., Zimmerman, M. and Stangl, D. (1994) Structured Interview for DSM-IV personality (SIDP-IV). University of Iowa Department of Psychiatry, Iowa City.

Phelan, M., Slade, M., Thornicroft, G. *et al.* (1995) The Camberwell Assessment of Need: the validity and reliability of an instrument to assess the needs of people with severe mental illness. *British Journal of Psychiatry*, **167**, 589–595.

Phillips, K. A., Gunderson, J. G., Triebwasser, J. *et al.* (1998) Reliability and validity of depressive personality disorder. *American Journal of Psychiatry*, **155**, 1044–1048.

Phillips, S. L., Heads, T. C., Taylor, P. J. and Hill, G. M. (1999) Sexual offending and antisocial sexual behavior among patients with schizophrenia. *Journal of Clinical Psychiatry*, **60**, 170–175.

Pierce, D. W. (1977) Suicidal intent and self injury. *British Journal of Psychiatry*, **130**, 377–385.

Pilgrim, J. A., Mellers, J. D., Boothby, H. A. and Mann, A. H. (1993) Inter-rater and temporal reliability of the Standardized Assessment of Personality and the influence of informant characteristics. *Psychological Medicine*, **23**, 779–786.

Pinel, P. (1801) A Treatise of Insanity. Translated from French by D. D. Davis, 1962. New York: Hafner Publishing Co.

Piper, W. E., Joyce, A. S., Azim, H. F. and Rosie, J. S. (1994) Patient characteristics and success in day treatment. *Journal of Nervous and Mental Disease*, **182**, 381–386.

Piven, J., Wzorek, M., Landa, R. *et al.* (1994) Personality characteristics of the parents of autistic individuals. *Psychological Medicine*, **24**, 783–795.

Pomeroy, J. C. and Ricketts, B. (1985) Long-term attendance in the psychiatric out-patient department for non-psychotic illness. *British Journal of Psychiatry*, **147**, 508–516.

Pope, H. G., Jonas, J. M., Hudson, J. I., *et al.* (1983) The validity of DSM-III borderline personality disorder: a phenomenologic, family history, treatment response, and long-term follow-up study. *Archives of General Psychiatry*, **40**, 23–30.

Porter, R. (1987) *Mind-forg'd manacles: a history of madness in England from the Restoration to the Regency*. London: Athlone Press.

Prescott, C. A. and Kendler, K. S. (1999) Genetic and environmental contributions to alcohol abuse and dependence in a population-based sample of male twins. *American Journal of Psychiatry*, **156**, 34–40.

Presly, A. J. and Walton, H. J. (1973) Dimensions of abnormal personality. *British Journal of Psychiatry*, **122**, 269–276.

Prichard, J. C. (1837) *A treatise on insanity and other diseases affecting the mind*. Philadelphia: Harwell, Barrington and Harwell.

Puccinelli, M. and Wilkinson, G. (1994) Outcome of depression in psychiatric settings. *British Journal of Psychiatry*, **164**, 297–304.

Quaersell, R. (1985) Locked up or put to bed: psychiatry in the treatment of the mentally ill in Sweden 1800–1920. *The Anatomy of Madness*, Vol. 2, 86–97. Edited by Bynum, W., Porter, R. and Shepherd, M. Tavistock, London.

Rado, S. (1956) Dynamics and classification of disordered behaviour. In *Psychoanalysis of Behaviour*, vol. 1, pp. 268–285. New York: Grune and Stratton.

Rao, V. (1975) In *World History of Psychiatry*, edited by J. G. Howells. London: Baillière Tindall.

Rapoport, R. N. (1960) *Community as doctor: new perspectives on a therapeutic community*. London: Tavistock Publications.

Rees, A., Hardy, G. E. and Barkham, M. (1997) Covariance in the measurement of depression/anxiety and three Cluster C personality disorders (avoidant, dependent, obsessive-compulsive). *Journal of Affective Disorders*, **45**, 143–153.

Reich, J. (1987) Instruments measuring DSM-III and DSM-III-R personality disorders. *Journal of Personality Disorders*, **1**, 220–240.

Reich, J. H. (1989) Update on instruments to measure DSM-III and DSM-III-R personality disorders. *Journal of Nervous and Mental Disease*, **177**, 366–370.

Reich, J. H. and Green, A. I. (1991) Effect of personality disorders on outcome of treatment. *Journal of Nervous and Mental Disease*, **179**, 74–82.

Reich, J. and Vasile, R. (1993) Effect of personality disorders on the treatment outcome of Axis 1 conditions: An update. *Journal of Nervous and Mental Disease*, **181**, 475–484.

Reich, J., Noyes, R., Jr, Coryell, W. and O'Gorman, T. W. (1986) The effect of state anxiety on personality measurement. *American Journal of Psychiatry*, **143**, 760–763.

Reich, J. and Thompson, W. D. (1987) DSM-III personality disorder clusters in three populations. *British Journal of Psychiatry*, **150**, 471–475.

Reich, J., Noyes, R., Jr and Troughton, E. (1987) Dependent personality disorders associated with phobic avoidance in patients with panic disorder. *American Journal of Psychiatry*, **144**, 323–326.

Reich, J., Noyes, R., Jr and Troughton, E. (1988) Lack of agreement between instruments assessing DSM-III personality disorders. *Proceedings of the first Millon Clinical Multiaxial Inventory Conference*, USA.

Reich, J. H., Yates, W. and Nduaguba, M. (1989) Prevalence of DSM-111 personality disorders in the community. *Social Psychiatry*, **24**, 12–16.

Reich, J., Lyons, M. and Cai, B. (1996) Familial vulnerability factors to post-traumatic stress disorder in male military veterans. *Acta Psychiatrica Scandinavica*, **93**, 105–112.

Reich, W. (1933) *Charakter Analyse*. Leipzig: Sexpol Verlag.

Rennie, T. A. C. (1939) Follow-up study of 500 patients

with schizophrenia admitted to hospital from 1913 to 1923. *Archives of Neurology Psychiatry (Chicago)*, **42**, 877–891.

Rey, E. R., Bailer, J., Brauer, W., Handel, M., Laubenstein, D. and Stein, A. (1994) *Acta. Psychiatrica Scandinavica*, **90**, 405–412.

Roberts, J. (1997) How to recognise a therapeutic community. *Prison Service Journal*, **111**, 4–7.

Robertson, G. (1987) Mentally abnormal offenders: manner of death. *British Medical Journal*, **295**, 632–634.

Robins, L., Helzer, J., Weissman, M., *et al.* (1984) Lifetime prevalence of specific psychiatric disorders in three sites. *Archives of General Psychiatry*, **41**, 949–958.

Robins, J. (1986) *Fools and Mad: a history of the insane in Ireland*. Dublin: Institute of Public Administration.

Robins, L. N. (1966) *Deviant Children Grown Up*. Baltimore: Williams and Wilkins.

Robins, L., Helzer, J., Croughan, J., *et al.* (1979) The National Institute of Mental Health Diagnostic Interview Schedule. Rockville, Md: NIMH.

Rogers, J. H., Widiger, T. A. and Krupp, A. (1995) Aspects of depression associated with borderline personality disorder. *American Journal of Psychiatry*, **152**, 268–270.

Ronningstam, E. (1996) Pathological narcissism and narcissistic personality disorder. *Harvard Review of Psychiatry*, **3**, 326–340.

Rosenthal, D., Wender, P. H., Ket-Y., S. S. *et al.* (1971) The adopted-away offspring of schizophrenics. *American Journal of Psychiatry*, **128**, 307–311.

Rost, K. M., Akins, R. N., Brown, F. W. and Smith, G. R. (1992) The comorbidity of DSM-III-R personality disorders in somatization disorder. *General Hospital Psychiatry*, **14**, 322–326.

Rounsaville, B. J., Kranzler, H. R., Ball, S. *et al.* (1998) Personality disorders in substance abusers: relation to substance use. *Journal of Nervous and Mental Disease*, **186**, 87–95.

Runeson, B. and Beskow, J. (1991) Borderline personality disorder in young Swedish suicides. *Journal of Nervous and Mental Disease*, **179**, 153–156.

Rutherford, M. J., Cacciola, J. S., Alterman, A. I. and Cook, T. G. (1997) Social competence in opiate-addicted individuals: gender differences, relationship to psychiatric diagnoses, and treatment response. *Addictive Behavior*, **22**, 419–425.

Rutter, M. (1987) Temperament, personality and personality disorder. *British Journal of Psychiatry*, **150**, 443–458.

Rutter, M., Birch, H., Thomas, A. and Chess, S. (1964) Temperamental characteristics in infancy and later development of behavioural disorders. *British Journal of Psychiatry*, **110**, 651–661.

Ryle, A. (1997a) The structure and development of borderline personality disorder: a proposed model. *British Journal of Psychiatry*, **170**, 82–87.

Ryle, A. (1997b) *Cognitive analytic therapy and borderline personality disorder*. John Wiley: Chichester.

Salzman, C., Wolfson, A. N., Schatzberg, A. *et al.* (1995) Effect of fluoxetine on anger in symptomatic volunteers

with borderline personality disorder. *Journal of Clinical Psychopharmacology*, **15**, 23–29.

Samuels, J., Nestadt, G., Romanoski, A. *et al.* (1994) DSM-111 personality disorders in the community. *American Journal of Psychiatry*, **151**, 1055–1062.

Sanderson, W. C., Wetzler, S., Beck, A. T. and Betz, F. (1994) Prevalence of personality disorders among patients with anxiety disorders. *Psychiatry Research*, **51**, 167–174.

Sargant, W. and Slater, E. (1962) An Introduction to Physical Methods of Treatment in Psychiatry, 5th edn. Edinburgh: Churchill Livingstone.

Sartorius, N., Kaelber, C. T., Cooper, J. E. *et al.* (1993) Progress toward achieving a common language in psychiatry. Results from the field trial of the clinical guidelines accompanying the WHO classification of mental and behavioral disorders in ICD-10. *Archives of General Psychiatry*, **50**, 115–124.

Schneider, K. (1923) *Die Psychopathischen Personlichkeiten*. Berlin: Springer.

Schotte, C. K., De Doncker, D., Vankerckhoven, C. *et al.* (1998) Self-report assessment of the DSM-IV personality disorders. Measurement of trait and distress characteristics: the ADP-IV. *Psychological Medicine*, **28**, 1179–1188.

Schroeder, M. L. and Livesley, W. J. (1991) An evaluation of DSM-III-R personality disorders. *Acta Psychiatrica Scandinavica*, **84**, 512–519.

Schroeder, M. L., Wormsworth, J. A. and Livesley, W. J. (1992) Dimensions of personality disorder and their relationships to the big five dimensions of personality. *Psychological Assessment*, **4**, 47–53.

Schuckit, M. A. and Gunderson, E. K. E. (1977) Accident and assault deaths in the United States Navy: demography and preliminary interpretations. *Military Medicine*, **142**, 607–610.

Schulsinger, F. (1972) Psychopathy, heredity and environment. *International Journal of Mental Health*, **1**, 190–206.

Sears, R. R. (1936) Experimental studies of projection: 1, attribution of traits. *Journal of Social Psychology*, **7**, 151–163.

Seivewright, H., Tyrer, P., Casey, P. and Seivewright, N. (1991) A three-year follow-up of psychiatric morbidity in urban and rural primary care. *Psychological Medicine*, **21**, 495–503.

Seivewright, N. (1987) Relationship between life events and personality in psychiatric disorder. *Stress Medicine*, **3**, 163–168.

Seivewright, N. (1988) *Personality disorder, life events and the onset of mental illness*. In: Personality Disorder. Diagnosis, Management & Course, ed. P. Tyrer. Wright, London, pp. 82–92.

Seivewright, N. (1999) Personality disorder and the occurrence of adverse life events. MD Thesis, University of Nottingham.

Seivewright, N. and Tyrer, P. (1990) Relationship of dysthymia to anxiety and other neurotic disorders. In *Dysthymic disorder*, ed. S. W. Burton and H. S. Akiskal, pp. 24–36. London: Gaskell Books, Royal College of Psychiatrists.

Seivewright, N. and Daly, C. (1997) Personality disorder

and drug use: a review. *Drug & Alcohol Review*, **16**, 235–250.

Seivewright, H., Tyrer, P. and Johnson, T. (1998) Prediction of outcome in neurotic disorder: a five year prospective study. *Psychological Medicine*, **28**, 1149–1157.

Seivewright, N., Tyrer, P., Ferguson, B. *et al.* (2000). A logitudinal study of the influence of life events and personality status on diagnostic change in three neurotic disorders. *Depression and Anxiety*, (in press).

Shawcross, C. R. and Tyrer, P. (1985) Influence of personality on response to monoamine oxidase inhibitors and tricyclic antidepressants. *Journal of Psychiatric Research*, **19**, 557–562.

Shea, M. T., Widiger, T. A. and Klein, M. H. (1992) Comorbidity of personality disorders and depression: implications for treatment. *Journal of Consulting and Clinical Psychology*, **60**, 857–868.

Shea, M. T., Pilkonis, P. A., Beckham, E. *et al.* (1990) Personality disorder and treatment outcome in the NIMH Treatment of Depression Collaborative Research Program. *American Journal of Psychiatry*, **147**, 711–718.

Sheard, M. H., Marini, J. L., Bridges, C. I. and Wagner, E. (1976) The effect of lithium on impulsive aggressive behavior in man. *American Journal of Psychiatry*, **133**, 1409–1413.

Sheehy, M., Goldsmith, L. and Edward, C. (1980) A comparative study of borderline patients in a psychiatric out-patient clinic. *American Journal of Psychiatry*, **137**, 1374–1379.

Shepherd, M., Cooper, B., Brown, A. C. and Kalton, G. W. (1966) *Psychiatric Illness in General Practice.* Oxford: Oxford University Press.

Shields, J. and Slater, E. (1960) Hereditary and psychological abnormality. In *Handbook of Abnormal Psychology*, edited by H. J. Eysenck, pp. 298–343. London: Pitman Medical.

Siever, L. J. and Davis, K. L. (1991) A psychobiologic perspective on the personality disorders. *American Journal of Psychiatry*, **148**, 1647–1658.

Silverman, J. M., Siever, L. J., Horvath, *et al.* (1993) Schizophrenia-related and affective personality disorder traits in relatives of probands with schizophrenia and personality disorders. *American Journal of Psychiatry*, **150**, 435–442.

Simons, R. C. (1987) Self-defeating and sadistic personality disorders: needed additions to the diagnostic nomenclature. *Journal of Personality Disorders*, **1**, 161–167.

Simonsen, E. (1994) The borderline conditions: an introduction from a Scandinavian perspective. *Acta Psychiatrica Scandinavica Supplement*, **379**, 6–11.

Sims, A. (1975) Factors predictive of outcome in neurosis. *British Journal of Psychiatry*, **127**, 45–62.

Sims, A. and Prior, P. (1978) The pattern of mortality in severe neurosis. *British Journal of Psychiatry*, **133**, 299–305.

Singleton, N., Meltzer, H., Gatward, R. *et al.* (1998) *Psychiatric morbidity among prisoners in England and Wales.* London: Statistical Office.

Sjöbring, H. (1973) Personality structure and development. *Acta Psychiatrica Scandinavica, Supplementum*, 244.

Skodol, A. E., Oldham, J. M., Hyler, S. E. *et al.* (1993) Comorbidity of DSM-III-R eating disorders and personality disorders. *International Journal of Eating Disorders*, **14**, 403–416.

Skodol, A. E., Rosnick, L., Kellman, D. *et al.* (1988) Validating structured DSM-III-R personality disorder assessments with longitudinal data. *American Journal of Psychiatry*, **145**, 1297–1299.

Slater, E. and Cowie, V. (1971) *The Genetics of Mental Disorders.* London: Oxford University Press.

Slater, E. (1948) Book review of Eysenck's Dimensions of Personality. *British Medical Journal*, **2**, 657.

Small, L. F., Small, J. C., Alig, V. B. and Moore, D. F. (1970) Passive-aggressive personality disorders: a search for a syndrome. *American Journal of Psychiatry*, **126**, 973–983.

Smith, G. E. (1916) Shock and the soldier. *Lancet i*, 853–857.

Snaith, R. P. (1976) Personality and depressive illness. *British Journal of Psychiatry*, **128**, 101–102.

Soloff, P. H., George, A., Nathan, R. S. *et al.* (1986). Progress in pharmacotherapy of personality disorders: a double blind study of amitriptyline, haloperidol and placebo. *Arch Gen Psychiatry*, **43**, 691–697.

Soloff, P. H. (1994) Is there any drug treatment of choice for the borderline patient? *Acta Psychiatrica Scandinavica*, **89** (suppl 379): 50–55.

Soloff, P. H., Cornelius, J., and Georege, A. (1991). The depressed borderline: one disorder or two? *Psychopharmacological Bulletin*, **27**, 23–30.

Soloff, P. H., George, A., Nathan, R. S. and Schulz, P. M. (1987) Characterizing depression in borderline patients. *Journal of Clinical Psychiatry*, **48**, 155–157.

Southwick, S. M., Yehuda, R. and Giller, E. L. (1995). Psychological dimensions of depression in borderline personality disorder. *American Journal of Psychiatry*, **152**, 789–791.

Spielberger, C. D., Gorsuch, R. L. and Lushene, R. E. (1970) Manual for the State-trait Anxiety Inventory. Palo Alto, California: Consulting Psychologists Press.

Spitzer, R. L. (1983). Psychiatric diagnosis: are clinicians still necessary? *Comprehensive Psychiatry*, **24**, 399–411.

Spitzer, R. and Endicott, J. (1979) Justification for separating schizotypal and borderline personality disorders. *Schizophrenia Bulletin*, **5**, 95–100.

Spitzer, R. and Endicott, J. (1983) Schedule for Affective Disorders and Schizophrenia (SADS). New York: New York State Psychiatric Institute.

Spitzer, R. L., Endicott, J. and Gibbon, M. (1979) Crossing the border into borderline personality and border schizophrenia. *Archives of General Psychiatry*, **36**, 17–24.

Spitzer, R., Endicott, J. and Robins, E. (1978) Research diagnostic criteria: rationale and reliability. *Archives of General Psychiatry*, **35**, 773–782.

Spitzer, R., Williams, J. B. W. and Gibbon, M. (1987) Structured Interview for DSM-III-R personality disorders. New York: Biometrics Research Department, New York State Psychiatric Institute.

Srole, L., Langer, T., Michael, S. *et al.* (1962). *Mental Health in the Metropolis.* New York: McGraw Hill.

Standage, K. F. (1978) The diagnosis of personality disorders: a pilot study. *Canadian Psychiatric Association Journal*, **23**, 15–22.

Standage, K. F. (1979) The use of Schneider's typology for the diagnosis of personality disorders – an examination of reliability. *British Journal of Psychiatry*, **135**, 238–242.

Stangl, D., Pfohl, B., Zimmerman, M. *et al.* (1985) Structured Interview for DSM-III personality disorders. *Archives of General Psychiatry*, **42**, 591–596.

Stein, G. (1998). *Anxiety disorders*. In: Seminars in General Adult Psychiatry Vol 1, eds G. Stein & G. Wilkinson. London: Gaskell, pp. 554–622.

Stein, G. S. (1992) Drug treatment of the personality disorders. *British Journal of Psychiatry*, **161**, 167–184.

Stern, A. (1938) Psychoanalytic investigation of and therapy in the borderline group of neuroses. *Psychiatric Quarterly*, **7**, 467–489.

Stern, J., Murphy, M. and Bass, C. (1993) Personality disorders in patients with somatisation disorder: a controlled study. *British Journal of Psychiatry*, **163**, 785–789.

Stone, M. H., Hurt, S. W., Stone, D. K. (1987) The PI 500: long-term follow-up of borderline patients meeting DSM-III criteria – 1. Global outcome. *Journal of Personality Disorders*, **1**, 291–298.

Stone, M. H. (1993) Long-term outcome in personality disorder. *British Journal of Psychiatry*, **162**, 299–313.

Strain, J. J., Smith, G. C., Hammer, J. S. *et al.* (1998) Adjustment disorder: a multisite study of its utilization and interventions in the consultation-liaison psychiatry setting. *General Hospital Psychiatry*, **20**, 139–149.

Strauss, J., Bartko, J. J. and Carpenter, W. T. (1973) The use of clustering techniques for the classification of psychiatric patients. *British Journal of Psychiatry*, **122**, 531–540.

Stuart, S., Pfohl, B., Battaglia, M. *et al.* (1998) The cooccurrence of DSM-III-R personality disorders. *Journal of Personality Disorders*, **12**, 302–315.

Swartz, M., Blazer, D., George, L. and Winfield, I. (1990) Estimating the prevalance of borderline personality disorder in the community. *Journal of Personality Disorders*, **4**, 257–272.

Tantam, D., Holmes, D. and Cordess, C. (1993) Nonverbal expression in autism of Asperger type. *Journal of Autism and Devleopmental Disorder*, **23**, 111–133.

Taylor, P. J. and Gunn, J. (1984) Violence and psychosis. 1 – risk of violence among psychotic men. *British Medical Journal*, **288**, 1945–1949.

Tellegen, A. (1985) Structures of mood and personality and their relevance to assessing anxiety, with an emphasis on self report. In *Anxiety and the Anxiety Disorders*, edited by A. H. Tuema and J. D. Maser, pp. 681–706. Hillsdale, NJ: Erlbaum.

Thompson, D. J. and Goldberg, D. (1987) Hysterical personality disorder. The process of diagnosis in clinical and experimental settings. *British Journal of Psychiatry*, **150**, 241–245.

Thornton, C. and Russell, J. (1997) Obsessive compulsive comorbidity in the dieting disorders. *International Journal of Eating Disorders*, **21**, 83–87.

Trull, T. J., Widiger, T. A. and Frances, A. (1987) Covariation of criteria sets for avoidant, schizoid and dependent personality disorders. *American Journal of Psychiatry*, **144**, 767–771.

Tupin, J. P., Mahar, D. and Smith, D. (1973a) Two types of violent offenders with psychosocial disorders. *Diseases of the Nervous System*, **34**, 356–363.

Tupin, J. P., Smith, D. B., Clanon, T. L. *et al.* (1973b) The long-term use of lithium in aggressive prisoners. *Comprehensive Psychiatry*, **14**, 311–317.

Turkat, I. D. and Maisto, S. A. (1985) Personality disorders: application of the experimental method to the formulation and modification of personality disorders. In D. H. Barlow (ed.) *Clinical handbook of psychological disorders: a step by step treatment manual*. New York: Guilford Press.

Tyrer, P. (1985) Neurosis divisible? *Lancet*, **i**, 685–688.

Tyrer, P. (1989) *Classification of Neurosis*. Chichester: John Wiley.

Tyrer, P. (1992) Flamboyant, erratic, dramatic, borderline, antisocial, sadistic, narcissistic, histrionic and impulsive personality disorders: who cares which? *Criminal Behaviour and Mental Health*, **2**, 95–104.

Tyrer, P. (1994) What are the borders of borderline personality disorder? *Acta Psychiatrica Scandinavica*, **89**, supplement 257, 38–44.

Tyrer, P. (1996) Comorbidity or consanguinity. *British Journal of Psychiatry*, **168**, 669–671.

Tyrer, P. (1998a) Drug treatment of personality disorder. *Psychiatric Bulletin*, **22**, 242–244.

Tyrer, P. (1998b) Conference report: III European Congress on Personality Disorders, July 8–11, 1998, University of Sheffield, UK. *Journal of Personality Disorders*, **12**, 373–374.

Tyrer, P. (1999) Borderline personality disorder: a motley diagnosis in need of reform. *Lancet*, **354**, 2095–2096.

Tyrer, P. and Alexander, J. (1979) Classification of personality disorder. *British Journal of Psychiatry*, **135**, 163–167.

Tyrer, P. and Ferguson, B. (1987) Problems in the classification of personality disorder. *Psychological Medicine*, **17**, 15–20.

Tyrer, P. and Alexander, J. (1988) Personality Assessment Schedule. In: *Personality Disorders: Diagnosis, Management and Course*, ed. P Tyrer. London: Wright, pp. 43–62.

Tyrer, P. and Seivewright, H. (1988). Studies of Outcome. In: *Personality Disorders. Diagnosis, Management and Course*, ed. P. Tyrer. London: Wright, pp. 119–136.

Tyrer, P., Alexander, M. S., Cicchetti, D. *et al.* (1979) Reliability of a schedule for rating personality disorders. *British Journal of Psychiatry*, **135**, 168–174.

Tyrer, P. and Johnson, T. (1996) Establishing the severity of personality disorder. *American Journal of Psychiatry*, **153**, 1593–1597.

Tyrer, J. and Tyrer, P. (1997) Personality Assessment Schedule Program for rating severity and type of personality disturbance. London: Department of Public Mental Health, Division of Neuroscience and Psychological Medicine, Imperial College School of Medicine.

Tyrer, P., Strauss, J. and Cicchetti, D. (1983a) Temporal reliability of personality in psychiatric patients. *Psychological Medicine*, **13**, 393–398.

Tyrer, P., Casey, P. and Gall, J. (1983b) The relationship between neurosis and personality disorder. *British Journal of Psychiatry*, **142**, 404–408.

Tyrer, P., Owen, R. and Dawling, S. (1983c) Gradual withdrawal of diazepam after long-term therapy. *Lancet*, **i**, 1402–1406.

Tyrer, P., Cicchetti, D. V., Casey, P. R., Fitzpatrick, K. *et al.* (1984) Cross-national reliability study of a schedule for assessing personality disorders. *Journal of Nervous and Mental Diseases*, **172**, 718–721.

Tyrer, P., Owen, R. and Cicchetti, D. (1984b) The brief scale for anxiety: A sub-division of the comprehensive psychopathological rating scale. *Journal of Neurology, Neurosurgery and Psychiatry*, **47**, 970–975.

Tyrer, P., Alexander, J., Remington, M. and Riley, P. (1987) Relationship between neurotic symptoms and neurotic diagnosis: longitudinal study. *Journal of Affective Disorders.*, **13**, 13–21.

Tyrer, P., Seivewright, N., Murphy, S. *et al.* (1988a) The Nottingham Study of Neurotic Disorder: comparison of drug and psychological treatments *Lancet*, **ii**, 235–240.

Tyrer, P., Alexander, J. and Ferguson, B. (1988b). Personality Assessment Schedule (PAS). In: *Personality Disorders: Diagnosis, Management and Course*, ed P. Tyrer. London: Wright, pp. 140–167.

Tyrer, P., Casey, P. and Ferguson, B. (1988c) Personality disorder and mental illness. In: Tyrer, P., ed. *Personality disorders: diagnosis, management and course.* London: Wright, 1988: 93–104.

Tyrer, P., Ferguson, B., Fowler-Dixon, R. and Kelemen, A. (1990a). A plea for the diagnosis of hypochondriacal personality disorder. *Journal of Psychosomatic Research*, **34**, 637–642.

Tyrer, P., Seivewright, N., Ferguson, B. *et al.* (1990b). The Nottingham Study of Neurotic Disorder: relationship between personality disorder and symptoms. *Psychological Medicine*, **20**, 423–431.

Tyrer, P., Murphy, S. and Riley, P. (1990c) The Benzodiazepine Withdrawal Symptom Questionnaire. *Journal of Affective Disorders*, **19**, 53–61.

Tyrer, P., Seivewright, N., Ferguson, B. and Tyrer, J. (1992) The general neurotic syndrome: a coaxial diagnosis of anxiety, depression and personality disorder. *Acta Psychiatrica Scandinavica*, **85**, 201–206.

Tyrer, P., Seivewright, N., Ferguson, B. *et al.* (1993) The Nottingham Study of Neurotic Disorder: effect of personality status on response to drug treatment, cognitive therapy and self-help over two years. *British Journal of Psychiatry*, **162**, 219–226.

Tyrer, P., Merson, S., Onyett, S. and Johnson, T. (1994) The effect of personality disorder on clinical outcome, social networks and adjustment: a controlled clinical trial of psychiatric emergencies. *Psychological Medicine*, **24**, 731–740.

Tyrer, P., Gunderson, J., Lyons, M. and Tohen, M. (1997) Extent of comorbidity between mental state and personality disorders. *Journal of Personality Disorders*, **11**, 242–259.

Tyrer, P., Seivewright, N. and Seivewright, H. (1999) Long term outcome of hypochondriacal personality disorder. *Journal of Psychosomatic Research*, **46**, 177–185.

UK700 Group (Creed, F., Burns, T., Butler, T. *et al.* (1999) Comparison of intensive and standard case management for patients with psychosis: rationale of the trial. *British Journal of Psychiatry*, **174**, 74–78.

UK700 Group (Burns, T., Creed, F., Fahy, T. *et al.* (1999) Intensive versus standard case management for severe psychotic illness: a randomised trial. *The Lancet*, **353**, 2185–2189.

Urwin, P. and Gibbons, J. L. (1979) Psychiatric diagnosis in self-poisoning patients. *Psychological Medicine*, **9**, 501–507.

Vaillant, G. E. (1964) Prospective predictors of schizophrenic remission. *Archives of General Psychiatry*, **11**, 509–518.

Van Velzen, C. J. M. and Emmelkamp, P. M. G. (1996) The assessment of personality disorder: implications for cognitive and behavior therapy. *Behaviour Research and Therapy*, **34**, 655–668.

Verkes, R. J., Van der Mast, R. C., Hengeveld, M. W., Tuyl, J. P., Zwinderman, A. H. and Van Kempen, G. M. (1998a) Reduction by paroxetine of suicidal behavior in patients with repeated suicide attempts but not major depression. *American Journal of Psychiatry*, **155**, 543–547.

Verkes, R. J., Van der Mast, R. C., Kerkhof, A. J. *et al.* (1998b) Platelet serotonin, monoamine oxidase activity, and [3H] paroxetine binding related to impulsive suicide attempts and borderline personality disorder. *Biological Psychiatry*, **43**, 740–46.

Vernon, P. E. (1963) *Personality assessment: a critical survey.* London: Methuen and Co Ltd.

Vize, C. and Tyrer, P. (1994) The relationship between personality and psychiatric disorders. *Current Opinion in Psychiatry*, **7**, 123–128.

Von Knorring, L., Perris, C., Eisemann, M. *et al.* (1983) Pain as a symptom in depressive disorders. II. Relationship to personality traits as assessed by means of KSP. *Pain*, **17**, 377–384.

Walker, N. (1968) *Crime and Insanity in England, Vol. 1: The historical perspective.* Edinburgh University Press.

Walker, L. C. A. (1987) Inadequacies of the masochistic personality disorder diagnosis for women. *Journal of Personality Disorders*, **1**, 183–189.

Walton, H. J. and Presly, A. S. (1973) Use of a category system in the diagnosis of abnormal personality. *British Journal of Psychiatry*, **122**, 259–268.

Walton, H. J., Foulds, G. A., Littmann, S. K. and Presly, A. S. (1970) Abnormal personality. *British Journal of Psychiatry*, **116**, 497–510.

Watson, D. and Clark, L. A. (1984) Negative affectivity:

the disposition to experience aversive emotional states. *Psychological Bulletin*, **96**, 465–490.

Watson, D., Clark, L. A. and Harkness, A. R. (1994) Structures of personality and their relevance to psychopathology. *Journal of Abnormal Psychology*, **103**, 18–31.

Weinryb, R. M., Rössel, R. J. (1991) Karolinska Psychodynamic Profile – KAPP. *Acta Psychiatrica Scandinavica*; **83** (suppl 363): 1–23.

Weinryb, R. M., Rössel, R. J., Gustavsson, J. P. *et al.* (1997) The Karolinska Psychodynamic Profile (KAPP): Studies of character and well-being. *Psychoanalytic Psychology*, **14**, 495–515.

Weinryb, R. M., Gustavsson, J. P., Åsberg, M. and Rössel, R. J. (1992) Stability over time of character assessment using a psychodynamic instrument and personality inventories. *Acta Psychiatrica Scandinavica*, **86**, 179–184.

Weissman, M. M., and Klerman, G. L. (1977) The chronic depressive in the community: unrecognised and poorly treated. *Comprehensive Psychiatry*, **18**, 523–532.

Weissman, M. M., Myers, J. K. and Harding, P. S. (1978) Psychiatric disorders in a US urban community: 1975 to 1976. *American Journal of Psychiatry*, **135**, 459–462.

Weissman, M. M. and Myers, J. K. (1980) Psychiatric disorders in a US community. *Acta Psychiatrica Scandinavica*, **62**, 99–111.

West, D. (1974) Criminology, deviant behaviour and mental disorder. *Psychological Medicine*, **4**, 1–3.

Westen, D. and Shedler, J. (1999) Revising and assessing axis II, Part I: developing a clinically and empirically valid assessment method. *American Journal of Psychiatry*, **156**, 258–272.

Westen, D., Moses, J., Silk, K. R. *et al.* (1992) Quality of depressive experience in borderline personality disorder and major depression: when depression is not just depression. *Journal of Personality Disorders*, **6**, 382–393.

Whiteley, J. S. (1970) The response of psychopaths to a therapeutic community. *British Journal of Psychiatry*, **116**, 517–529.

Whitelock, P. R., Overall, J. E. and Patrick, J. H. (1971) Personality patterns and alcohol abuse in a state hospital population. *Journal of Abnormal Psychology*, **78**, 9–16.

Widiger, T. A. and Frances, A. (1985) The DSM-III personality disorders: perspectives from psychology. *Archives of General Psychiatry*, **42**, 615–623.

Widiger, T. A., Mangine, S., Corbitt, E. M. *et al.* (1995). Personality Disorder Interview-IV: A Semistructured Interview for the Assessment of Personality Disorders. Odessa, FL: Psychological Assessment Resources.

Williams, A. F. (1976) The alcoholic personality. In *The Biology of Alcoholism, vol. 4, Social Aspects of Alcoholism*. New York: Plenum Press.

Williams, P. (1979) Deciding how to treat – the relevance of psychiatric diagnosis. *Psychological Medicine*, **9**, 179–86.

Wing, J. K. (1982) Course and prognosis of schizophrenia. In *Handbook of Psychiatry*, edited by J. K. Wing and L. Wing, vol. 3, pp. 33–41. Cambridge: Cambridge University Press.

Wing, J. K., Cooper, J. E. and Sartorius, N. (1974) *The Measurement and Classification of Psychiatric Symptoms*. Cambridge: Cambridge University Press.

Winokur, G. (1972) Depression spectrum disease: description of family study. *Comprehensive Psychiatry*, **13**, 328.

Winston, A., Pollack, J., McCullough, L. *et al.* (1991) Brief psychotherapy of personality disorders. *American Journal of Psychiatry*, **151**, 190–194.

Wolff, S. (1991) 'Schizoid' personality in child and adult life. *British Journal of Psychiatry*, **159**, 615–635.

Wolff, S. and Chick, J. (1980) Schizoid personality in childhood: a controlled follow-up study. *Psychological Medicine*, **10**, 85–100.

World Health Organization (1949) *International Classification of Disease*. 7th revision. Geneva: World Health Organization.

World Health Organization (1968) *International Classification of Disease*. 8th revision. Geneva: World Health Organization.

World Health Organization (1978) *Mental Disorders: Glossary and Guide to the Classification in accordance with the Ninth Revision of the International Classification of Diseases* Geneva: World Health Organization.

World Health Organization (1979) *International Classification of Disease*, 9th revision. Geneva: World Health Organization.

World Health Organization (1987) *International Classification of Disease*, draft of 10th revision. Geneva: World Health Organization.

World Health Organization (1992) ICD-10: Classification of Mental and Behavioural Disorders. Geneva: World Health Organization.

World Health Organization. (1993) *The ICD-10: Classification of Mental and Behavioural Disorders: Diagnostic Criteria for Research*. Geneva: World Health Organization.

Yates, W. R., Sieleni, B., Reich, J. and Brass, C. (1989). Comorbidity of bulimia nervosa and personality disorder. *Journal of Clinical Psychiatry*, **50**, 57–59.

Young, J. E. (1990) *Cognitive therapy for personality disorders: a schema-focused approach*. Professional Resource Exchange Inc: Sarasota, Florida.

Young, J. E. (1994) *Cognitive therapy for personality disorders: a schema-focused approach*. (Revised edition). Practitioner's Resource Series. Professional Resource Press, Sarasota, Florida.

Zanarini, M., Frankenburg, F., Chauncey, D. and Gunderson, J. (1987) The Diagnostic Interview for Personality Disorders (DIPD): Interrater and test-retest reliability. *Comprehensive Psychiatry*, **28**, 467–480.

Zanarini, M., Gunderson, J., Marino, M. *et al.* (1989). Childhood experiences of borderline patients. *Comprehensive Psychiatry*, **30**, 18–25.

Zanarini, M. C., Frankenburg, F. R., Sickel, A. E. and Yong, L. (1994) Diagnostic Interview for DSM-IV Personality Disorders (DIPD-IV). Massachusetts: McLean Hospital, 115 Mill Street, Belmont.

Zanarini, M. C., Frankenburg, F. R., Dubo, E. D. *et al.* (1998) Axis I comorbidity of borderline personality disorder. *American Journal of Psychiatry*, **155**, 1733–1739.

Zanarini, M. C., Frankenburg, F. R., Reich, D. B. *et al.* (1999) Violence in the lives of adult borderline patients. *Journal of Nervous and Mental Disease*, **187**, 65–71.

Zersson, D. von and Akiskal, H. S. (1998) Personality factors in affective disorders: historical developments and current issues with special reference to the concepts of temperament and character. *Journal of Affective Disorders*, **51**, 1–5.

Zersson, D. von (1982) Personality and affective disorders. In *Handbook of Affective Disorders*, edited by E. S. Paykel, pp. 212–228. Edinburgh: Churchill Livingstone.

Zerssen, D. von, Possl, J., Hecht, H. *et al.* (1998) The Biographical Personality Interview (BPI)—a new approach to the assessment of premorbid personality in psychiatric research. Part I: Development of the instrument. *Journal of Psychiatric Research*, **32**, 19–25.

Zimmerman, M. (1994) Diagnosing Personality Disorders: A review of issues and research methods. *Archives of General Psychiatry*, **51**, 225–245.

Zimmerman, M. and Coryell, W. H. (1990) Diagnosing personality disorders in the community. *Archives of General Psychiatry*, **47**, 527–531.

Zimmerman, M., Coryell, W., Pfohl, B., Corenthal, C. and Stangl, D. (1986) ECT response in depressed patients with and without a DSM-III personality disorder. *American Journal of Psychiatry*, **143**, 1030–1032.

Zimmerman, M., Pfohl, B., Coryell, W. *et al.* (1988). Diagnosing personality disorder in depressed patients: a comparison of patient and informant interviews. *Archives of General Psychiatry*, **45**, 733–737.

Index

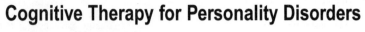
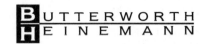
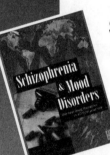